Data Science in Healthcare

Data Science in Healthcare

Editor

Tim Hulsen

MDPI • Basel • Beijing • Wuhan • Barcelona • Belgrade • Manchester • Tokyo • Cluj • Tianjin

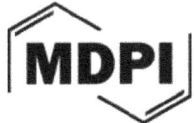

Editor
Tim Hulsen
Philips Research
The Netherlands

Editorial Office
MDPI
St. Alban-Anlage 66
4052 Basel, Switzerland

This is a reprint of articles from the Special Issue published online in the open access journal *International Journal of Environmental Research and Public Health* (ISSN 1660-4601) (available at: https://www.mdpi.com/journal/ijerph/special_issues/DSH).

For citation purposes, cite each article independently as indicated on the article page online and as indicated below:

LastName, A.A.; LastName, B.B.; LastName, C.C. Article Title. *Journal Name* **Year**, *Volume Number*, Page Range.

ISBN 978-3-0365-3983-6 (Hbk)
ISBN 978-3-0365-3984-3 (PDF)

Cover image courtesy of Tim Hulsen
Licensed by Aleksandr Khakimullin/Shutterstock

© 2022 by the authors. Articles in this book are Open Access and distributed under the Creative Commons Attribution (CC BY) license, which allows users to download, copy and build upon published articles, as long as the author and publisher are properly credited, which ensures maximum dissemination and a wider impact of our publications.

The book as a whole is distributed by MDPI under the terms and conditions of the Creative Commons license CC BY-NC-ND.

Contents

About the Editor ix

Tim Hulsen
Data Science in Healthcare: COVID-19 and Beyond
Reprinted from: *Int. J. Environ. Res. Public Health* **2022**, *19*, 3499, doi:10.3390/ijerph19063499 . . . 1

Jennifer Pan, Joseph Marie St. Pierre, Trevor A. Pickering, Natalie L. Demirjian, Brandon K.K. Fields, Bhushan Desai and Ali Gholamrezanezhad
Coronavirus Disease 2019 (COVID-19): A Modeling Study of Factors Driving Variation in Case Fatality Rate by Country
Reprinted from: *Int. J. Environ. Res. Public Health* **2020**, *17*, 8189, doi:10.3390/ijerph17218189 . . . 5

Ebtesam Alomari, Iyad Katib, Aiiad Albeshri and Rashid Mehmood
COVID-19: Detecting Government Pandemic Measures and Public Concerns from Twitter Arabic Data Using Distributed Machine Learning
Reprinted from: *Int. J. Environ. Res. Public Health* **2021**, *18*, 282, doi:10.3390/ijerph18010282 . . . 17

Francesco Bellocchio, Paola Carioni, Caterina Lonati, Mario Garbelli, Francisco Martínez-Martínez, Stefano Stuard and Luca Neri
Enhanced Sentinel Surveillance System for COVID-19 Outbreak Prediction in a Large European Dialysis Clinics Network
Reprinted from: *Int. J. Environ. Res. Public Health* **2021**, *18*, 9739, doi:10.3390/ijerph18189739 . . . 51

Tim Hulsen
Sharing Is Caring—Data Sharing Initiatives in Healthcare
Reprinted from: *Int. J. Environ. Res. Public Health* **2020**, *17*, 3046, doi:10.3390/ijerph17093046 . . . 69

Shital S. Muke, Deepak Tugnawat, Udita Joshi, Aditya Anand, Azaz Khan, Ritu Shrivastava, Abhishek Singh, Juliana L. Restivo, Anant Bhan, Vikram Patel and John A. Naslund
Digital Training for Non-Specialist Health Workers to Deliver a Brief Psychological Treatment for Depression in Primary Care in India: Findings from a Randomized Pilot Study
Reprinted from: *Int. J. Environ. Res. Public Health* **2020**, *17*, 6368, doi:10.3390/ijerph17176368 . . . 81

Yongseok Seo, Seungyeon Lee, Joung-Sook Ahn, Seongho Min, Min-Hyuk Kim, Jang-Young Kim, Dae Ryong Kang, Sangwon Hwang, Phor Vicheka and Jinhee Lee
Association of Metabolically Healthy Obesity and Future Depression: Using National Health Insurance System Data in Korea from 2009–2017
Reprinted from: *Int. J. Environ. Res. Public Health* **2021**, *18*, 63, doi:10.3390/ijerph18010063 103

Veronica Rojas-Mendizabal, Cristián Castillo-Olea, Alexandra Gómez-Siono and Clemente Zuñiga
Assessment of Thoracic Pain Using Machine Learning: A Case Study from Baja California, Mexico
Reprinted from: *Int. J. Environ. Res. Public Health* **2021**, *18*, 2155, doi:10.3390/ijerph18042155 . . . 113

Xialv Lin, Xiaofeng Wang, Yuhan Wang, Xuejie Du, Lizhu Jin, Ming Wan, Hui Ge and Xu Yang
Optimized Neural Network Based on Genetic Algorithm to Construct Hand-Foot-and-Mouth Disease Prediction and Early-Warning Model
Reprinted from: *Int. J. Environ. Res. Public Health* **2021**, *18*, 2959, doi:10.3390/ijerph18062959 . . . 125

Ricardo Peralta, Mario Garbelli, Francesco Bellocchio, Pedro Ponce, Stefano Stuard, Maddalena Lodigiani, João Fazendeiro Matos, Raquel Ribeiro, Milind Nikam, Max Botler, Erik Schumacher, Diego Brancaccio and Luca Neri
Development and Validation of a Machine Learning Model Predicting Arteriovenous Fistula Failure in a Large Network of Dialysis Clinics
Reprinted from: *Int. J. Environ. Res. Public Health* **2021**, *18*, 12355, doi:10.3390/ijerph182312355 . **151**

Francesco Bellocchio, Caterina Lonati, Jasmine Ion Titapiccolo, Jennifer Nadal, Heike Meiselbach, Matthias Schmid, Barbara Baerthlein, Ulrich Tschulena, Markus Schneider, Ulla T. Schultheiss, Carlo Barbieri, Christoph Moore, Sonja Steppan, Kai-Uwe Eckardt, Stefano Stuard and Luca Neri
Validation of a Novel Predictive Algorithm for Kidney Failure in Patients Suffering from Chronic Kidney Disease: The Prognostic Reasoning System for Chronic Kidney Disease (PROGRES-CKD)
Reprinted from: *Int. J. Environ. Res. Public Health* **2021**, *18*, 12649, doi:10.3390/ijerph182312649 . **163**

Abdur Rasool, Chayut Bunterngchit, Luo Tiejian, Md. Ruhul Islam, Qiang Qu and Qingshan Jiang
Improved Machine Learning-Based Predictive Models for Breast Cancer Diagnosis
Reprinted from: *Int. J. Environ. Res. Public Health* **2022**, *19*, 3211, doi:10.3390/ijerph19063211 . . . **181**

About the Editor

Tim Hulsen

Tim Hulsen is a bioinformatician and data scientist with a broad experience in both academia and the industry, working on a wide range of oncology projects. After receiving his MSc in biology in 2001, he obtained a PhD in bioinformatics in 2007 from a collaboration between the Radboud University Nijmegen and the pharma company N.V. Organon.

After a two year post-doc at the Radboud University Nijmegen, he moved to Philips Research in 2009, where he worked on biomarker discovery for one year, before moving to the Translational Research IT field, working on big data projects in oncology, such as Prostate Cancer Molecular Medicine (PCMM), Translational Research IT (TraIT), Movember Global Action Plan 3 (GAP3), and the European Randomized Study of Screening for Prostate Cancer (ERSPC).

His current projects are Liquid Biopsies and Imaging (LIMA), which is concerned with the use of Liquid Biopsies and Imaging data in breast cancer and rectal cancer, and ReIMAGINE, which studies the use of imaging to prevent unnecessary biopsies in prostate cancer. He is the author of several publications in the area of big data, data management, precision medicine, and personalized healthcare.

Editorial

Data Science in Healthcare: COVID-19 and Beyond

Tim Hulsen

Department of Hospital Services & Informatics, Philips Research, 5656AE Eindhoven, The Netherlands; tim.hulsen@philips.com

Citation: Hulsen, T. Data Science in Healthcare: COVID-19 and Beyond. *Int. J. Environ. Res. Public Health* **2022**, *19*, 3499. https://doi.org/10.3390/ijerph19063499

Received: 2 December 2021
Accepted: 14 March 2022
Published: 16 March 2022

Publisher's Note: MDPI stays neutral with regard to jurisdictional claims in published maps and institutional affiliations.

Copyright: © 2022 by the author. Licensee MDPI, Basel, Switzerland. This article is an open access article distributed under the terms and conditions of the Creative Commons Attribution (CC BY) license (https://creativecommons.org/licenses/by/4.0/).

Data science is an interdisciplinary field that applies numerous techniques, such as machine learning (ML), neural networks (NN) and artificial intelligence (AI), to create value, based on extracting knowledge and insights from available 'big' data [1]. The recent advances in data science and AI have had a major impact on healthcare already, as can be seen in the recent biomedical literature [2]. Improved sharing and analysis of medical data results in earlier and better diagnoses, and more patient-tailored treatments. This increased data sharing, in combination with advances in health data management, works hand-in-hand with trends such as increased patient-centricity (with shared decision making), self-care (e.g., using wearables), and integrated healthcare delivery. Using data science and AI, researchers can deliver new approaches to merge, analyze, and process complex data and gain more actionable insights, understanding, and knowledge at the individual and population level [3]. AI can be applied in all three major areas of early detection and diagnosis, treatment, as well as outcome prediction and prognosis evaluation [4]. ML algorithms can make predictions on how a disease will develop or respond to treatment, deep learning algorithms can find malignant tumors in magnetic resonance (MR) images and digital pathology images, and natural language-processing (NLP) algorithms can analyze unstructured documents with high speed and accuracy. These are just a few examples of what data science can do. This Special Issue focuses on how data science and AI are used in healthcare, and on related topics such as data sharing and data management. Since this Special Issue contains papers from 2020 to 2022, naturally there are a few papers about the COVID-19 pandemic: one on the determination of potential risk factors for the case fatality rate, one on the analysis of Arabic Twitter data to detect government pandemic measures and public concerns, and one on an enhanced sentinel surveillance system for outbreak prediction. There are also papers about data-sharing initiatives, depression treatment, the relationship between depression and metabolic status, cardiac thoracic pain, hand-foot-and-mouth disease infection, arteriovenous fistula (AVF) failure, chronic kidney disease (CKD) and breast cancer diagnosis.

"Coronavirus Disease 2019 (COVID-19): A Modeling Study of Factors Driving Variation in Case Fatality Rate by Country" by Pan et al. [5], "COVID-19: Detecting Government Pandemic Measures and Public Concerns from Twitter Arabic Data using Distributed Machine Learning" by Alomari et al. [6] and "Enhanced Sentinel Surveillance System for COVID-19 Outbreak Prediction in a Large European Dialysis Clinics Network" by Bellocchio et al. [7] all present research around the COVID-19 pandemic. Pan et al. [5] identified 24 potential risk factors driving variation in SARS-CoV-2 case fatality rate (CFR). Their model predicted an increased CFR for countries that waited over 14 days to implement social distancing interventions after the 100th reported case. Smoking prevalence and the percentage population over the age of 70 years were also associated with higher CFR. Hospital beds per 1000 and CT scanners per million were identified as possible protective factors associated with decreased CFR. Alomari et al. [6] proposes a software tool comprising a collection of unsupervised Latent Dirichlet Allocation (LDA) ML and other methods for the analysis of Twitter data in Arabic with the aim to detect government pandemic measures and public concerns during the COVID-19 pandemic. Using the tool, they collected a dataset comprising 14 million tweets from the Kingdom of Saudi Arabia (KSA) for the period 1 February to 1 June 2020. They detected 15 government pandemic measures and public concerns, and six macro-concerns (economic sustainability, social sustainability, etc.), and formulated their information-structural, temporal, and spatio-temporal relationships. Bellocchio et al. [7] present a sentinel surveillance system supported by an ML prediction model, whereby the occurrence of COVID-19 cases in a clinic propagates distance-weighted risk estimates to adjacent dialysis units. The system allows for a prompt risk assessment and a timely response to the challenges posed by the COVID-19 epidemic throughout Fresenius Medical Care (FMC) European dialysis clinics.

"Sharing Is Caring-Data Sharing Initiatives in Healthcare" by Hulsen [8] shows an analysis of the current literature around data sharing, and discusses five aspects of data sharing in the medical domain, namely publisher requirements, data ownership, growing support for data sharing, data sharing initiatives and how the use of federated data might be a solution. With federated data, there is no need for a centralized source database (with all its privacy issues), because the algorithm is brought to the data instead of the other way around. The author also discusses some potential future developments around data sharing, such as medical crowdsourcing and data generalists.

"Digital Training for Non-Specialist Health Workers to Deliver a Brief Psychological Treatment for Depression in Primary Care in India: Findings From a Randomized Pilot Study" by Muke et al. [9] evaluates the feasibility and acceptability of a digital program for training non-specialist health workers to deliver a brief psychological treatment for depression. This study, performed in Sehore (a rural district in Madhya Pradesh, India) adds to mounting efforts aimed at leveraging digital technology to increase the availability of evidence-based mental health services in low-resource primary care settings in.

"Association of Metabolically Healthy Obesity and Future Depression; Using National Health Insurance System Data in Korea from 2009–2017" by Seo et al. [10] investigates if depression and metabolic status are relevant by classifying them into the following four categories by their metabolic status and body mass index: (1) metabolically healthy non-obese (MHN); (2) metabolically healthy obese (MHO); (3) metabolically unhealthy non-obese (MUN); and (4) metabolically unhealthy obese (MUO). Their results show that the MHN ratio in women is higher than in men. In both men and women, depression incidence was the highest among MUO participants. In female participants, MHO is also related to a higher risk of depressive symptoms. This indicates that MHO is not an entirely benign condition in relation to depression in women. Therefore, reducing the number of metabolic syndrome and obesity patients in Korea will likely reduce the incidence of depression.

"Assessment of Thoracic Pain Using Machine Learning: A Case Study from Baja California, Mexico" by Rojas-Mendizabal et al. [11] aims to determine the correlated variables with thoracic pain of cardiac origin. Their analysis of 258 geriatric patients from Medical Norte Hospital in Tijuana (Baja California, Mexico) uses two ML techniques, i.e., tree classification and cross-validation. Their results suggest that among the main factors related to cardiac thoracic pain are dyslipidemia, chronic kidney failure, hypertension, diabetes, smoking habits, and troponin levels at the time of admission.

"Optimized Neural Network Based on Genetic Algorithm to Construct Hand-Foot-and-Mouth Disease Prediction and Early-Warning Model" by Lin et al. [12] discusses the high number of recent infections of hand-foot-and-mouth disease (HFMD). Previous research on the prevalence of HFMD mainly predicts the number of future cases based on the number of historical cases in various places, and the influence of many related factors that affect the prevalence of this disease is ignored. Existing early-warning research of HFMD mainly uses direct case report, which uses statistical methods in time and space to provide early-warnings of outbreaks separately. It leads to a high error rate and low confidence in the early-warning results. This paper uses ML methods to establish an HFMD epidemic prediction model with a high accuracy. Both incidence data and environmental (mostly weather) data are used.

"Development and Validation of a Machine Learning Model Predicting Arteriovenous Fistula Failure in a Large Network of Dialysis Clinics" by Ricardo et al. [13] derived and validated an arteriovenous fistula failure model (AVF-FM) based on ML. The model was trained in the derivation set (70% of initial cohort) by exploiting the information routinely collected in the Nephrocare European Clinical Database (EuCliD; 13,369 patients). Model performance was tested by concordance statistic and calibration charts in the remaining 30% of records. Feature importance was computed using the SHapley Additive exPlanations (SHAP) method. The model achieved good discrimination and calibration properties by combining routinely collected clinical and sensor data, requiring no additional effort by healthcare staff. Therefore, it can potentially facilitate risk-based personalization of AVF surveillance strategies.

In "Validation of a Novel Predictive Algorithm for Kidney Failure in Patients Suffering from Chronic Kidney Disease: The Prognostic Reasoning System for Chronic Kidney Disease (PROGRES-CKD)" by Ricardo et al. [14] a novel algorithm predicting end-stage kidney disease (ESKD) is described, named PROGRES-CKD. This Naïve-Bayes classifier accurately predicts kidney failure onset among chronic kidney disease (CKD) patients. Contrary to equation-based scores, PROGRES-CKD extends to patients with incomplete data and allows for the explicit assessment of prediction robustness in case of missing values. The algorithm may efficiently assist physicians' prognostic reasoning in real-life applications.

Finally, Rasool et al. [15] discuss in "Improved Machine Learning-based Predictive Models for Breast Cancer Diagnosis" four different predictive models to improve breast-cancer diagnostic accuracy, as well as data exploratory techniques (DET) such as feature distribution, correlation, elimination and hyperparameter optimization. The Wisconsin Diagnostic Breast Cancer (WDBC) and Breast Cancer Coimbra Dataset (BCCD) datasets were used as input. They report a significant improvement in the models' diagnostic capability with their DET. Therefore, the techniques can help to improve breast cancer diagnosis.

The manuscripts in this Special Issue give us only a brief overview of the wide use of data science in healthcare, and offer a glimpse into the future, where even faster computers and more advanced AI algorithms will make many more applications possible. For example, whereas many AI algorithms only use data from specific data types, this can be expanded to a combination of a wide range of patient-related (structured or unstructured) data, including clinical data, imaging data, digital pathology data, genomics data, data from wearables, and much more, to optimize the result for the patient. AI systems will not replace clinicians on a large scale, but rather will support their care for patients [16]. For example, AI can also be used to optimize the workflow in the hospital, or to create intelligent chatbots to help patients while reducing the workload for the clinicians. Furthermore, AI algorithms created in these times of COVID-19 might be of good use when managing similar pandemics in the future. It is probably safe to say that in ten years from now, there will not be a 'Data Science in Healthcare' Special Issue, because by that time almost everything in healthcare will be influenced by data science.

Funding: This research received no external funding.

Conflicts of Interest: The author declares no conflict of interest.

References

1. Hulsen, T.; Jamuar, S.S.; Moody, A.R.; Karnes, J.H.; Varga, O.; Hedensted, S.; Spreafico, R.; Hafler, D.A.; McKinney, E.F. From Big Data to Precision Medicine. *Front. Med.* **2019**, *6*, 34. [CrossRef] [PubMed]
2. Hulsen, T. Literature analysis of artificial intelligence in biomedicine. *Pharm. Res. Pers. Med.* **2021**. [CrossRef]
3. Hulsen, T. Challenges and solutions for big data in personalized healthcare. In *Big Data in Psychiatry & Neurology*; Moustafa, A.A., Ed.; Academic Press: London, UK, 2021; pp. 69–94. [CrossRef]
4. Jiang, F.; Jiang, Y.; Zhi, H.; Dong, Y.; Li, H.; Ma, S.; Wang, Y.; Dong, Q.; Shen, H.; Wang, Y. Artificial intelligence in healthcare: Past, present and future. *Stroke Vasc. Neurol.* **2017**, *2*, 230–243. [CrossRef] [PubMed]

5. Pan, J.; St Pierre, J.M.; Pickering, T.A.; Demirjian, N.L.; Fields, B.K.K.; Desai, B.; Gholamrezanezhad, A. Coronavirus Disease 2019 (COVID-19): A Modeling Study of Factors Driving Variation in Case Fatality Rate by Country. *Int. J. Environ. Res. Public Health* **2020**, *17*, 8189. [CrossRef] [PubMed]
6. Alomari, E.; Katib, I.; Albeshri, A.; Mehmood, R. COVID-19: Detecting Government Pandemic Measures and Public Concerns from Twitter Arabic Data Using Distributed Machine Learning. *Int. J. Environ. Res. Public Health* **2021**, *18*, 282. [CrossRef] [PubMed]
7. Bellocchio, F.; Carioni, P.; Lonati, C.; Garbelli, M.; Martínez-Martínez, F.; Stuard, S.; Neri, L. Enhanced Sentinel Surveillance System for COVID-19 Outbreak Prediction in a Large European Dialysis Clinics Network. *Int. J. Environ. Res. Public Health* **2021**, *18*, 9739. [CrossRef] [PubMed]
8. Hulsen, T. Sharing Is Caring-Data Sharing Initiatives in Healthcare. *Int. J. Environ. Res. Public Health* **2020**, *17*, 3046. [CrossRef] [PubMed]
9. Muke, S.S.; Tugnawat, D.; Joshi, U.; Anand, A.; Khan, A.; Shrivastava, R.; Singh, A.; Restivo, J.L.; Bhan, A.; Patel, V.; et al. Digital Training for Non-Specialist Health Workers to Deliver a Brief Psychological Treatment for Depression in Primary Care in India: Findings from a Randomized Pilot Study. *Int. J. Environ. Res. Public Health* **2020**, *17*, 6368. [CrossRef] [PubMed]
10. Seo, Y.; Lee, S.; Ahn, J.S.; Min, S.; Kim, M.H.; Kim, J.Y.; Kang, D.R.; Hwang, S.; Vicheka, P.; Lee, J. Association of Metabolically Healthy Obesity and Future Depression: Using National Health Insurance System Data in Korea from 2009–2017. *Int. J. Environ. Res. Public Health* **2020**, *18*, 63. [CrossRef] [PubMed]
11. Rojas-Mendizabal, V.; Castillo-Olea, C.; Gómez-Siono, A.; Zuñiga, C. Assessment of Thoracic Pain Using Machine Learning: A Case Study from Baja California, Mexico. *Int. J. Environ. Res. Public Health* **2021**, *18*, 2155. [CrossRef] [PubMed]
12. Lin, X.; Wang, X.; Wang, Y.; Du, X.; Jin, L.; Wan, M.; Ge, H.; Yang, X. Optimized Neural Network Based on Genetic Algorithm to Construct Hand-Foot-and-Mouth Disease Prediction and Early-Warning Model. *Int. J. Environ. Res. Public Health* **2021**, *18*, 2959. [CrossRef] [PubMed]
13. Peralta, R.; Garbelli, M.; Bellocchio, F.; Ponce, P.; Stuard, S.; Lodigiani, M.; Fazendeiro Matos, J.; Ribeiro, R.; Nikam, M.; Botler, M.; et al. Development and Validation of a Machine Learning Model Predicting Arteriovenous Fistula Failure in a Large Network of Dialysis Clinics. *Int. J. Environ. Res. Public Health* **2021**, *18*, 12355. [CrossRef] [PubMed]
14. Bellocchio, F.; Lonati, C.; Titapiccolo, J.; Nadal, J.; Meiselbach, H.; Schmid, M.; Baerthlein, B.; Tschulena, U.; Schneider, M.; Schultheiss, U.T.; et al. Validation of a novel predictive algorithm for kidney failure in patients suffering from chronic kidney disease: The Prognostic Reasoning System for Chronic Kidney Disease (PROGRES-CKD). *Int. J. Environ. Res. Public Health* **2021**, *18*, 12649. [CrossRef] [PubMed]
15. Rasool, A.; Bunterngchit, C.; Tiejian, L.; Islam, M.R.; Qu, Q.; Jiang, Q. Improved Machine Learning-Based Predictive Models for Breast Cancer Diagnosis. *Int. J. Environ. Res. Public Health* **2022**, *19*, 3211. [CrossRef]
16. Davenport, T.; Kalakota, R. The potential for artificial intelligence in healthcare. *Future Healthc. J.* **2019**, *6*, 94. [CrossRef] [PubMed]

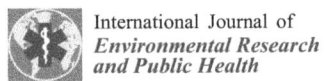

Article

Coronavirus Disease 2019 (COVID-19): A Modeling Study of Factors Driving Variation in Case Fatality Rate by Country

Jennifer Pan [1,†], Joseph Marie St. Pierre [1,†], Trevor A. Pickering [1,2], Natalie L. Demirjian [1,3], Brandon K.K. Fields [1], Bhushan Desai [1,4] and Ali Gholamrezanezhad [1,4,*]

1. Keck School of Medicine, University of Southern California, Los Angeles, CA 90033, USA; panjenni@usc.edu (J.P.); jstpierr@usc.edu (J.M.S.P.); tpickeri@usc.edu (T.A.P.); ndemirji@usc.edu (N.L.D.); bkfields@usc.edu (B.K.K.F.); bhushan.desai@med.usc.edu (B.D.)
2. Department of Preventive Medicine, Keck School of Medicine, University of Southern California, Los Angeles, CA 90033, USA
3. Department of Integrative Anatomical Sciences, Keck School of Medicine, University of Southern California, Los Angeles, CA 90033, USA
4. Department of Radiology, Keck School of Medicine, University of Southern California, Los Angeles, CA 90033, USA
* Correspondence: ali.gholamrezanezhad@med.usc.edu; Tel.: +443-839-7134
† These authors contributed equally to the work and should be considered as co-first authors.

Received: 21 September 2020; Accepted: 2 November 2020; Published: 5 November 2020

Abstract: *Background:* The novel Severe Acute Respiratory Syndrome Coronavirus-2 has led to a global pandemic in which case fatality rate (CFR) has varied from country to country. This study aims to identify factors that may explain the variation in CFR across countries. *Methods:* We identified 24 potential risk factors affecting CFR. For all countries with over 5000 reported COVID-19 cases, we used country-specific datasets from the WHO, the OECD, and the United Nations to quantify each of these factors. We examined univariable relationships of each variable with CFR, as well as correlations among predictors and potential interaction terms. Our final multivariable negative binomial model included univariable predictors of significance and all significant interaction terms. *Results:* Across the 39 countries under consideration, our model shows COVID-19 case fatality rate was best predicted by time to implementation of social distancing measures, hospital beds per 1000 individuals, percent population over 70 years, CT scanners per 1 million individuals, and (in countries with high population density) smoking prevalence. *Conclusion:* Our model predicted an increased CFR for countries that waited over 14 days to implement social distancing interventions after the 100th reported case. Smoking prevalence and percentage population over the age of 70 years were also associated with higher CFR. Hospital beds per 1000 and CT scanners per million were identified as possible protective factors associated with decreased CFR.

Keywords: COVID-19; SARS-CoV-2; pneumonia; computed tomography; case fatality rate; social distancing; smoking

1. Introduction

On 31 December 2019, a pneumonia of increasing incidence and unknown etiology in Wuhan, China was reported to the World Health Organization (WHO). Investigations led to the discovery of a novel coronavirus, later dubbed Severe Acute Respiratory Syndrome Coronavirus-2 (SARS-CoV-2), which causes the pathology known as Coronavirus Disease 2019 (COVID-19) [1]. Despite initial containment measures recommended by the WHO in early January 2020, COVID-19 spread rapidly to other countries in the following weeks and was eventually classified as a global pandemic on 11 March

2020 [2,3]. Since then, it has posed major challenges to healthcare systems in affected countries around the world while crippling the global economy. At the time of our analysis, epidemiological data indicates that COVID-19 had since spread to 205 countries with over 3.1 million reported cases and over 227,000 deaths worldwide [4].

As effective antiviral therapies and vaccines remain unavailable, current efforts to halt the transmission of COVID-19 rely on social distancing, individual quarantine and isolation, and community containment measures [5]. Yet there has been great variation worldwide in the implementation of such measures. As demonstrated in China, the spread of the disease was slowed by effectively combining the largest quarantine ever implemented—over 200,000 people were either tracked via contact tracing or received medical observation as of 30 January 2020—with stringent community facemask use, limitations on social gatherings, isolation of affected workplace institutions, and lockdown of multiple public transportation outlets to isolate communities and towns with outbreaks [6,7]. However, this approach is resource-intensive and is less likely to be emulated by more liberal democracies [8]. Therefore, it may be useful to examine the differences in implementation of quarantine policies in different countries and their impact on disease mortality.

Numerous studies have examined the daily and cumulative number of confirmed cases by country and have analyzed variation in case-fatality rate (CFR), defined as number of deaths relative to number of confirmed cases. Estimates of CFR are placed at 2.3% in China, while estimates of infection-fatality ratio (IFR), which attempt to account for proportions of mild and asymptomatic disease, sits markedly lower at 0.1–0.94% [7,9–11]. However, because the exact proportions of mild and asymptomatic cases are variable and reliant on estimations in lieu of confirmatory testing, IFR-based metrics have yet to produce a reliable model [10,11]. Therefore, CFR remains a more concrete measure of describing and identifying predictive factors associated with disease mortality. CFR varies from country to country and, while multiple studies have found links to possible underlying factors driving changes in case mortality, a complete explanation of this variation remains unclear. Using country-specific data from global organizations, our study aims to identify factors that best explain differences in CFR among 39 highly impacted countries during the first five months of the COVID-19 pandemic. To the best of our knowledge, this is the first study to investigate multiple factors affecting CFR using country-specific data to drive our modeling.

2. Materials and Methods

2.1. Data Collection

We began by conducting a targeted literature search for potential risk factors for COVID-19 mortality through Pubmed, using variations on terms including "COVID-19 mortality risk factors" and "pandemic mortality risk factors". Our approach was similar to a study conducted by Morales et al., investigating H1N1 influenza risk factors that varied by country [12]. In our review of studies on the current pandemic as well as past SARS and influenza pandemics, we identified 24 risk factors (Table S1) for COVID-19 fatality that were worth investigating, including quarantine policies, air travel activity, age distribution, comorbidities, healthcare access, availability of diagnostic tests, cumulative and daily testing data, and environmental factors such as air pollution and climate [5–7,13–22]. Regarding quarantine policies, government responses varied by country. For purposes of this study, we defined this intervention as the first date per international news sources when recommendations were made or legislation was passed limiting gathering size, closing non-essential business, or encouraging social distancing (Table S2). School closures and international travel bans were not considered as they only applied to certain individuals within each country's population.

To calculate CFR, we used the total confirmed cases and deaths for a given country from Our World in Data [4]. As higher testing rates per capita could be associated with an increased record of mild cases, we included total cumulative tests and tests per 1000 to explore the relationship between CFR and testing capacity per capita. Additionally, we included socioeconomic factors such as GDP, level of education, and scientific production. To examine healthcare-related factors, we included hospital beds, physicians per 1000, and per capita healthcare expenditure. We also looked at the availability of CT scanners and radiologists per one million population, as CT chest imaging represents a possibly limited resource that can increase the diagnostic accuracy. This was particularly true during the first wave of the pandemic, during which reverse transcription polymerase chain reaction (RT-PCR) kits were limited and imaging was relied upon by multiple countries for diagnosis of the disease [23]. Finally, given recent data linking the comorbidities of obesity and chronic lung disease to increased disease severity and poorer outcomes in cases of COVID-19 [16,19,24], we included prevalence of obesity, chronic obstructive pulmonary disease (COPD), and tobacco use, along with particulate matter as a measure of air pollution.

We decided to include in our analysis all countries with over 5000 COVID-19 deaths at the time of writing [4]. This cutoff was chosen to generate a set of at least 20 countries located in all hemispheres with diverse quarantine measures, GDPs, and geographic locations. 39 countries were found to meet this criterion and were included in the study. For each country, data was generated for the 24 variables from the following sources: Our World in Data project [4], World Bank database [25], OECD database [26], United Nations World Population Prospects [27], Global Health Data Exchange [28], and various international news sources (Table S2).

2.2. Statistical Analysis

We began by examining the distributions of and correlations among all variables. We found that population density, GDP in 2017, scientific production, total tests, air travel, percentage illiterate, and air pollution were highly positively skewed. To reduce the influence of extreme observations, we transformed these variables on the log scale, except for population density for which a square root transformation was sufficient. We next examined the univariable relationships between independent variables and case fatality rates to find candidate variables for our final multivariable model. We found the negative binomial model for case fatality rate to be appropriate, as the overdispersion parameter α was statistically significant in each of these models. We noted the significance of each variable in these univariable models and selected variables for a preliminary multivariable model at $p < 0.15$. We additionally wanted to examine whether the effect of candidate predictors was moderated by population density and time to quarantine. We therefore examined models with each independent variable and (1) an interaction with population density and (2) an interaction with days from 100th case to quarantine (dichotomized as >14 days). Days from 100th case to quarantine was dichotomized as it showed a nonlinear relationship with CFR, with higher CFR rates in the highest quartile (>14 days). Our preliminary multivariable model was created by including all univariable candidate predictors and then adding all significant interaction terms. A hands-on guided approach was used to check for any anomalies that arose when adding or removing variables from the final model. Our preliminary final model contained all multivariable predictors significant at $p < 0.05$. Before arriving at our final model, each variable excluded in the univariable step was added back one-by-one to ensure they were still nonsignificant predictors of case fatality rate. All analyses were performed in Stata (v15.0).

3. Results

Case fatality rate varied widely by country, as low as 0.6% and as high as 17.7% (M = 5.4%, SD = 4.3%). Means and standard deviations of candidate predictors are shown in Table 1, along with rate ratios from the univariable negative binomial model for each individual predictor. We found that percent population >70 years old, general mortality per 1000 individuals, percentage of population illiterate, percentage of population with HIV, and air pollution were significantly associated with case fatality rate in these univariable models. In addition, tests per 1000 individuals, percentage of population obese, smokers, tobacco users, and with HIV significantly interacted with population density.

Table 1. Descriptive statistics (mean & SD) for candidate predictor variables, rate ratios (SE) for univariable relationships between predictors and case fatality rate, and p-value for the interaction of each predictor variable with population density (square root transformed). For comparability, all rate ratios reflect the effect of the standardized predictor on case fatality rate.

Variable	Mean (SD)	Rate Ratio (SE)	p (Density Interaction)
Percent population >70 years old [†]	8.9 (4.7)	1.33 (0.16) *	-
Population density	158.7 (148.2)	1.14 (0.32)	-
Population size [†]	135.4×10^6 (310×10^6)	1.07 (0.14)	-
GDP in 2017 ($) [†]	1.82×10^{12} (3.57×10^{12})	1.23 (0.16)	-
GDP per capita in 2017	29761 (22379)	1.11 (0.15)	-
Healthcare expenditure per capita	2849 (2735)	1.17 (0.16)	-
Scientific production [†]	53393 (91189)	1.20 (0.15)	-
Hospital beds per 1000	3.95 (2.91)	0.92 (0.14)	-
Physicians per 1000	2.78 (1.26)	1.16 (0.14)	-
General mortality per 1000	7.82 (2.62)	1.44 (0.21) *	-
Life expectancy	78.7 (4.3)	1.21 (0.14)	-
CT scanners per 1 million	26.6 (22.2)	0.75 (0.13)	-
Radiologists [†]	5863 (14180)	1.20 (0.20)	-
Radiologists per 1 million	64.1 (43.2)	1.25 (0.20)	-
Total tests [†]	330013 (325817)	1.15 (0.14)	-
Tests per 1000	12.0 (9.4)	1.04 (0.15)	0.04
Median age	36.3 (6.8)	1.23 (0.14)	-
Days from 100th case to quarantine	9.5 (8.4)	1.26 (0.18)	-
Air travel [†]	93587 (165381)	1.05 (0.13)	-
Education	73.5 (19.2)	0.88 (0.14)	-
Percent Illiterate [†]	4.5 (8.1)	0.75 (0.09) *	-
Percent Obese	21.1 (8.5)	0.99 (0.15)	0.005
Percent Smokers	20.3 (6.2)	1.08 (0.14)	0.03
Percent Tobacco Users	23.3 (8.0)	1.11 (0.15)	0.06
Percent HIV	0.2 (0.3)	1.30 (0.18) *	0.001
Percent COPD	5.4 (2.3)	1.23 (0.15)	-
Air pollution [†]	27.2 (34.0)	0.68 (0.09) **	-

[†] Log-transformed variable was used for Rate Ratio, * $p < 0.05$, ** $p < 0.01$.

We also found several instances of collinearity. For example, we found high correlations between: smoking prevalence and tobacco use prevalence (r = 0.92, $p < 0.001$); air travel and GDP (r = 0.96, $p < 0.001$); and percentage of population >70 years old was correlated with several variables such as general mortality (r = 0.80, $p < 0.001$), prevalence of COPD (r = 0.71, $p < 0.001$), life expectancy (r = 0.74, p < 0.001), physicians per capita (r = 0.73, $p < 0.001$), tests per capita (r = 0.88, $p < 0.001$), and GDP (r = 0.71, $p < 0.001$). When collinear variables were included in the model, we sequentially added them in one-by-one and evaluated the model fit; the variable producing the best fit was retained in the model.

Our final model included time from 100th case to quarantine (dichotomized >14 days), hospital beds per 1000 individuals, percentage population over 70 years, CT scanners per 1 million individuals (log-transformed), and interaction between smoking prevalence and population density. This model had good agreement between observed and predicted CFR values (Figure 1). We found that countries waiting over 14 days from the 100th case to quarantine had 1.5 times the case fatality rate of those that did not wait as long ($p = 0.045$), and each percentage increase in the population over 70 years was associated with 1.15-time increase in the case fatality rate ($p < 0.001$). Though proportion of population over 70 years was correlated with a slew of health-related variables, there were some that were predictive of case fatality rate above and beyond the proportion of the population that is elderly. We found that each additional hospital bed per 1000 individuals reduced the case fatality rate by 15% (RR = 0.85, $p < 0.001$), and that a 1-unit increase in the log number of CT scanners per million was associated with half the case fatality rate (RR = 0.49, $p < 0.001$). The deleterious effect of smoking on case fatality rate was significant, but only in countries with higher density (p-interaction < 0.001). To aid in interpretation, we calculated the rate ratio at the mean, and 0.5 SD below and above the mean, of square root transformed population density. These results are presented in Table 2 (Model 1).

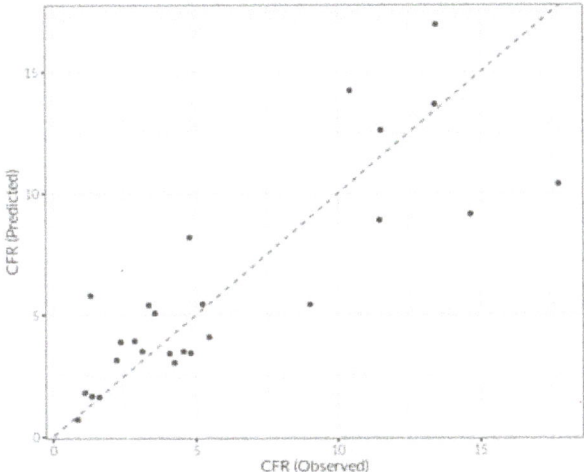

Figure 1. Final model (Model 1) of predicted values plotted against observed values of case fatality rate. These two variables were correlated at r = 0.84.

Table 2. Final multivariable negative binomial model predicting case fatality rate. Rate ratios and 95% confidence intervals are presented. Smoking prevalence is evaluated at the mean of (square root transformed) population density, 0.5 SD below (low, approximately 65 per km^2), and 0.5 SD above (high, approximately 200 per km^2). Model I contains our final estimates without imputation ($n = 26$), Model II additionally adjusts for date of 100th case, and Model III shows the results from our final model on imputed CT scanner data ($n = 39$).

Variable	Model I RR (95% CI)	Model II RR (95% CI)	Model III RR (95% CI)
Prevalence smoking (10% population increase)			
at low population density	1.00 (0.69, 1.44)	1.13 (0.80, 1.61)	0.96 (0.69, 1.33)
at mean population density	1.59 (0.99, 2.56)	1.72 (1.12, 2.65)	1.33 (0.90, 1.96)
at high population density	2.53 (1.32, 4.87)	2.62 (1.46, 4.70)	1.83 (1.09, 3.07)
>14 days from 100th case to quarantine	1.54 (1.01, 2.35)	1.23 (0.78, 1.92)	1.57 (1.01, 2.43)
Hospital beds per 1000 individuals	0.85 (0.78, 0.92)	0.84 (0.77, 0.90)	0.58 (0.45, 0.74)
Percent population >70 years	1.15 (1.08, 1.23)	1.12 (1.03, 1.20)	1.13 (1.07, 1.20)
CT scanners per 1 million individuals (log)	0.49 (0.34, 0.67)	0.44 (0.32, 0.60)	0.67 (0.46, 0.98)
Date of 100th case (days)	-	0.96 (0.92, 0.99)	-

We performed additional sensitivity analyses to explore the effect of (1) date of country being impacted by COVID-19 and (2) missing covariate data. First, we created a new model by including date of 100th case to examine any change in coefficients (Table 2, Model 2). It was suspected that CFR may be lower in countries that reached their 100th case later, as they may not have had sufficient time for the virus to act on individuals. We examined the correlation between date of 100th case and days-to-quarantine and found a negative relationship (r = −0.47, $p = 0.003$) after excluding China, which was impacted early but also had quick quarantine implementation (Figure 2). We also note that

13 countries were missing data on CT scanners in our model. To determine possible impacts of this missing data, we performed multiple imputation with 25 data sets using all complete variables in the data that were not included in our final models. Our final model changed slightly but not appreciably (Table 2, Model 3). Date of 100th case was not significant when added to this model ($p = 0.66$; model not shown).

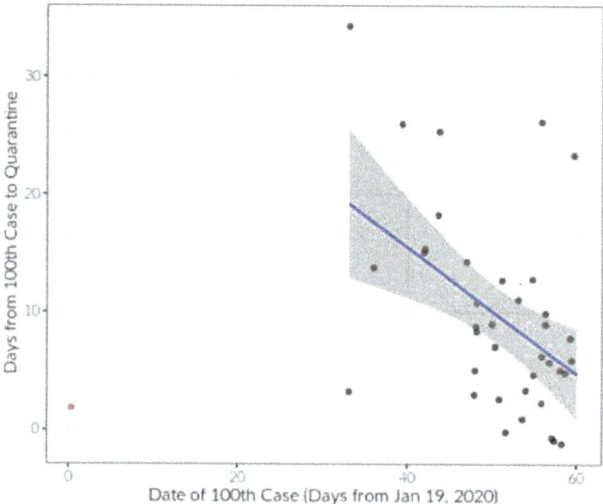

Figure 2. Days from 100th case to quarantine plotted against date of 100th case (in days from 19 January 2020; China's 100th case). The two variables are correlated (r = −0.47, $p = 0.003$) after removing China (red square).

4. Discussion

Our analysis of 24 variables relative to COVID-19 mortality across 39 countries suggests that the case fatality rate is related to a variety of country-specific factors, including time to implement social distancing measures after the 100th case, hospital beds per 1000 individuals, percentage population over 70 years, CT scanners per 1 million individuals, and smoking prevalence with high population density.

Social distancing interventions, such as increased case isolation and community contact reduction, have been shown to be highly effective in slowing the spread of the virus [29]. According to our model, countries that waited over 14 days to implement social distancing interventions after their 100th reported case saw an increased CFR (RR = 1.54, $p = 0.045$), consistent across all population densities. As COVID-19 spread has been shown to occur during the asymptomatic incubation period [30,31], the promptness of local and national government response in implementing quarantine policies may have played a crucial role in limiting human-to-human transmission. As respiratory failure from Acute Respiratory Distress Syndrome appears to be the leading cause of mortality [32], surges in severe COVID-19 cases have the potential to overwhelm the capacity of a country's healthcare system to provide mechanical ventilation and other intensive resources [33,34]. Thus, timely implementation of social distancing measures may, in many cases, have delayed epidemic peak in regard to CFR by reducing exponential growth of cases [29]. However, we did see this effect attenuated when including date of 100th case in the model. While it may be possible that countries that were affected more recently may not have had time to fully experience the true extent of COVID-related deaths, we did find that countries affected by COVID-19 later were quicker to implement quarantine measures. Because of this, we cannot truly disentangle the effect of time-to-quarantine from date of 100th case.

With regards to comorbidities, our model predicts that a 10% increase in smoking prevalence more than doubles the CFR in countries with high population density (RR = 2.53, $p < 0.001$). There is a growing body of evidence associating increased risk of both increased severity of disease, ICU admission, and death among infected patients with smoking history, particularly active smokers [35,36]. Yet, it is unclear why our model correlated smoking prevalence with increased CFR strongly in high-density populations only. One possible explanation is that high density areas are more likely to suffer outbreaks sufficient to overwhelm the local hospital and ICU capacity, triggering mass casualty protocols with possible triaging of resource allocation in favor of patients with more favorable prognostic indicators [37,38]. Smoking history is often associated with other medical comorbidities, notably cardiovascular disease, which may contribute to a poorer overall prognostic presentation and thus less priority in a resource-poor scenario [36,39]. Finally, the effect that smoking may have as a potential risk factor is likely to be more exaggerated in densely populated regions where these vulnerable individuals interact with others in closer proximity and with higher frequency. Smoking prevalence may also be related to other factors that are impacted by population density. It will be necessary to further explore the effects of smoking and its sequalae on disease course to determine the additional considerations that should be given to patients with a history of smoking, particularly in areas of high population density.

Case fatality rate was reduced by 15% (RR = 0.85, $p < 0.001$) for each additional hospital bed per 1000 individuals, a reflection of resources available for delivering inpatient medical services. Studies on past influenza pandemics have shown that scarcity of healthcare resources and clinical infrastructure, particularly in rural or developing areas, is a major limitation to pandemic preparedness [40–42]. It is important to note that the capacity of a healthcare system is tied not only to infrastructure but also to the availability of providers; in order to increase capacity, it will be necessary to build a larger healthcare workforce to support more hospital beds and higher patient volume [41]. CT scanners represent another limited resource that appears to be a protective factor. Our model shows that a 1-unit increase in the log number of CT scanners per million was associated with half the case fatality rate (RR = 0.49, $p < 0.001$). A possible explanation for this protective effect is that CT scans have led to earlier detection of the disease, as early reports describe characteristic imaging features that are helpful in aiding diagnosis [43]. This may have been particularly advantageous in developing countries, where the capacity to develop and mass-distribute testing was limited during the first months of the pandemic [43–45], as well as for frontline providers in any country irrespective of testing ability as a means of providing earlier diagnosis [46,47]. Countries with more radiologists and CT scanners per capita are also likely to have increased availability of other health resources, and thus the variables may serve as proxy for other factors that reflect the robustness of a nation's healthcare system.

Our model also suggests a positive relationship between CFR and percentage of the population over age 70, with every added percent increasing the CFR by a factor of 1.15. This variable is highly associated with general mortality ($r = 0.80$, $p < 0.001$), life expectancy ($r = 0.74$, $p < 0.001$), and COPD ($r = 0.71$, $p < 0.001$) at the country level and could potentially be viewed as a proxy for indicating a country with older, more vulnerable population. Observations on age and increased case mortality are consistent with multiple retrospective studies identifying advanced age as a potential risk factor for more severe disease and worsened prognosis [48,49]. There are multiple possible explanations for this observation. In addition to frailty and increased risk of having multiple co-morbidities, some studies suggest age-related declines in T and B cell function alongside preserved innate immunity may be contributory, with the resultant cytokine 2-dominant response triggering a pro-inflammatory state which increases mortality [50,51].

Limitations and Future Directions

This modeling study used a cross-sectional, ecological dataset taken during the pandemic's first wave. As such, most of our model's limitations stem from the weaknesses of this approach. As with most data gathered in the first several months of the pandemic, accuracy was limited by the information available at that time and capacity to report cases in a timely manner may vary from country to country. This limitation affects estimates of CFR, which has been shown to require an assessment of the delay between infection and the reporting of case data as well as the extent to which death-related cases are underreported. Furthermore, CFR itself is best modeled as a continuous variable which changes over time as the disease spreads to areas which vary in risk due to population density and demographic, as well as how healthcare systems and government policies adapt to disease burden [52]. Finally, given the ecological nature of our study, it should be noted that our findings and discussion of risk factors do not necessarily reflect a relationship between these variables and probability of survival at the individual level.

In addition, our study was limited by the availability of datasets used for country-specific data. Some of the datasets used to generate data for the 24 variables did not include all countries. For example, although our univariate analysis did not find a significant correlation between CFR and total radiologists or radiologists per one million, our data on radiologists per country was limited to one study from 2008 that included only 26 of the 39 countries analyzed [53]. More data is needed on this subject, as early reports on the global response to COVID-19 have shown that computerized tomography (CT) of the chest may serve an integral role in the timely diagnosis of the disease, as well as in severity staging and monitoring of clinical course [43,44,47,54,55]. Another limitation arises from utilizing data pertaining to entire countries for risk factors that may vary within each country on a geographically smaller scale-among cities, for example. This is especially true for large countries such as the United States and China with wide variations in population density, resource availability, and environmental characteristics based on region. For the timing of isolation and quarantine measures, our study relied on multiple secondary news sources for specific dates (Table S2), which, despite a standardized and systematic approach, is inherently less reliable than documentation from a single primary source.

Future studies are also needed to evaluate the effect and timing of government interventions on disease spread and CFR. While our results suggest a possible relationship between early government implementation of social distancing measures and reduced CFR, it remains unclear whether differences in the type or stringency of these measures appreciably influences CFR. Timing of quarantine measures is also important, and a comparison of specific state-imposed measures as well as their timing relative to the date of first confirmed case and other milestones of cumulative case growth could represent a strong follow-up to our findings. We also suggest a closer look at the relationship between smoking and its association with severe disease, as well as the extent to which such risk factors affect comprehensive care under triage protocols in resource-restricted circumstances.

5. Conclusions

Using country-based multivariate modeling, our study found significant correlations between increased CFR and smoking prevalence, percentage of a population over the age of 70 years, increased time to implementation of social distancing or stay-at-home measures, as well as decreased CFR and hospital beds per 1000 and CT scanners per million. Notably, CFR appears to increase significantly for every day after the 100th documented case where governmental precautions are not put in place. More research is needed on the relationship between the timing and effectiveness of government precautions and case fatality rate, as well as the role that hospital bed capacity and CT scanner availability play in reducing case fatality. The relationship between population density and smoking prevalence, as well as the influence smoking has on disease course, is also worth further exploration.

Supplementary Materials: The following are available online at http://www.mdpi.com/1660-4601/17/21/8189/s1, Table S1: 24 country-level risk factors with potential influence on COVID-19 case fatality rates, Table S2: Date of first government intervention per aggregation of secondary news sources as indicated.

Author Contributions: J.P. and J.M.S.P. generated the dataset. B.K.K.F. and N.L.D. provided feedback and guidance during the data collection. T.A.P. performed the statistical analysis. B.D. coordinated interdepartmental outreach. J.P., J.M.S.P., and T.A.P. drafted the manuscript with support from A.G., who conceived the idea.

All authors reviewed the manuscripts and provided edits prior to submission. J.P. and J.M.S.P. contributed equally to the work and should be considered as co-first authors. All authors have read and agreed to the published version of the manuscript.

Funding: This work was supported by grants UL1TR001855 and UL1TR000130 from the National Center for Advancing Translational Science (NCATS) of the U.S. National Institutes of Health. The content is solely the responsibility of the authors and does not necessarily represent the official views of the National Institutes of Health.

Conflicts of Interest: The authors declare no conflict of interest.

References

1. World Health Organization. *Novel Coronavirus (2019-nCoV) Situation Report—1 (2020)*; World Health Organization: Geneva, Switzerland, 2020.
2. World Health Organization. *Novel Coronavirus (2019-nCoV) Situation Report—12 (2020)*; World Health Organization: Geneva, Switzerland, 2020.
3. WHO. *Director-General's Opening Remarks at the Media Briefing on COVID-19—11 March 2020*; World Health Organization: Geneva, Switzerland, 2020.
4. Roser, M.; Ritchie, H.; Ortiz-Ospina, E. *Coronavirus Disease (COVID-19)—Statistics and Research (2020)*; Our World in Data: Oxford, UK, 2020; Available online: https://ourworldindata.org/coronavirus (accessed on 15 April 2020).
5. Wilder-Smith, A.; Freedman, D.O. Isolation, quarantine, social distancing and community containment: Pivotal role for old-style public health measures in the novel coronavirus (2019-nCoV) outbreak. *J. Travel Med.* **2020**, *27*. [CrossRef] [PubMed]
6. Wilder-Smith, A.; Chiew, C.J.; Lee, V.J. Can we contain the COVID-19 outbreak with the same measures as for SARS? *Lancet Infect. Dis.* **2020**. [CrossRef]
7. Anderson, R.M.; Heesterbeek, H.; Klinkenberg, D.; Hollingsworth, T.D. How will country-based mitigation measures influence the course of the COVID-19 epidemic? *Lancet* **2020**, *395*, 931–934. [CrossRef]
8. Lee, A. Wuhan novel coronavirus (COVID-19): Why global control is challenging? *Public Health* **2020**, *179*, A1–A2. [CrossRef] [PubMed]
9. World Health Organization. *Coronavirus Disease 2019 (COVID-19) Situation Report—30 (2020)*; World Health Organization: Geneva, Switzerland, 2020.
10. Jung, S.; Akhmetzhanov, A.; Hayashi, K.; Linton, N.M.; Yang, Y.; Yuan, B.; Kobayashi, T.; Kinoshita, R.; Nishiura, H. Real-Time Estimation of the Risk of Death from Novel Coronavirus (COVID-19) Infection: Inference Using Exported Cases. *J. Clin. Med.* **2020**, *9*, 523. [CrossRef] [PubMed]
11. Famulare, M. *2019-nCoV: Preliminary Estimates of the Confirmed-Case-Fatality-Ratio and Infection-Fatality-Ratio, and Initial Pandemic Risk Assessment*; Institute for Disease Modeling: Bellevue, WA, USA, 2020.
12. Morales, K.F.; Paget, J.; Spreeuwenberg, P. Possible explanations for why some countries were harder hit by the pandemic influenza virus in 2009—A global mortality impact modeling study. *BMC Infect Dis.* **2017**, *17*. [CrossRef] [PubMed]
13. Hosseini, P.; Sokolow, S.H.; Vandegrift, K.J.; Kilpatrick, A.M.; Daszak, P. Predictive Power of Air Travel and Socio-Economic Data for Early Pandemic Spread. *PLoS ONE* **2010**, *5*. [CrossRef] [PubMed]
14. World Health Organization. *Report of the WHO-China Joint Mission on Coronavirus Disease 2019 (COVID-19)*; World Health Organization: Geneva, Switzerland, 2020.
15. Richardson, S.; Hirsch, J.S.; Narasimhan, M.; Crawford, J.M.; McGinn, T.; Davidson, K.W.; Barnaby, D.P.; Becker, L.B.; Chelico, J.D.; Cohen, S.L.; et al. Presenting Characteristics, Comorbidities, and Outcomes Among 5700 Patients Hospitalized With COVID-19 in the New York City Area. *J. Am. Med.* **2020**. [CrossRef]
16. Adams, M.; Katz, D.; Grandpre, J. Population-Based Estimates of Chronic Conditions Affecting Risk for Complications from Coronavirus Disease. *J. Emerg. Infect. Dis.* **2020**, *26*. [CrossRef]
17. Lau, H.; Khosrawipour, V.; Kocbach, P.; Mikolajczyk, A.; Ichii, H.; Schubert, J.; Bania, J.; Khosrawipour, T. Internationally lost COVID-19 cases. *J. Microbiol. Immunol. Infect.* **2020**. [CrossRef]
18. Shin, H.J.; Kim, M.H.; Lee, S.; Kim, H.S.; Myoung, J.; Kim, B.T.; Kim, S.J. Current Status of Epidemiology, Diagnosis, Therapeutics, and Vaccines for Novel Coronavirus Disease 2019 (COVID-19). *J. Microbiol. Technol.* **2020**, *30*, 313–324.

19. Martelleti, L.; Martelleti, P. Air Pollution and the Novel Covid-19 Disease: A Putative Disease Risk Factor. *SN Compr. Clin. Med.* **2020**. [CrossRef] [PubMed]
20. Ogen, Y. Assessing nitrogen dioxide (NO2) levels as a contributing factor to coronavirus (COVID-19) fatality. *Sci. Total Environ.* **2020**. [CrossRef] [PubMed]
21. Monami, M.; Silverii, A.; Mannucci, E. Potential Impact of Climate on Novel CoronaVirus (COVID-19) Epidemic. *J. Occup. Environ. Med.* **2020**, *62*, e371–e372. [CrossRef] [PubMed]
22. Liu, J.; Zhou, J.; Yao, J.; Zhang, X.; Li, L.; Xu, X.; He, X.; Wang, B.; Fu, S.; Niu, T.; et al. Impact of meteorological factors on the COVID-19 transmission: A multi-city study in China. *Sci. Total Environ.* **2020**, *726*, 138513. [CrossRef]
23. Pascarella, G.; Strumia, A.; Piliego, C.; Bruno, F.; Del Buono, R.; Costa, F.; Scarlata, S.; Agrò, F. COVID-19 diagnosis and management: A comprehensive review. *J. Intern. Med.* **2020**, *288*, 192–206. [CrossRef]
24. Stefan, N.; Birkenfeld, A.L.; Schulze, M.B. Obesity and impaired metabolic health in patients with COVID-19. *Nat. Rev. Endocrinol.* **2020**, *16*, 341–342. [CrossRef] [PubMed]
25. The World Bank. World Bank Open Data. Available online: https://data.worldbank.org/ (accessed on 25 April 2020).
26. Organisation for Economic, Co-operation and Development. OECD Data. Available online: http://data.oecd.org (accessed on 25 April 2020).
27. World Population Prospects—Population Division—United Nations. Available online: https://population.un.org/wpp/DataQuery/ (accessed on 29 April 2020).
28. Global Health Data Exchange. GHDx. Available online: http://ghdx.healthdata.org/ (accessed on 29 April 2020).
29. Milne, G.; Xie, S. The Effectiveness of Social Distancing in Mitigating COVID-19 Spread: A modelling analysis. *MedRxiv* **2020**. [CrossRef]
30. CDC. Coronavirus Disease 2019 (COVID-19). *Cent. Dis. Control Prev.* 2020. Available online: https://www.cdc.gov/coronavirus/2019-ncov/prevent-getting-sick/social-distancing.html (accessed on 26 April 2020).
31. Li, Q.; Guan, X.; Wu, P.; Wang, X.; Zhou, L.; Tong, Y.; Ren, R.; Leung, K.S.; Lau, E.H.; Wong, J.Y.; et al. Early Transmission Dynamics in Wuhan, China, of Novel Coronavirus-Infected Pneumonia. *N. Engl. J. Med.* **2020**, *382*, 1199–1207. [CrossRef]
32. Ruan, Q.; Yang, K.; Wang, W.; Jiang, L.; Song, J. Clinical predictors of mortality due to COVID-19 based on an analysis of data of 150 patients from Wuhan, China. *Intensive Care Med.* **2020**. [CrossRef]
33. Ranney, M.L.; Griffeth, V.; Jha, A.K. Critical Supply Shortages—The Need for Ventilators and Personal Protective Equipment during the Covid-19 Pandemic. *N. Engl. J. Med.* **2020**, *382*. [CrossRef]
34. Vergano, M.; Bertolini, G.; Giannini, A.; Gristina, G.R.; Livigni, S.; Mistraletti, G.; Riccioni, L.; Petrini, F. Clinical Ethics Recommendations for the Allocation of Intensive Care Treatments in exceptional, resource-limited circumstances. *Crit. Care.* **2020**, *24*, 165. [CrossRef]
35. Vardavas, C.I.; Nikitara, K. COVID-19 and smoking: A systematic review of the evidence. *Tob. Induc. Dis.* **2020**, *18*. [CrossRef]
36. Guo, F.R. Active smoking is associated with severity of coronavirus disease 2019 (COVID-19): An update of a meta-analysis. *Tob. Induc. Dis.* **2020**, *18*, 37. [CrossRef] [PubMed]
37. Phua, J.; Weng, L.; Ling, L.; Egi, M.; Lim, C.M.; Divatia, J.V.; Shrestha, B.R.; Arabi, Y.M.; Ng, J.; Gomersall, C.D.; et al. Intensive care management of coronavirus disease 2019 (COVID-19): Challenges and recommendations. *Lancet Respir. Med.* **2020**. [CrossRef]
38. Riccioni, L.; Bertolini, G.; Giannini, A.; Vergano, M.; Gristina, G.; Livigni, S.; Mistraletti, G.; Flavia Petrini Gruppo di Lavoro Siaarti-Società Italiana di Anestesia Analgesia Rianimazione E Terapia Intensiva. Clinical ethics recommendations for the allocation of intensive care treatments, in exceptional, resource-limited circumstances. *Recenti Prog. Med.* **2020**, *111*, 207–211.
39. Guan, W.J.; Ni, Z.Y.; Hu, Y.; Liang, W.H.; Ou, C.Q.; He, J.X.; Liu, L.; Shan, H.; Lei, C.L.; Hui, D.S.; et al. Clinical Characteristics of Coronavirus Disease 2019 in China. *N. Engl. J. Med.* **2020**, *382*, 1708–1720. [CrossRef]
40. Oshitani, H.; Kamigaki, T.; Suzuki, A. Major Issues and Challenges of Influenza Pandemic Preparedness in Developing Countries. *Emerg. Infect. Dis.* **2008**, *14*, 875–880. [CrossRef] [PubMed]
41. Krumkamp, R.; Kretzschmar, M.; Rudge, J.W.; Ahmad, A.; Hanvoravongchai, P.; Westenhoefer, J.; Stein, M.; Putthasri, W.; Coker, R. Health service resource needs for pandemic influenza in developing countries: A linked transmission dynamics, interventions and resource demand model. *Epidemiol. Infect.* **2011**, *139*, 59–67. [CrossRef] [PubMed]

42. Hanvoravongchai, P.; Adisasmito, W.; Chau, P.N.; Conseil, A.; De Sa, J.; Krumkamp, R.; Mounier-Jack, S.; Phommasack, B.; Putthasri, W.; Shih, C.S.; et al. Pandemic influenza preparedness and health systems challenges in Asia: Results from rapid analyses in 6 Asian countries. *BMC Public Health* **2010**, *10*, 322. [CrossRef]
43. Yang, W.; Sirajuddin, A. The role of imaging in 2019 novel coronavirus pneumonia (COVID-19). *Eur. Radiol.* **2020**. [CrossRef]
44. Fields, B.K.K.; Demirjian, N.L.; Gholamrezanezhad, A. Coronavirus Disease 2019 (COVID-19) diagnostic technologies: A country-based retrospective analysis of screening and containment procedures during the first wave of the pandemic. *Clin. Imaging* **2020**, *67*, 219–225. [CrossRef]
45. Davarpanah, A.H.; Mahdavi, A.; Sabri, A.; Langroudi, T.F.; Kahkouee, S.; Haseli, S.; Kazemi, M.A.; Mehrian, P.; Mahdavi, A.; Falahati, F.; et al. Novel Screening and Triage Strategy in Iran During Deadly Coronavirus Disease 2019 (COVID-19) Epidemic: Value of Humanitarian Teleconsultation Service. *J. Am. Coll. Radiol.* **2020**, *17*, 734–738. [CrossRef]
46. Ai, T.; Yang, Z.; Hou, H.; Zhan, C.; Chen, C.; Lv, W.; Tao, Q.; Sun, Z.; Xia, L. Correlation of Chest CT and RT-PCR Testing in Coronavirus Disease 2019 (COVID-19) in China: A Report of 1014 Cases. *Radiology* **2020**, *296*, E32–E40. [CrossRef] [PubMed]
47. Fang, Y.; Zhang, H.; Xie, J.; Lin, M.; Ying, L.; Pang, P.; Ji, W. Sensitivity of Chest CT for COVID-19: Comparison to RT-PCR. *Radiology* **2020**, *296*, E115–E117. [CrossRef] [PubMed]
48. Zhou, F.; Yu, T.; Du, R.; Fan, G.; Liu, Y.; Liu, Z.; Xiang, J.; Wang, Y.; Song, B.; Gu, X.; et al. Clinical course and risk factors for mortality of adult inpatients with COVID-19 in Wuhan, China: A retrospective cohort study. *Lancet Lond. Engl.* **2020**, *395*, 1054–1062. [CrossRef]
49. Grasselli, G.; Zangrillo, A.; Zanella, A.; Antonelli, M.; Cabrini, L.; Castelli, A.; Cereda, D.; Coluccello, A.; Foti, G.; Fumagalli, R.; et al. Baseline Characteristics and Outcomes of 1591 Patients Infected with SARS-CoV-2 Admitted to ICUs of the Lombardy Region, Italy. *JAMA* **2020**. [CrossRef] [PubMed]
50. Opal, S.M.; Girard, T.D.; Ely, E.W. The immunopathogenesis of sepsis in elderly patients. *Clin. Infect. Dis. Off. Publ. Infect. Dis. Soc. Am.* **2005**, *41*, S504–S512. [CrossRef]
51. Weiskopf, D.; Weinberger, B.; Grubeck-Loebenstein, B. The aging of the immune system. *Transpl. Int.* **2009**, *22*, 1041–1050. [CrossRef]
52. Khafaie, M.A.; Rahim, F. Cross-Country Comparison of Case Fatality Rates of COVID-19/SARS-COV-2. *Osong Public Health Res. Perspect.* **2020**, *11*, 74–80. [CrossRef]
53. Nakajima, Y.; Yamada, K.; Imamura, K.; Kobayashi, K. Radiologist supply and workload: International comparison: Working Group of Japanese College of Radiology. *Radiat. Med.* **2008**, *26*, 455–465. [CrossRef]
54. Salehi, S.; Balakrishnan, S.; Gholamrezanezhad, A. Coronavirus Disease 2019 (COVID-19): A Systematic Review of Imaging Findings in 919 Patients. *Am. J. Roentgenol.* **2020**. [CrossRef]
55. Xie, X.; Zhong, Z.; Zhao, W.; Zheng, C.; Wang, F.; Liu, J. Chest CT for Typical 2019-nCoV Pneumonia: Relationship to Negative RT-PCR Testing. *Radiology* **2020**, *296*, E41–E45. [CrossRef]

Publisher's Note: MDPI stays neutral with regard to jurisdictional claims in published maps and institutional affiliations.

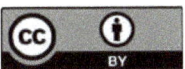 © 2020 by the authors. Licensee MDPI, Basel, Switzerland. This article is an open access article distributed under the terms and conditions of the Creative Commons Attribution (CC BY) license (http://creativecommons.org/licenses/by/4.0/).

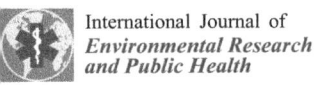

Article

COVID-19: Detecting Government Pandemic Measures and Public Concerns from Twitter Arabic Data Using Distributed Machine Learning

Ebtesam Alomari [1], Iyad Katib [1], Aiiad Albeshri [1] and Rashid Mehmood [2,*]

[1] Department of Computer Science, Faculty of Computing and Information Technology, King Abdulaziz University, Jeddah 21589, Saudi Arabia; EAlomari0011@stu.kau.edu.sa (E.A.); IAKatib@kau.edu.sa (I.K.); AAAlbeshri@kau.edu.sa (A.A.)
[2] High Performance Computing Center, King Abdulaziz University, Jeddah 21589, Saudi Arabia
* Correspondence: RMehmood@kau.edu.sa

Citation: Alomari, E.; Katib, I.; Albeshri, A.; Mehmood, R. COVID-19: Detecting Government Pandemic Measures and Public Concerns from Twitter Arabic Data Using Distributed Machine Learning. *Int. J. Environ. Res. Public Health* **2021**, *18*, 282. https://doi.org/10.3390/ijerph18010282

Received: 22 November 2020
Accepted: 28 December 2020
Published: 1 January 2021

Publisher's Note: MDPI stays neutral with regard to jurisdictional claims in published maps and institutional affiliations.

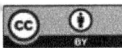

Copyright: © 2021 by the authors. Licensee MDPI, Basel, Switzerland. This article is an open access article distributed under the terms and conditions of the Creative Commons Attribution (CC BY) license (https://creativecommons.org/licenses/by/4.0/).

Abstract: Today's societies are connected to a level that has never been seen before. The COVID-19 pandemic has exposed the vulnerabilities of such an unprecedently connected world. As of 19 November 2020, over 56 million people have been infected with nearly 1.35 million deaths, and the numbers are growing. The state-of-the-art social media analytics for COVID-19-related studies to understand the various phenomena happening in our environment are limited and require many more studies. This paper proposes a software tool comprising a collection of unsupervised Latent Dirichlet Allocation (LDA) machine learning and other methods for the analysis of Twitter data in Arabic with the aim to detect government pandemic measures and public concerns during the COVID-19 pandemic. The tool is described in detail, including its architecture, five software components, and algorithms. Using the tool, we collect a dataset comprising 14 million tweets from the Kingdom of Saudi Arabia (KSA) for the period 1 February 2020 to 1 June 2020. We detect 15 government pandemic measures and public concerns and six macro-concerns (economic sustainability, social sustainability, etc.), and formulate their information-structural, temporal, and spatio-temporal relationships. For example, we are able to detect the timewise progression of events from the public discussions on COVID-19 cases in mid-March to the first curfew on 22 March, financial loan incentives on 22 March, the increased quarantine discussions during March–April, the discussions on the reduced mobility levels from 24 March onwards, the blood donation shortfall late March onwards, the government's 9 billion SAR (Saudi Riyal) salary incentives on 3 April, lifting the ban on five daily prayers in mosques on 26 May, and finally the return to normal government measures on 29 May 2020. These findings show the effectiveness of the Twitter media in detecting important events, government measures, public concerns, and other information in both time and space with no earlier knowledge about them.

Keywords: COVID-19; coronavirus; machine learning; big data; social media; apache spark; Twitter; Arabic language; distributed computing; smart cities; smart healthcare; smart governance; Triple Bottom Line (TBL)

1. Introduction

The level of digital and physical connectedness of today's societies has never been seen before. We are able to see and talk to people on the other side of the planet as if they are with us. We are able to control machines in the farthest continents using our smartphones. We are able to physically travel across the world in a day. We travel a lot to distant lands and frequently share gifts and viruses with each other.

Unfortunately, the COVID-19 pandemic has exposed the vulnerabilities of this unprecedentedly connected world. The COVID-19 pandemic, or coronavirus pandemic (COVID-19 is the name of the disease), is caused by the virus SARS-CoV-2 (Severe Acute

Respiratory Syndrome CoronaVirus 2) [1]. As of 19 November 2020, over 56 million people have been infected with nearly 1.35 million deaths, and the numbers are growing [1]. Social, economic, and environmental sustainability has been severely affected throughout the world. There is a growing consensus that the post-pandemic societies and world may take a different course for living, work, education, and other spheres of life. If (partial or full) remote working, businesses, and education are to become the norm, many people may choose to move and live in suburban or rural areas, and this will shift the course of urbanization.

There is a need to understand what is happening around the world during and after the pandemic, what measures are being taken to fight the pandemic by the government and authorities, what the needs of the people are, and what people's concerns and priorities are, etc. This information can help us to understand the implications of various pandemic measures (e.g., social isolation), manage the pandemic, address people's concerns, understand the impact of various policies for the post-pandemic future, and more.

Traditional methods of data collection and analysis using surveys and other means cannot capture such timely and large-scale data, alongside them having other disadvantages. Researchers in recent years have increasingly used social media including Twitter to study different issues in many application domains and sectors [2–5]. Naturally, social media has also been used during the COVID-19 pandemic times even more so, because the use of social media and virtual platforms by the public has increased due to social isolation and reduced mobility. A detailed literature review has revealed that the state-of-the-art research on social media analytics for COVID-19-related studies is limited. Many more studies are needed to improve the breadth and depth of the research on the subject in several aspects (Section 2 elaborates the research gap, novelty, and contributions of our work).

1.1. Description of the Proposed Work

In this paper, we propose a software tool comprising a collection of machine learning and other methods for the analysis of Twitter data in Arabic with the aim to detect government pandemic measures and public concerns during the COVID-19 pandemic. The methods used in the tool include an unsupervised Latent Dirichlet Allocation (LDA) topic modeling algorithm, natural language processing (NLP), correlation analysis, and other spatio-temporal information extraction and visualization methods. The tool was built using a range of technologies including MongoDB, Parquet, Apache Spark, Spark SQL, and Spark ML. The tool comprises five software components (see Section 3). The Data Collection and Storage Component (DCSC) uses various search queries and geo-coordinates to collect data using Twitter REST (Representational State Transfer) API (Application Programming Interface) and stores it using MongoDB and Apache Spark DataFrame (DF), a distributed data collection organized into named columns. The Data Pre-Processing Component (DPC) removes noise from the text and provides cleaned, normalized, and stemmed tokens. The Measures and Concerns Detector Component (MCDC) uses an unsupervised LDA model to cluster the tweets and detect government and public measures and concerns. The correlations in data are also computed here. The Spatio-Temporal Information Component (STIC) performs spatial and temporal analysis by extracting the date, time, location, and other information from the tweets. The Validation and Visualization Component (VVC) visualizes the results spatially and temporally using maps and other tools and validates the detected measures and concerns using internal or external sources such as news media. The Twitter dataset used in this specific study comprises 14 million tweets. It was collected using the Twitter API from 1 February 2020 to 1 June 2020 for the Kingdom of Saudi Arabia.

The software developed for this work is part of the tool Iktishaf [6–9] that we have been developing for the last few years. Earlier work on this tool has focused mainly on mobility-related event detection using supervised learning. We have also developed other tools for big data social media analytics in healthcare [10], logistics [11,12], and public opinion mining for government services [13]. These works have used Twitter data in Arabic or English.

1.2. Findings

We formulate and analyze the findings of this paper from three relationship perspectives: information-structural, temporal, and spatio-temporal.

Information-Structural Perspective: Using the tool, in terms of the information-structural (or subject matters) perspective, we have detected 15 government pandemic measures and public concerns (quarantine, loan, salary, mobility, etc.) and have grouped them into six macro-concerns (economic sustainability, social sustainability, contain the virus, etc.). For the **pandemic measures** implemented by the Saudi government in relation to the COVID-19 pandemic, we detect curfew and restrictions on mobility in the country, quarantine and fines, restrictions on praying in the mosques, campaigns to stay home, COVID-19 prevention, and cleaning services provided to curb the coronavirus spread. For **economic sustainability**, we detected that the government provided financial incentives including loans and private-sector salaries. Businesses increased offers to increase their sales. People moved to or increased their online economic activities, such as the activities related to prize draws for income earnings. For health, well-being, and **social sustainability**, we detected that blood donation and treatment at hospitals have been a major cause of concern. People also actively talked about the new number of cases. The **daily livelihood** issues in Saudi Arabia include five daily congregational prayers at the mosques that were suspended by the government. This was a major concern because praying five daily prayers in congregations is compulsory in Islam (with certain exceptions). People usually pray in mosques in congregations, standing close to each other and aligning shoulders and ankles with the person on the right and left, which is risky in the pandemic situation. People also increased in supplications for the safety of people. Roads were found to be empty or with abnormally low traffic during the corona times, and this was also vigorously discussed. A significant reduction in mobility was noted across the country that was related to **environmental sustainability**, health, and well-being due to the reduction in traffic congestion and air pollution. The detected events in Kingdom of Saudi Arabia (KSA) are also aligned with **international concerns**, such as various lockdown measures [14], reduced mobility [15], reduction in blood donations [16], financial difficulties and related government incentives [17,18], and worries related to returning to normal times [19].

Temporal Perspective: Regarding the temporal perspective of the various pandemic-related events within the time period of the dataset (1 February 2020–1 June 2020), we are able to see timely relationships in the progression of various events. Figure 1 shows the timeline of some of the detected government measures and public concerns. Some of these events in the Twitter activity that remained high for a period are shown with their start and end times. The earliest detected events in the data are related to virus infection, prevention, curfew, and stay home. Between **mid-March 2020** and the **end of May** (with some intermittent gaps), people also increased their Twitter activity related to the virus infection concern (spread of coronavirus and the increase in the number of cases). The curfew (7 a.m.–6 p.m.) in Saudi Arabia was ordered firstly on **22 March** and applied from the next day. The events related to loans were detected with the highest peak on **22 March** (Saudi Arabian Monetary Agency (SAMA) announced it on the same day [20]). The activities on Twitter related to the quarantine event (we use "measure", "concern", and "event" interchangeably, as appropriate) remained high during **the initial period** of the curfew to around **mid-April**. The "No Mobility" event (empty roads) was vigorously discussed on **24 March**, two days after the curfew was ordered. The curfew situation and the reduction in government services along with people's fear of getting infected by the virus had caused a reduction in blood donations and blood supplies. The activity on this topic requesting blood donations was seen to be increased from **late March** to **mid-April**. On **2 April**, a 24 h curfew was enforced in Makkah and Medina (the two holiest cities in KSA and the Muslim world), which stirred heavy Twitter activity. The events for the salary events were detected on the **3 April** the day King Salman of Saudi Arabia ordered to contribute towards 60% of the salaries of Saudi private-sector employees with a financial incentive of 9 billion Riyals in total (this was verified through external sources [21]). A peak activity related to the Five Daily Prayers concern was found on **26 May** when the Ministry of Interior announced that they would allow daily prayers to be held in all mosques of the Kingdom (except the mosques in Makkah city). Finally, we detected the "Back to Normal" government measure on **29 May 2020**.

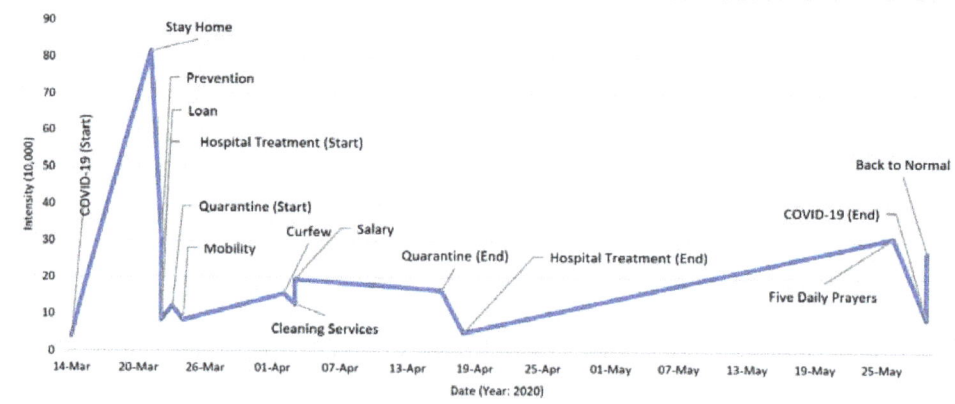

Figure 1. The timeline of some of the detected government pandemic measures and public concerns.

Spatio-Temporal Perspective: We extracted location information using different approaches including tweet text and hashtags, geo-coordinate attributes, and user profiles. We were able to detect important events in over 50 cities around the kingdom with major activities related to COVID-19 cases, curfew, etc., in the Makkah, Riyadh, and Eastern provinces.

We validated the detected government measures and public concerns and their spatial and temporal nature through external validation by searching online news media or through internal validation by checking tweets. These findings show the effectiveness of the Twitter media in detecting important events, government measures, public concerns, and other information in both time and space with no earlier knowledge about them.

The organization of the paper is as follows. Section 2 reviews the related works and elaborates on the research gaps. Section 3 explains our methodology and the design of the tool. Section 4 discusses the results and analysis. Section 5 gives the conclusions and directions for future work.

2. Literature Review

Smart cities and societies are driven by the need to provide highly competitive, productive, and smarter environments through the innovation and optimization of urban processes and life [22,23]. Artificial intelligence has taken us by storm [24], and has led to the emergence of concepts such as artificially intelligent cities [25]. A key to providing smartness for emerging urban and rural environments is to continuously sense and analyze these environments and make timely and effective decisions [6,10,24,26]. Social media analysis using machine learning has become a key method to provide the pulse for sensing and engaging with the environments [6] and is expected to provide smarter solutions for our fight against COVID-19 and future pandemics as well as during peace times.

We review here the literature relevant to the topic of this paper, which is the detection of COVID-19-related public concerns from social media (big) data in the Arabic language using machine learning, specifically the LDA topic modelling method. Firstly, in Section 2.1, we provide a background on the pre-COVID-19 use of social media in various application domains. Subsequently, we review in Section 2.2 the works about COVID-19 analysis that have used social media data without limiting the reviewed works to any analysis method or a language. In Section 2.3, we review the works about COVID-19 analysis and social media that have specifically used topic modelling for analysis purposes; these works are not limited to any language. We focus on the Arabic language in Section 2.4 and review the works related to COVID-19 analysis that use Twitter data. Finally, Section 2.5 discusses the research gap.

2.1. Use of Social Media in Research (Pre-COVID-19)

Digital societies could perhaps be characterized by their increasing desire to express themselves and interact with others, and this is done through various digital platforms such as social media. It is reported that roughly 58% of the global "eligible population" (70% of the eligible population in 100 countries around the world) uses social media [10,27]. Social media could provide a two-way communication channel for individuals, governments, businesses, and others to engage with their friends, communities, stakeholders, etc. [10]. The traditional methods of data collection and analysis using surveys and other means cannot capture such timely and large-scale data, alongside them having other disadvantages. Researchers in recent years have increasingly used social media including Twitter to study different issues in many application domains and sectors, and this trend has been ramping up in COVID-19-related research and other studies. Social media and Internet of Things (IoT) provide the pulse for sensing and engaging with the environments [10]. Sentiment analysis, or opinion mining, that utilizes social and other textual media is a vital tool in natural language processing (NLP), defined as "the field of study that analyzes people's opinions, sentiments, evaluations, appraisals, attitudes, and emotions toward entities such as products, services, organizations, individuals, issues, events, topics, and their attributes" [10,28]. Many of the notable works on sentiment analysis rely on machine learning and social media, with applications in logistics and urban planning [12,25,29–31]; categorizing tweets about road conditions into useful, nearly useful, and irrelevant complaint tweets [2]; identifying sources of noise pollution [32]; extracting traffic-related information from tweets [3]; general and traffic-related event detection [6,9,11,33–35]; public opinion mining for government services [13]; detecting health-related topics from the stream of tweets (without aiming to detect a particular illness) [36]; tracking the side effects of certain medications [37]; the detection of top symptoms, diseases, and medications and related awareness activities [10]; tracking flu infections on Twitter [38], influenza surveillance from social media data [39–41]; and many more.

2.2. COVID-19 and Social Media (General)

We review here the works about COVID-19 analysis that have used social media data without regard to any modelling method or a language. Singh et al. [42] analyzed tweets about coronavirus in different languages including English, French, German, Italian, and others. Furthermore, they have performed spatiotemporal analysis of the data. They focused on three countries, which are the United States, Italy, and China, and showed the time series of tweets and the daily confirmed COVID-19 cases. They found that the countries that had a higher number of COVID-19 cases also had a higher number of tweets about COVID-19. Gencoglu [43] applied supervised classification to capture COVID-19-related discourse during the pandemic. They collected around 26 million tweets using Twitter streaming API with keyword filtering. They trained classifiers using k-nearest neighbor, logistic regression, and support vector machine (SVM) to classify the tweets into 11 categories including donate, prevention, reporting, share, speculation, symptoms, and others. For training the machine learning classifiers, they utilized two annotated datasets of questions and comments related to COVID-19. The dataset consisted of several languages, including English, French, and Spanish, and was generated by native-speaker annotators based on an ontology. Then, they employed language-agnostic BERT (Bidirectional Encoder Representations) sentence embeddings to obtain a pre-trained model. To extract embeddings, they used the TensorFlow framework on a 64-bit Linux machine with an NVIDIA Titan Xp GPU. They found that Twitter activity increased due to the increase in the spread of COVID-19 across the world.

Several other works on the use of social media for COVID-19 analysis have been reported. These include studies on American and Chinese peoples' views on COVID-19 [44], the mood of Indian people during the pandemic [45], the spread of anti-Asian hate speech [46], the political tension between Brazil and China [47], and the identification of emotional valence and predominant emotions [48]. Moreover, others have looked into modelling social media data for COVID-19-related analysis to study the spread of misinformation about the coronavirus [49–51], discovering political conspiracies in the U.S. that were posted by Twitter automated accounts during the COID-19 outbreak [52], identifying the causal relationship of the daily Twitter activity and sentiments during the pandemic [53], and studying the frequency of the phrases "Chinese virus" and "China virus" before and after the outbreak in the United States [54].

None of the works reported in this subsection have a focus or methods similar to our research reported in this paper. None of them have used the distributed big data computing framework Apache Spark. The discussed works did not support social media in the Arabic language, which, as mentioned earlier, has its own challenges, particularly since it is not based on the Latin script. Moreover, the size and period of the used data are also different.

2.3. COVID-19 and Topic Modeling

We review here the works about COVID-19 analysis using social media that have specifically used topic modelling as the modelling method. These works are not limited to any language. Liu et al. [55] studied the role of the Chinese mass media during the COVID-19 crisis using news articles from the WiseSearch database. They applied LDA and extracted 20 topics and then classified them into nine themes. The topics include prevention and control policy, prevention and control measures, medical affiliation and staff, epidemiologic study, and others. The themes include confirmed cases, prevention and control procedures, medical treatment and research, detection at public transportation, and others. Kaila and Prasad [56] applied LDA analysis and found the topics related to the coronavirus from 18,000 tweets. Besides, they applied sentiment analysis and found that most of the tweets were negative. Abd-Alrazaq et al. [57] identified twelve topics from 167,073 tweets, collected for the period 2 February 2020 to 15 March 2020, using LDA and grouped them into four themes: the origin of COVID-19, the source of the novel coronavirus, the impact of COVID-19 on people and countries, and the methods for decreasing the spread of COVID-19. Then, they used a simple string-matching technique to find tweets that contain the selected keywords of the topics. Additionally, they calculated the interaction rate for each topic after calculating the sentiment score and the number of retweets, likes, and followers for each topic. None of the works discussed in this paragraph have applied temporal or spatial analysis, supported social media in the Arabic language, or used distributed big data computing platforms such as Apache Spark.

Med [58] collected 94,467 posts from the Reddit website in the period between 3 March and 31 March. Then, they applied LDA and found 50 topics, 10 of them were assigned to one of the following categories: public health measures, daily life impact, and sense of pandemic severity. After that, they measured daily changes in the frequency of topics. Ordun et al. [59] applied keyword analysis to find the most frequent words. They analyzed around 5.5 million tweets in different languages that are based on Latin script. Arabic, Chinese, and other languages that are based on non-Latin scripts were not included. They used term-frequency inverse-document-frequency (TF-IDF) and defined the max_features to 10,000. In addition, they performed topic modeling and identified twenty topics using the default parameters of the Gensim LDA MultiCore model. For each topic, they extracted the top twenty terms and used the first three terms to label the topic. Further, they used Uniform Manifold Approximation and Projection (UMAP) to visualize how the 20 topics grouped together. Additionally, they performed a temporal analysis to examine the trend of topics over time. Additionally, they applied time-to retweet analysis and measure the time between the tweet and the retweets. None of the works discussed in this paragraph have used distributed big data computing platforms such as Apache Spark, supported social media in the Arabic language, or applied spatial analysis.

Mackey et al. [60] applied the Biterm Topic Model (BTM) to detect topics related to COVID-19 symptoms, experiences with access to testing, and disease recovery. They collected around 4 million tweets after filtering by keywords. The data was collected for the period 3 March 2020 to 20 March 2020. Then, the tweets were grouped into five main thematic categories: "conversations about first and secondhand reports of symptoms", "symptom reporting concurrent with lack of testing", "discussion of recovery", "confirmation of negative diagnosis", and "discussion about recalling symptoms". For the analysis, they used python packages and R-studio. Additionally, they analyzed the time and location for the geotagged tweets (in our work, we use multiple methods for the location extraction of tweets). Li et al. [61] detected stress symptoms related to COVID-19 in the United States. They integrated a Correlation Explanation (CorEx) learning algorithm and clinical Patient Health Questionnaire (PHQ) lexicon and proposed a CorExQ9 algorithm. They collected 80 million tweets for the period of January 2020 to April 2020 and used a Jupyter computing environment deployed on the Texas A&M High Performance Computer. They compared CorExQ9 with LDA and non-negative matrix factorization (NMF). Moreover, they visualized the symptoms of COVID-19 related stress at the county level for multiple two-week periods. These works differ from our work in multiple aspects, including the differences in the foci of the studies, the overall methodology, the specifics of analysis, the time period of the data used, and particularly the processing of social media in the Arabic language.

2.4. COVID-19 and Twitter (Arabic Language)

We review the works related to COVID-19 analysis that use Twitter data with a focus on the tweets in the Arabic language. Alam et al. [62] analyzed Arabic and English tweets during the COVID-19 pandemic to find whether the tweets contained a factual claim. They defined annotation guidelines for manual annotation. Alshaabi et al. [63] collected tweets in 24 languages including Arabic. They created time series for the top thousand 1 g for each language. Then, they applied basic observations about some of the time series data, including the use of the word "virus" in the tweets of all languages. Alsudais and Rayson [64] collected around 1 million tweets about coronavirus for the period December 2019 to April 2020 and clustered them using the K-means algorithm with the Python Scikit-learn package. They found five topics; these are "COVID-19 statistics", "prayers for God", "COVID-19 locations", "advice and education for prevention", and "advertising". Besides this, to identify rumors, they applied supervised classification and labeled 2000 tweets as false information, correct information, and unrelated. The review of the works on COVID-19 analysis using Twitter data in the Arabic language shows that the works on the topic are scarce and are limited in their variety and the depth of the technologies, methods, and analysis used in those works. For example, none of these works have used big data platforms, and none have reported spatio-temporal analysis.

2.5. Research Gap, Novelty, and Contributions

The literature review provided in this section clearly establishes the enormous potential of social media analytics for COVID-19-related studies. The traditional methods of data collection and analysis using surveys and other means cannot capture such timely and large-scale data, alongside them having other disadvantages. The state-of-the-art social media analytics for COVID-19-related studies is limited. Many more studies are needed to improve the breadth and depth of the research on the subject with regard to the focus of the studies, the size and diversity of the data, the applicability and performance of the machine learning methods, the diversity of the social media languages, the scalability of the computing platforms, etc. The maturity of research in this area will allow the development, commercialization, and wide adoption of the tools for pandemic-related and general surveillance and other purposes.

The research reported in this paper is different from the existing works on social media analytics for COVID-19-related studies in several respects, including the focus of the studies, the methodology, the size of the data, the time/period of the social media data, support for the social media in the Arabic language, whether the studies have used big data distributed computing platforms, the breadth and the depth of the reported analysis such as spatial and temporal analysis, the geographical focus of the studies, and the specific findings. None of the existing works have reported a similar COVID-19 analysis of Twitter data in the Arabic language with regard to the modelling method used and the depth of the analysis. The Twitter data we have used, its time period, and the methodology of its collection and analysis are different. The methods used for the validation of the findings are also different. None of the existing works on the COVID-19 analysis has used big data technologies for social media in Arabic. Even the works that use big data distributed computing platforms for the analysis of text in languages other than Arabic are very limited and differ in several aspects. The scalability of the software systems for COVID-19 analysis is critical and is being hampered due to the challenges related to the management, integration, and analysis of big data (the 4V challenges). We have developed a novel architecture and pipeline (see Figure 2) for big data management and analysis using distributed machine learning. We have also provided an analysis of the execution time complexity for LDA algorithms for a different number of iterations (between 5 and 1000 iterations) on a varying number of computing cores (see Section 4.4). The use of big data distributed computing technologies is important, because it will allow the scalability and integration of COVID-19-related software with each other and with other healthcare and smart city systems.

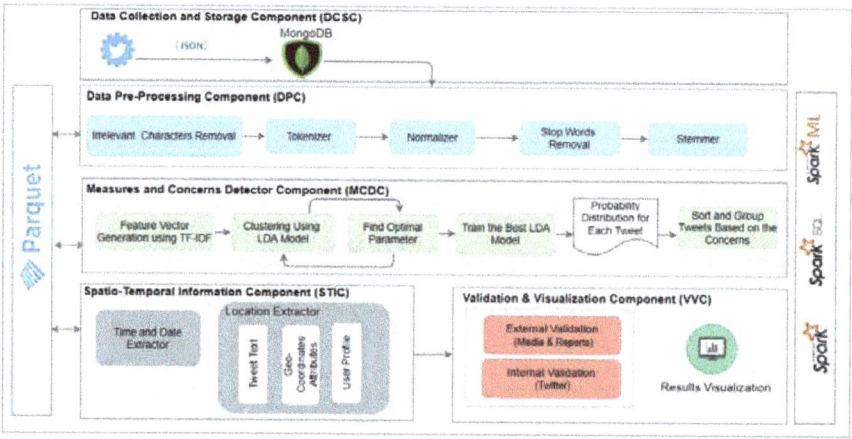

Figure 2. The tool architecture.

3. The System Methodology and Design

The architecture of the proposed system is depicted in Figure 2. It comprises five components that are depicted in the figure as five separate blocks and discussed in the following subsections subsequent to the overview below.

3.1. The System Overview

We built our tool in Apache Spark, which is a big data platform for in-memory computations on distributed data. Apache Spark provides the Spark ML package for machine learning and Spark SQL for data handling. Spark SQL acts as a distributed SQL engine. Additionally, it offers a programming abstraction called DataFrames, which is conceptually equivalent to a table in a relational database but is immutable, parallel, and distributed to handle big data. Moreover, the proposed tool was developed using Python and runs over Aziz supercomputer, which supports running Spark with YARN. Aziz consists of 380 regular computer nodes, 112 compute nodes with large memory, as well as 2 additional GPU compute nodes and 2 additional MIC compute nodes. All the computer nodes run CentOS 6.4 with dual Intel E5-2695v2 processors. Each node has 24 cores. Regular nodes provide 96 GB memory, while large memory nodes provide 256 GB memory. Further, they provided the Fujitsu Exabyte File System (FEFS) which offers high-speed storage to store input/output data for the running jobs. It provides 7 petabytes of memory.

Algorithm 1 shows the master algorithm. The inputs are the search queries and the geo-coordinates, which are required for the Data Collection and Storage Component (DCSC) in addition to the location dictionary, which will be used during spatio-temporal information extraction. The dataset was collected using the Twitter REST API and stored in MongoDB. Then, the tweets will be loaded into Spark DataFrame (DF), which is a distributed data collection organized into named columns. After that, the tweet Dataframe will be passed to the Data Pre-Processing Component (DPC), which removes noise from the text and provides cleaned, normalized, and stemmed tokens. Furthermore, the major concerns will be discovered using the Measures and Concerns Detector Component (MCDC), which applies an unsupervised LDA model to cluster the tweets. Subsequently, to perform spatial and temporal analysis, the date, time, and location information are extracted using a Spatio-Temporal Information Component (STIC). Finally, in the Validation and Visualization Component (VVC), the results are visualized and validated against external or internal sources.

Algorithm 1: Master
Input: search_query; geo_coordinate; location_d   **Output:** The discovered concerns and their space and time information
1   *tweets* ← DCSC(search_query, geo_coordinate)   2   *spark* ← createSparkSession()   3   *tweets_DF* ← spark.read(tweets)   4   *tweets_p_DF* ← DPC(tweets_DF)   5   *tweets_g_DF* ← CDC(tweets_p_DF)   6   *tweets_st_DF* ← STEC(tweets_g_DF, location_d)   7   *VVC*(tweets_g_DF, tweets_st_DF)

3.2. Data Collection and Storage Component (DCSC)

The experimental dataset contains Arabic tweets collected using Twitter REST API during the period from 1 February to 1 June 2020. The total number of fetched tweets are approximately 14.8 million tweets. The tweets were acquired using two methods. First, we use keywords and hashtags related to coronavirus, such as #corona and #<كورونا>, #covid19, as well as official accounts that post about it, such as the account of the Saudi Ministry of Health (@SaudiMOH). The second method is fetching tweets without keyword filtering to make sure that we do not miss any important tweets because we want to see what are the topics that people were talking about and how the pandemic has changed their life. Subsequently, we used geolocation filtering to obtain only tweets posted in Saudi Arabia because our main focus in this work is to find the major concerns during the pandemic time in Saudi Arabia.

Algorithm 2 illustrates the algorithm of the data collection. To store the collected tweets, we searched for a storage method that supports flexible schemas. Therefore, we selected the NoSQL databases, particularly MongoDB, which is a document-oriented database. They enable storing various document data types, such as XML and JSON.

Moreover, to store the output of each component, we used Parquet file storage. One of the reasons for selecting Parquet is because it is supported by many data processing systems, including Apache Spark. Besides this, it automatically preserves the schema of the original data and provides a good performance for both storage and processing. The files were stored using the Fujitsu Exabyte File System (FEFS), which is a scalable parallel file system based on Lustre. Finally, the duplicated tweets were removed before passing them to the next stage, which is pre-processing.

Algorithm 2: Data Collection and Storage

Input: search_query; geo_coordinate
Output: The collected tweets
1   db ← connect_MongoDB()
2   api ← connect_Twitter_API()
3   collect_store_tweetsCOVID19(api, db, search_query, geo_coordinate)
4   collect_store_tweets(api, db, geo)

3.3. Data Pre-Processing Component (DPC)

The main pre-processing steps can be summarized as follows: (1) irrelevant character removal, (2) tokenizer, (3) normalizer (4) stop-word removal, and (5) stemmer. In the first step, we removed all the numbers, the English alphabet, and all punctuation marks. This means removing @, which every username started with, and # and _, which are used in hashtags. However, we leave the hashtag name itself if it is not in English because it might include useful information, such as the city name. Removing English and punctuation means also removing links and all punctuation including Arabic semi-colons (؛) and Arabic question marks (؟). Furthermore, we removed the thirteen forms of Arabic diacritics [65] which can be grouped under three categories: vowel, nunation and shadda diacritics. Vowel diacritics include the three main short vowels, called in Arabic Fatha (َ), Damma (ُ), and Kasra (ِ), as well as the Sukun diacritic (ْ), which indicates the absence of any vowel. Nunation diacritics represent the doubled version of the short vowels known in Arabic as Fathatan (ً), Dammatan (ٌ), Kasratan (ٍ). The last form of diacritics is Shadda (germination). It refers to the consonant-doubling diacritical (ّ). This also can be merged with diacritics from the two previous types and result in a new diacritic such as (َّ) or (ًّ).

The second step is dividing the text into tokens. We used the split() method in Python with the white-space separator. The third step is using the Normalizer to normalize the words (tokens) that contain different forms of Alif (أ, إ, آ), 'Yaa' (ى) and "TAA MARBUTAH/ ة" into the basic form. To clarify, the letter "Taa marbutah" (ة) will be replaced with "haa" (ه) while "Yaa" (ى) will be replaced with "dotless Yaa" (ي). Additionally, "Alif" with three forms (أ, إ, آ) will be replaced with "bare Alif" (ا).

The fourth step is removing stop-words. To do this, we modified the stop-words provided by the Natural Language Toolkit (NLTK) to include a new list of stop-words as well as normalize them. Since the NLTK stop-words list was designed for the formal Modern Standard Arabic, we modified the list to include words that usually used in dialectical Arabic, such as "ليش", "اللي", "ايش", and "ليه", in addition to that we consider the common grammar mistakes. For example, the preposition "على" might be written "علا" and "لكن" might be written "لاكن". Besides this, we included words that are usually used in Du'aa (prayer) such as "يارب", "اللهم", "الله". After that, we normalized the final stop-words list before using them because they will be extracted from a normalized text. This component is part of our earlier paper, Iktishaf. For further details, see the pre-processing algorithm in [6].

Finally, we stem the tokens using the Iktishaf Light Stemmer [6]. Unlike the existing Arabic light stemmers, Iktishaf stemmer was designed to minimize the number of letters removed and eliminate changes in the meaning. It used a predefined list of prefixes and suffixes. Then, based on the length of the word, the tool decides which affix can be removed.

That leads to minimizing the word confusion and losing or changing the word meaning. For further details, see the stemmer algorithm in [6].

3.4. Measures and Concerns Detector Component (MCDC)

To discover concerns, we used the Latent Dirichlet Allocation (LDA) topic modeling algorithm. It is a statistical model that is used to identify the main topics discussed in a collection of documents. It is an unsupervised method that models documents and topics based on dirichlet distribution. Each document is characterized by the probability distribution over various topics while each topic is modeled as a probability distribution over words. The model received a collection of documents and returned a set of topics. Each topic includes a set of words. This required defining the number of topics, denoted by k to model the distributions. In this work, the tweets are the documents and we refer to topics as concerns. Apache Spark supports LDA since Spark 1.3.0 in the MLlib package and it also supports it in ML package.

Algorithm 3 illustrates the algorithm of the Measures and Concerns Detector Component. The inputs for this component are the pre-processed tweets (tweet_p). The set concerns number ([K]), the set of iterations number ([R]), and the threshold value. The output of the DPC will be loaded from parquet files and stored in a Spark DataFrame (tweet_DF). For training the model, we need to pass the documents (tweets) as vectors of word counts. Thus, we used the CountVectorizer function. Then, we applied TF-IDF weight, which is a statistical measure used to evaluate how important a word is to a document (tweet) in a collection (tweets). This stands for term frequency-inverse document frequency. TF-IDF comprises of two parts Term Frequency (*TF*) and Inverse Document Frequency (*IDF*). *TF* measures how frequently a word occurs in a tweet. It is calculated using the following equation:

$$TF_{w,t} = \frac{f_{wt}}{n_t}, \quad (1)$$

where f_{wt} is the frequency of word w in tweet t and n_t is the total number of words in that tweet.

$$IDF_t = 1 + \log\frac{|T|}{|t : w \in t|} \quad (2)$$

where $|T|$ is the total number of tweets, and it is divided by the total number of tweets that contain the word w. Then, the multiplication of *TF* and *IDF* will represent the weight of the word w in tweet t.

$$TF - IDF_{w,t} = TF_{w,t} \times IDF_t. \quad (3)$$

After passing the collection of tweets as a vector to the LDA model, we need to specify the number of concerns (k), which also can be thought of as cluster centers. To find a suitable number of concerns, we tested different concerns numbers and calculated the perplexity. Perplexity is a statistical criterion of how well a probability model predicts a sample. It is a standard metric to measure generalization performance [66]. Lower perplexity score indicates a good model. Further, we tested different iteration numbers to find the best value.

Algorithm 3: Measures and Concerns Detector

Input: tweets_p; [K]; [R]; threshold
Output: concerns[][], tweets_g_DF

1   *spark* ← createSparkSession()
2   *tweets_DF* ← spark.read(tweets_p)
3   *features_DF* ← generate_TFIDF_vector(tweets_DF)
4   *LDAmodel* ← get_best_model(LDA_clustering(features_DF, [K], [R]))
5   *concernsProb_tw_DF* ← train_best_model(LDAmodel)
6   *concerns[][]* ← LDAmodel.describeTopics()
7   *concern_tw_DF* ← assign_tweets_to_concern(concernsProb_tw_DF)
8   *tweets_g_DF* ← group_filter_tweets(concern_tw_DF, threshold)

Figure 3 shows the perplexity score against the number of concerns, k. The perplexity score decreases with an increase in the value of k with some minor exceptions. The gain in the perplexity score after $k = 15$. is relatively insignificant. Therefore, we use 15 as the value of k—i.e., the number of concerns to be detected by our tool is set to 15. We also carried out an empirical analysis of the various concerns detected by different values of k and found that $k = 15$ produces the best results.

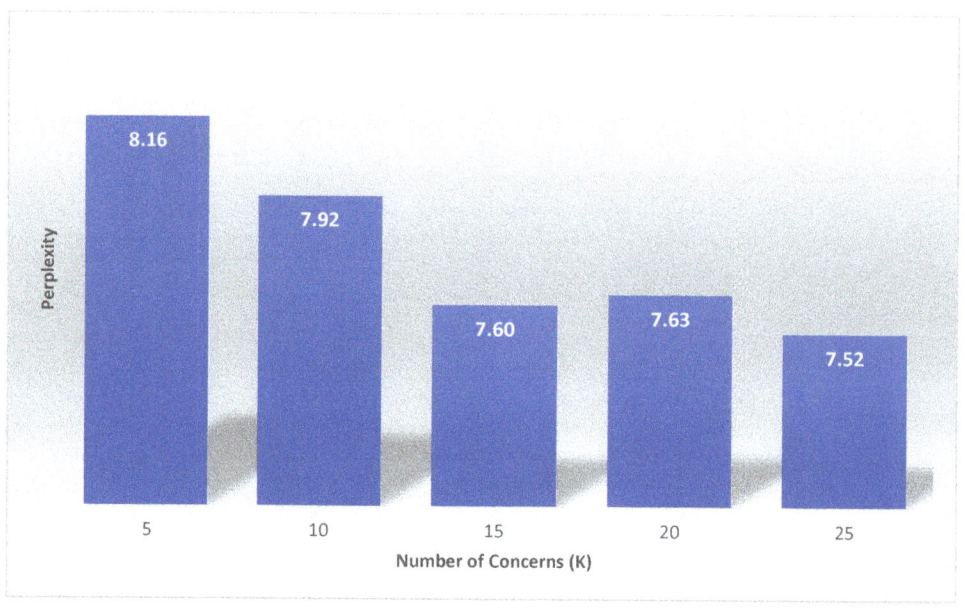

Figure 3. Perplexity score versus the number of concerns.

Moreover, the model that achieved the best results is trained to obtain a final concerns list. Furthermore, by calling the *describeTopics* function, we obtain a list of the top terms for each concern. From the list of terms, we can understand the concern and thus we define a label that represents it. For each tweet, we get an array of the probability distribution, which represents how much the tweet belongs to each cluster. The concerns probability as well as the tweets are stored in concernsProb_tw_DF. We need to make each tweet belong to one concern (cluster), so we pick the concern with the highest probability in the array and we consider it the best concern that represents the tweet. Thus, we get a group of tweets under each concern. Since we have a large number of tweets, we assume that some of them might be included under a specific concern because it represents the highest probability comparing to the other concerns but the probability value itself might be very low. To keep only tweets that are highly related to the concern, we decide to define a threshold and filter out the tweets that have a probability less than the threshold value. This value will depend on the data; in our particular case, we found that most of the tweets have a probability higher than 0.8 as shown in Figure 4. So, we set the threshold = 0.8. The outputs of this component are the lists of top keywords that explain each concern and the tweets grouped by the concerns. The detected concerns will be explained later in the results section (see Section 4).

In the MCDC component, we also compute the correlation matrix by calculating correlation coefficients between the keywords of the detected concerns. This helps in understanding relationships between the keywords. There are three main types of correlation coefficient formulas, which are Pearson, Kendall, and Spearman correlation. The Pearson correlation coefficient is the most commonly used. We selected it in this work. It measures the linear dependence between two variables. The Pearson correlation between two variables x and y is computed using Equation (4) below.

$$r = \frac{\sum(x_i - \bar{x})(y_i - \bar{y})}{\sqrt{\sum(x_i - \bar{x})^2 \sum(y_i - \bar{y})^2}},\qquad(4)$$

where x_i is the ith value of x variable, y_i is the ith value of y variable, $\bar{x}$ is the mean of the values of the x variable, and $\bar{y}$ is the mean of the values of the y variable.

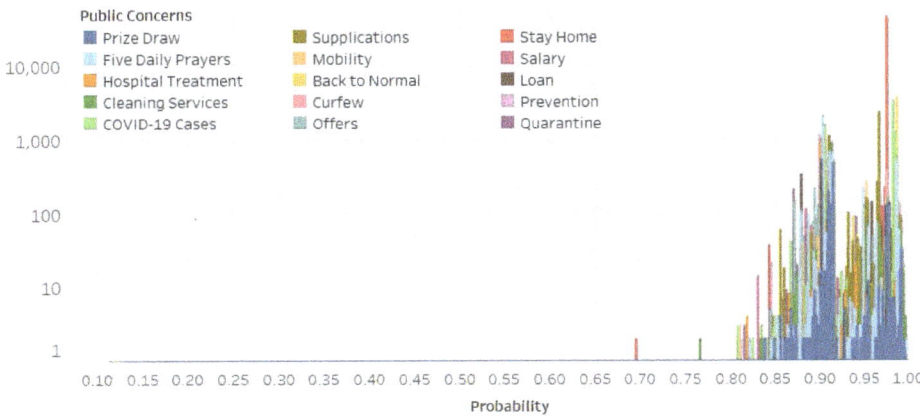

Figure 4. Tweet intensity versus probability of concerns.

The correlation matrix (see Section 4.1) is an asymmetrical (K × K) square matrix where AB entry is a cell in the matrix that shows the correlation between two keywords in row A and column B. Each cell has a value between 1 and −1, where 1 represents a strong positive correlation and −1 represents a strong negative correlation.

3.5. Spatio-Temporal Information Component (STIC)

In this work, we identify concerns, and then each tweet under each concern that has information about location or time, we call it an event. To apply spatio-temporal analysis, we need to know the time and the location of the extracted event.

The obtained data using the Twitter API are encoded using JavaScript Object Notation (JSON). Each tweet object we obtained can have over 150 attributes associated with it according to their documentation [67]. Each child object, such as users and place, encapsulates attributes to describe it.

We extracted time and date information from "created-at" attribute which shows UTC time when the tweet was created. For location extraction from the tweet object, we applied different techniques.

The first approach is extracting location names from the "text" attribute. It contains the tweet message. The location name might be explicitly mentioned in the text or it might be part of the hashtags. We generated a dictionary for Saudi cities in English and Arabic as well as their coordinates. Before using the dictionary to search for the cities' names in the text, we passed the Arabic names list to Iktishaf Light Stemmer because we extracted them from the text after applying pre-processing. However, if the city name is not found in the text, we move to the next approach, which is looking for geo coordinates information.

Therefore, the second approach is obtaining coordinates from "coordinate" or "place" child objects. The "place" child object includes several attributes, such as "place_type", "place_name", "country_code". The "place_type" can be either city or point of interest (poi). Moreover, we do not move to this approach unless we do not find the information in the text because the associate geo-coordinates within the tweet object represents the location where the user physically present at the time of posting the tweet and it does not necessarily be the actual location of the event that they are talking about. If users disable location services in their smartphones, the value of these attributes will be null.

Thus, the third approach we follow is extracting information from the "user" child object. This contains the user profile information such as the screen name and bio, which includes a short description as well as the country and city name. Users fill in the information manually so they can be written in English or Arabic and they might use different spelling such as Makkah can be written as Makah or mecca. Therefore, our location extractor was designed to extract both English and Arabic names as well as the common names for Saudi cities. However, users usually fill in this information when they create their account and do not change them when they travel to another country/city. That is why we leave this option to the end and we do not apply it unless we do not find the location information from the previous two approaches.

3.6. Validation and Visualization Component (VVC)

We followed two methods to validate the identified concerns as well as their spatial and temporal nature. The first method is based on searching against various official sources, reports, and news media on the web. We consider it an external validation. The second method is based on Twitter data we have, where it can give us the detailed information in addition to space and time information, particularly if it was posted by an official news account such as @spagov or the account of Ministry of Health.

After identifying the public concerns using the MCDC (see Section 3.4), we drew line charts to show changes of concerns overtimes. Further, to show the concerns for their spatial nature, we plotted them on top of the Saudi Arabia map. For this purpose, we used Power BI and Tableau.

4. Results and Analysis

We will now discuss the results of our proposed system. Section 4.1 describes the detected pandemic measures and concerns (topics) using LDA. Section 4.2 provides an analysis of the identified measures and concerns as regards their temporal nature (the date) as well as the validation process of the identified concerns using internal sources (Twitter) and external sources (online news media). Section 4.3 provides an analysis in terms of their spatio-temporal nature (the date and the cities). Section 4.4 provides an analysis of the model execution times using distributed computing. Finally, Section 4.5 discusses the relationship between the detected measures and concerns.

4.1. COVID-19: Pandemic Measures, Public Concerns, and Macro-Concerns

Table 1 lists the fifteen major pandemic measures and public concerns (hereon we refer to them as public concerns or concerns) discussed by the public on Twitter during the COVID-19 pandemic. These are grouped into six groups that we call macro-concerns (Column 1). These are virus infection, daily matters, contain the virus, social sustainability, economic sustainability, and back to normal. Column 2 gives the rank in terms of the importance of the concern based on the percentage of tweets for each concern (percentage is listed in Column 3). The concerns are listed, firstly, in groups (macro-concerns) and, within each macro-concern, by the descending order of the rank. The fifth column of the table shows the top ten keywords related to each concern. Primarily, these keywords are the clusters extracted by our tool using the LDA approach described in Section 3. Subsequently, we assigned a label (i.e., concern) to each cluster of keywords based on our understanding of the keywords in each cluster. For the purpose of gaining understanding about a cluster of keywords, we looked at the tweets that were associated with a cluster with the highest probabilities (we refer to these as the top-ranked tweets). We illustrate this in the following by example. The first row in the table lists the first public concern, which is **COVID-19 Cases**. This includes keywords including health, announce, new, case, register, and infection. These keywords are usually used by individuals and various organizations (e.g., the Ministry of Health in Saudi Arabia) when disseminating information related to the daily number of cases, deaths, etc. The following is one such tweet by the Ministry of Health (the number of cases, deaths, etc. would vary in these tweets).

الصحة تعلن تسجيل (382) حالة إصابة جديدة بفيروس كورونا الجديد 19 (كوفيد) وتسجل (23) حالة تعافي و (3) حالات وفاة رحمهم الله

The Ministry of Health announces the registration of (382) new cases of infection with the new Coronavirus (COVID 19) and records (35) cases of recovery and (5) cases of death, may God have mercy on them.

The second row lists the concern **Supplications** and its keywords. Supplication is an important part of Muslim beliefs and daily life. Muslims supplicate when they face difficulty or hear good news (they may also supplicate without any good or bad news). To illustrate, Muslims believe that a difficulty is a test from God (Allah), and thus they are encouraged to increase their supplications. During the pandemic, people might pray asking Allah to protect them and others from the virus. Muslims increase their supplications greatly during Ramadhan (the lunar month of fasting that comes once a year). The month of Ramadhan this year (2020) fell between 24 April and 23 May. The keywords for this concern are clearly representative of the label "Supplications".

The third concern is **Quarantine**. This is one of the methods that have been followed by various countries to prevent the spread of the virus by isolating healthy people from potentially unhealthy people who could have been infected with the SARS-CoV-2 virus. The fourth concern is about the **Five Daily Prayers**. Muslims pray in congregations, next to each other without gaps, at mosques five times a day. The Saudi government suspended all the congregational prayers across all mosques in the Kingdom to prevent the spread of the virus. We found tweets from individuals and organizations similar to the following top-ranked tweet.

عاجل ابتداءً من يوم الأحد 8 شوال 1441 وحتى نهاية يوم السبت 28 شوال 1441 سماح بأداء الصلوات الجمع في جميع مساجد المملكة ما عدا #مكة

Urgent starting from Sunday 8 Shawwal 1441 AH until the end of Saturday 28 Shawwal 1441 AH prayers are permitted to be performed in all mosques of the Kingdom, except for #Makkah

This explains the existence of the keywords Sunday, Saturday, and Shawwal in the clustered keywords. Shawal is the tenth month of the Islamic lunar calendar. The fifth identified concern is **Stay Home**. From the top keywords, we can see that people consider staying home a strong measure to stop the spread of COVID-19 and save lives. To increase awareness among people about the importance of their role in fighting the coronavirus outbreak, authorities used the slogan "We are all responsible", which is visible in the keywords of this concern. The sixth concern is **Loan**. The COVID-19 pandemic has severely affected people's financial situation globally due to reasons such as the loss of jobs. They are seeking loans or struggling to repay loans, which makes it one of the major pandemic concerns. The seventh concern is **Cleaning Services**. During the pandemic, the cleaning services were in high demand such as for cleaning public areas affected by virus-carrying people. The following tweet is an example of this concern.

أمانة #الرياض تواصل جولاتها بتعقيم وتنظيف طرق #الرياض #فترة #من عليك جولة بدفع وسط بيئة #صحية أمنة للمواطنين #واس_عام

#Riyadh_municipality continues its tours to sterilize and clean the roads of Riyadh during the period of #curfew to provide a safe and healthy environment for the residents # WAS_general

Table 1. COVID-19 pandemic: government measures and public concerns (1 February–1 June 2020).

Macro-Concern	Rank	%	Public Concern	Keywords
Virus Infection	1	10.46%	COVID-19 Cases	تعلن ,جديد ,صحه ,تسجيل ,وتسجيل ,بفيروس ,حالات ,جديده ,اصابه ,حاله Case, Infection, New, Cases, Virus, Register, Health, New, Announce
Daily Matters	2	8.86%	Supplications	اجعل ,رحمه ,وباء ,رمضان ,سبحان ,مسلم ,عافيه ,بلد ,عظيم ,امين Ameen, Great, Country, Health, Muslim, Glory to, Ramadan, Epidemic, Mercy, Make
	4	7.87%	Five Daily Prayers (Salah)	سبت ,مساجد ,جماعه ,صلاه ,جمعه ,نهايه ,شوال ,سلام ,حياه ,احد Sunday, Life, Shawwal, Peace, End, Friday, Prayer, Group, Mosque, Saturday
	11	5.81%	Mobility	حسب ,محلي ,وقت ,طرق ,مرور ,عبر ,طريق ,رياض ,جده Jeddah, Riyad, Road, Through, Traffic, Roads, Time, Local, Land, According to
Contain the Virus	3	8.38%	Quarantine	صح ,راح ,ممكن ,يعني ,حمدلل ,طيب ,شخص ,حجر ,شيء ,ناس People, Things, Quarantine, Person, Fine, Praise be to God, Means, Possible, Go, True
	5	6.53%	Stay Home	صحه ,دوره ,سلاحنا ,اقوى ,بقاء ,لمواجه ,كورونا ,منزل ,فايروس ,مسؤول Responsible, Virus, Home, Corona, Facing, Stay, Strong, Weapon, Circle, Health
	9	6.13%	Prevention (COVID-19)	للحد ,ساعه ,كورونا ,فيروس ,مساء ,انتشار ,ملك ,خادم ,شريف ,حرمين Haramain, Holy, Custodian, King, Spread, Evening, Virus, Corona, Hour, Reduce
	7	6.46%	Cleaning Services	امطار ,تواصل ,امانه ,نقل ,مدينه ,وسلم ,مكه ,تنظيف ,شركه ,رياض Riyadh, Company, Clean, Makkah, Peace, Medinah, Move, Municipality, Continue, Rains
	13	5.70%	Curfew	منوره ,فيديو ,جبيل ,قرار ,داخل ,مدينه ,مكرمه ,تجول ,مكه ,منع Prevent, Makkah, Wandering, Mukaramah, Medinah, Inside, Order, Jubail, Video, Munawarah
Social Sustainability	8	6.39%	Hospital Treatment	صاحب ,رقم ,تبرع ,دم ,فصيله ,صباح ,ملف ,بحاجه ,مستشفى ,خير Good, Hospital, Need, File, Morning, Type, Blood, Donation, Number, Owner
Economic Sustainability	6	6.48%	Loan	اهلي ,امن ,قادمه ,نور ,يوم ,سداد ,قروض ,حمد ,صباح ,رياض Riyadh, Morning, Thank, Loans, Pay, Day, Light, Coming, Security, My family
	10	5.92%	Prize Draw	موثق ,شروط ,يوم ,مواطن ,سحب ,فيروس ,هديه ,رتويت ,فيديو ,كورونا Corona, Video, Retweet, Gift, Virus, Withdraw, Citizen, Day, Terms, Documented
	12	5.80%	Salary	مجلس ,نظام ,اجتماع ,ازمه ,حكومه ,رواتب ,سعودي ,قطاع ,تم ,خاص Private, Done, Sector, Saudi, Salary, Government, Crisis, Meeting, System, Council
	14	4.74%	Offers	حقوق ,كوبون ,نون ,وتسجيل ,كورونا ,اولا ,تكون ,عكاظ ,كود ,خصم Discount, Code, Okaz, Be, First, Corona, Register, Noon, Coupon, Rights
Back to Normal	15	4.48%	Back to Normal	تعتمد ,امتثال ,كورونا ,احترازه ,مراحل ,دفاع ,رساله ,اولى ,بدايه ,عوده Back, Beginning, First, Message, Defense, Phase, Precaution, Corona, Compliance, Depend

The eighth concern is **Hospital Treatment**. From the top keywords, we can see that the need for blood donation became very high during the pandemic. This was an international concern because fewer people donated blood. It could be because they cannot visit hospitals/clinics because of the curfew or because they are worried about getting infected. Besides this, according to the Food and Drug Administration (FDA) [16] the number of blood donations dramatically declined during the pandemic time due to the implementation of social distancing as well as the cancellation of blood drives. We found several tweets in our dataset similar to the following, with differing patient file number and hospital name. We removed the file number from the tweet to protect the patient's identity.

عاجل صاحب الملف ----- بحاجة #تبرع #الفصيلة مقبول بالجميع لم يفصل اجل تشرف في الملف يصل #جدة

Urgent owner of the file —— needs #Blood #Donation type: accepts all blood types King Faisal Hospital #Jeddah

The ninth pandemic-related concern is about the **Prevention** of COVID-19. This is clear from the top keywords: reduce, spread, corona, virus, and others. The top tweets that we found for this concern have shown different prevention strategies applied by the government to instill a sense of responsibility and to increase awareness among people about the importance of their role in fighting the spread of this virus. One of the approaches is enforcing curfew. The following tweet was posted on 22 March by @spagov account, which is the official account of the official Saudi Press Agency (SPA) for the news of the royal decrees, orders, council of ministers, and official statements.

خادم الحرمين الشريفين يوصدر أمر بفرض حظر التجول للحد من انتشار #فيروس كورونا الجديد ابتداءً من الساعة 7 مساءً

The Custodian of the Two Holy Mosques issues a curfew order to limit the spread of the new #Corona_virus starting at 7 p.m.

Besides this, as another example, the Twitter account of the Ministry of Health (@SaudiMOH) has posted the following tweet on 22 March.

من أجل ؟؟سلامتكم نصيحتك تأجيل المواعيد و ؟الإجراءات الطبية غير العاجلة #الوقاية_من_كورونا

For your safety, we recommend postponing non-urgent medical appointments and procedures. #Coronavirus_prevention

Another tweet with the same hashtag, #Coronavirus_prevention, was posted by the official account of the Minister of Health Dr. Tawfiq Al-Rabiah (@tfrabiah) on 15 May before the end of the curfew and the return to normal. He encouraged people to wear masks before getting out of their houses.

انصح الجميع بضرورة استخدام الكمامة القماشية عند الخروج من المنزل #الوقاية_من_كورونا

I advise everyone to use a cloth mask when going out of the house #Coronavirus_prevention

Moreover, we found another tweet posted by @SaudiMOH on 30 March about the government order to treat all COVID-19 patients for free.

ونحن الصحي نحيي من عن أمر خادم الحرمين الشريفين حفظه الله □ ؟؟؟ لم جميع المصابين بفيروس #كورونا الجديد من المواطنين والمقيمين ومخالفي نظام الإقامة ؟؟

The Minister of Health announces the order of the Custodian of the Two Holy Mosques, may God preserve him for free treatment to all citizens and residents infected and violators of the residency system with the new #Coronavirus.

The tenth pandemic-related concern regards **Prize Draw**. Note in Table 1. the top keywords, such as withdrawal, documented, video, gift, and retweet. It is common on social media to see some users announce prizes that will be given to a randomly selected follower who retweets their tweet. This helps them to increase their popularity because they will get more followers and thus it would be a mean of earning. This can be done by individuals or companies. The following tweet is an example.

السحب الليلة موثق بالفيديو و.. والمتابعين رتويت وتابع

Withdrawal tonight is documented in the video . . . the gift is iPhone 11 retweet and follow

The 11th public concern includes the keywords roads and traffic, and therefore we named it **Mobility**. The levels of daily mobility have changed significantly during the

COVID-19 crisis throughout the world. All forms of transportation from road traffic flow to commercial flight activities have been reduced due to the fear of getting infected and the government lockdowns. The following tweet shows an example from Jeddah, the second largest Saudi city. This was posted on 19 March by the official account of the traffic department in Saudi Arabia, @eMoroor.

طرق جدة تشهد انخفاض في مستوى الحركة المرورية ، مما يعكس التزامها ؟ بإجراءات الوقاية و الاحترازي شاكراً لكم ونتمنى للجميع السلامة ؟؟؟

Jeddah roads are witnessing a decrease in the level of traffic, which reflects the commitment to preventive and precautionary procedures [.] Thank you and we wish everyone safety.

The 12th pandemic-related concern is **Salary**. The top keywords include salary, private, government, and sector. Many employees lost their jobs due to the government lockdown restrictions and the closure of shops. Besides this, small, medium, and large businesses were also severely affected. Many organizations cut down their employees' salaries and/or laid off their employees. The 13th concern is **Curfew**. The top keywords include prevent, wandering, and the names of some cities. The 14th public concern is **Offers**. Discount, code, and coupon are among the top keywords. Various vendors in order to compensate for their losses due to the business closures in physical spaces have provided offers to attract online shopping customers.

Finally, the 15th concern is **Back to Normal**. This is related to the issues that need to be addressed for returning to normal life (as opposed to the life during the pandemic). By the end of the curfew, the authorities in Saudi Arabia started a new awareness campaign under the slogan "العودة بحذر" (returning with caution). People were discussing and responding to this campaign on social media. This is the last concern in terms of the ranking, because we believe that it includes fewer tweets compared to the other concerns. The "Back to Normal" was a relatively recent public concern within the dataset this stage had started by the end of May and our dataset contains tweets until 1 June.

Figure 5 visualizes the correlation matrix. The correlation matrix is visualized as a heatmap using the Seaborn library in Python. We computed the correlation matrix by calculating the correlation coefficients between the keywords of the detected concerns to show the relationship between the keywords (see Section 3.5 for details on its computations). There are a total of 15 concerns with 10 keywords each. We remove the duplicates keywords that exist in multiple concerns and sort them based on the frequency and keep the top 50 keywords. The dark blue color represents the strongest positive relationship between keywords while the dark red represents the strongest negative correlation. For example, note the dark blue color between wandering and prevent, which are used when mentioning **Curfew**. Note the dark blue squares between the keywords facing, stay, home, and strong, which imply a strong positive relationship between them. As mentioned earlier, these keywords refer to the **Stay Home** concern. There also seems to be a strong positive correlation between custodian, holy, and Haramain, which are usually used when referring to the Custodian of the Two Holy Mosques, the King of Saudi Arabia. Besides, a strong positive correlation can also be noted between Makkah and Mukarramah, which is the full name of Makkah city, as well as Madinah and Munawwarah, which is the full name of Almadinah city, the two holiest cities in Islam. Additionally, note the light blue color between the Makkah and Madinah keywords that shows that these two words have a mild positive relationship, which makes sense because these two cities appear together in many tweets. Note also the positive correlation between case, health, announce, register, corona, and infection. As mentioned earlier, these keywords are used when posting about **COVID-19 cases**.

Note that the most distinctive horizontal or vertical line is the line for the corona keyword, indicating that it has a relatively distinctive relationship with most of the keywords even though the light colors indicate mild positive and negative correlations. The highest positive correlation appears to be between corona and virus, while the highest negative correlation is between corona and good. This makes sense, because good is a positive keyword. Finally, we note that there are not many dark red colors, implying that none of the keywords have strong negative correlations between them.

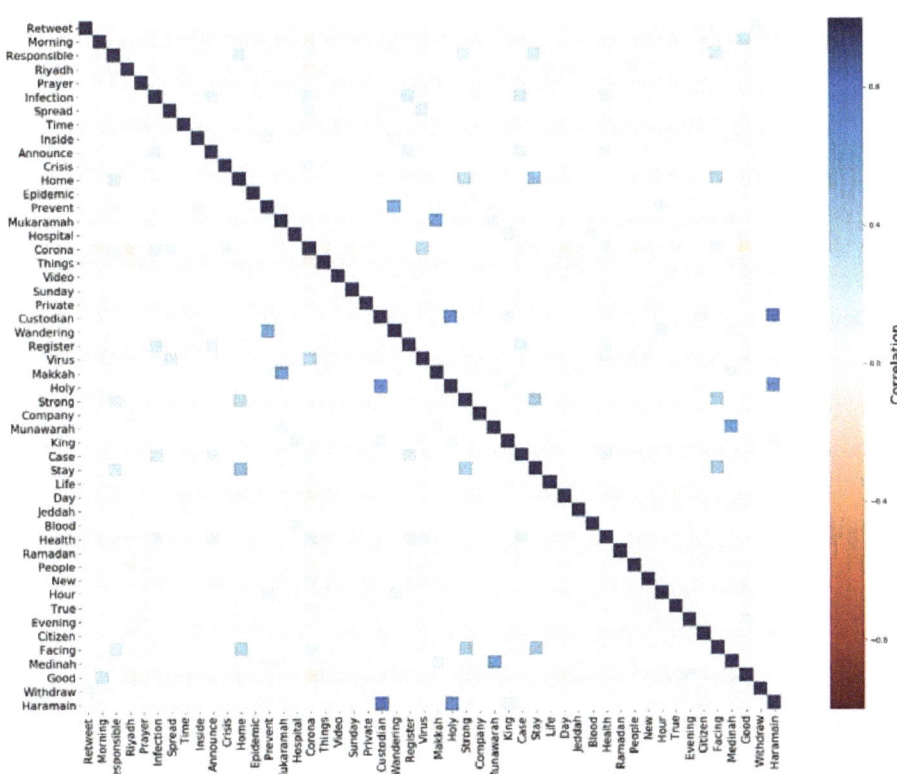

Figure 5. The correlation matrix of keywords.

4.2. Temporal Analysis

In this section, we will investigate how the public concerns have evolved over time during the pandemic. Figure 6 depicts the changes in the intensity of the tweets over time for the fifteen identified public concerns. We elaborate the data on these trends in Figure 6 using the following six figures, one for each of the six public macro-concerns.

Figure 7 depicts the intensity of tweets related to the public macro-concern **Contain the Virus**. The public concerns in this macro-class include curfew, stay home, quarantine, prevention, and cleaning services. The curfew was ordered on 22 March and applied from the next day between 7 a.m. and 6 p.m. It can be seen that the highest peak (for **Curfew**) was on 2 April. From external validation [68], we found that on that day the Makkah and Madinah cities were put under a 24 h curfew to prevent the spread of the virus and protect the health of residents. It appears that this 24 h curfew event was this detected highest peak because these are the two holiest cities in Saudi Arabia and for the whole Islamic world, and thus the lookdown of these two cities drew the attention of everyone.

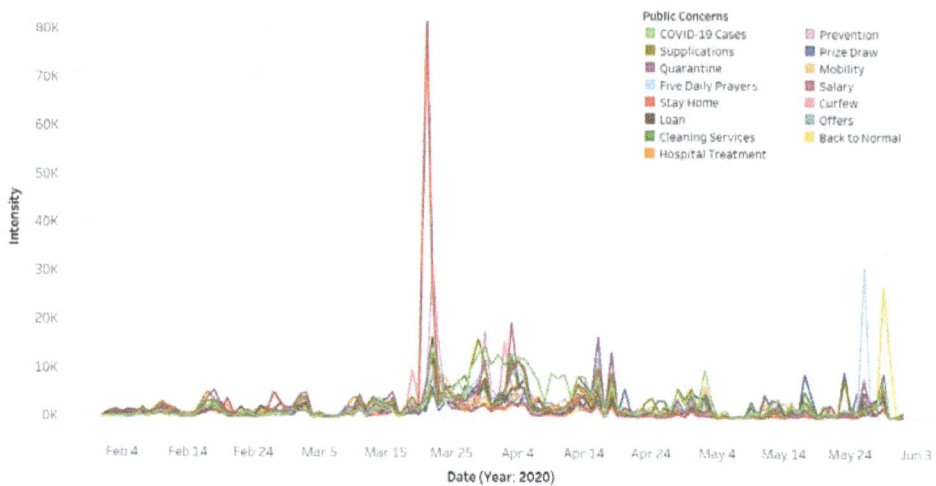

Figure 6. Daily Twitter activity of government measures and public concerns (all).

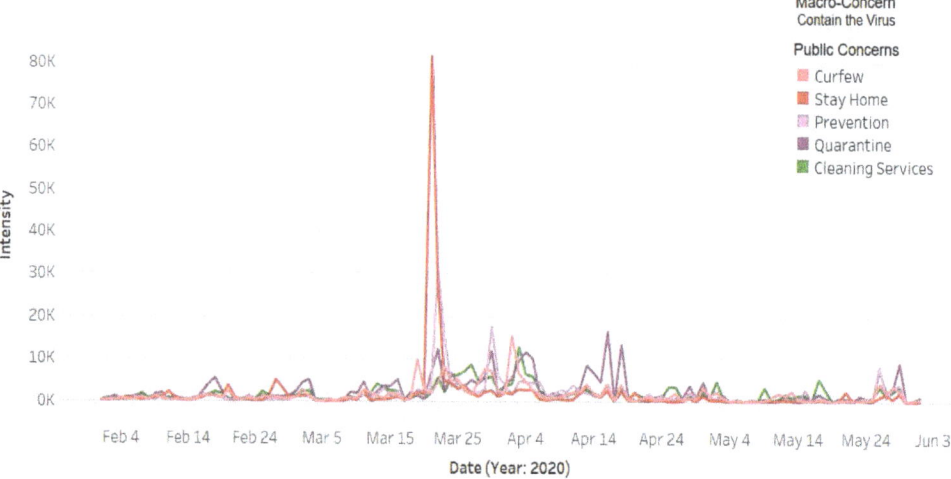

Figure 7. Daily Twitter activity for a macro-concern (**Contain the Virus**).

Figure 7 shows the Twitter activity for the **Stay at Home** public concern in red color. It can be seen that the highest peak for this concern was on 21 March. We found that on that day the Government Communication Center of the Information Ministry launched the new visual identity initiative for the awareness campaign for coronavirus under the slogan "كلنا مسؤول" (we are all responsible) to encourage people staying at home [69]. We believe that people interacted with this initiative and posted about it on Twitter using the hashtag #كلنا_مسؤول that explains a large Twitter activity related to the **Stay at Home** concern on that date. The **Prevention** concern is represented in Figure 7 using a light purple color. The highest detected peak for this concern was on 22 March and the second-highest peak was on 30 March. We found that many orders have been placed around the end of March to control the spread of the virus, including the order of curfew that has been announced on 22 March [70]. Further, as posted in the Ministry of Health website, on 30 March the King of Saudi Arabia ordered providing free treatment to all citizens, residents, and even those who violated the residency rules [71].

The line plot in purple color in Figure 7 represents the quarantine concern. There are several peaks between 22 March and 18 April. The posts about quarantine had increased after the spread of the virus in the country and the increase in the number of cases. As we mentioned earlier, the government enforced several actions, including lockdown and curfew, as well as closing mosques, schools, and shopping malls by the end of March. The public concern cleaning services is represented in Figure 7 in green color. Note in the graph that the number of tweets start increasing after 22 March and reach the highest point on 3 April. Generally speaking, individuals and organizations have become more careful and concerned with cleanliness. As mentioned in Section 4.1 using example tweets, the Riyadh municipality has been sterilizing and cleaning the roads of the Riyadh city to provide a safe and healthy environment. This tweet was posted on 26 March, which is in the same period that shows a surge in the discussion about this concern.

Figure 8 depicts the intensity of tweets related to the public macro-concern **Virus Infection** that includes one public concern, **COVID-19 Cases**. Note in the figure that between mid-March 2020 and the end of May (with some intermittent gaps), people have an increased Twitter activity related to the virus infection concern—i.e., the spread of coronavirus and the increase in the number of cases. Specifically, the top two highest peaks are on 22 and 30 March. We found from the external validation process that involves searching in online news media (see Section 3.6) that the number of daily cases increased on 22 March from 48 to 119, while on 30 March the number of cases increased from 96 to 154. This is a significant increase in the number of cases, considering that it was the beginning of the pandemic period in Saudi Arabia. This caught the attention of the people and increased the worries, leading to a peak in the Twitter activity on the subject.

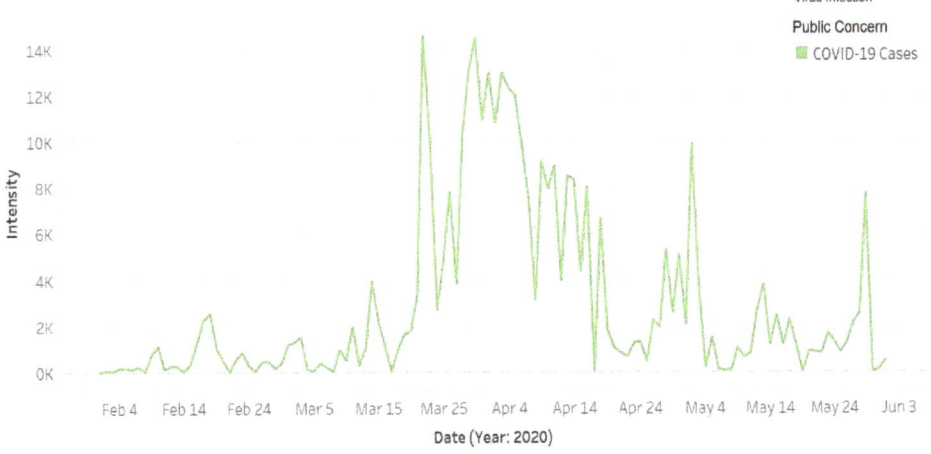

Figure 8. Daily Twitter activity for a macro-concern (virus infection).

Figure 9 shows the intensity of the tweets for the public macro-concern **Back to Normal** that includes one public concern with the same name **Back to Normal**. The highest peak was on 29 May. We found that on that date the Minister of Health posted the following tweet on Twitter:

نحن نبدأ مرحلة أولى من مراحل #العودة_بحذر ولذا نحن معتمدون على التزامكم. إن العودة ظنيا زيادة ؟؟ وزارة الصحة معتمدة على التزام على اتباع الاحتياطيات عبر زيارة باعك □ ؟إجراءات الوقائية

We are cautiously beginning the first stages of #returning_with_Caution, so we depend on your commitment. We hope that you follow the precautions.

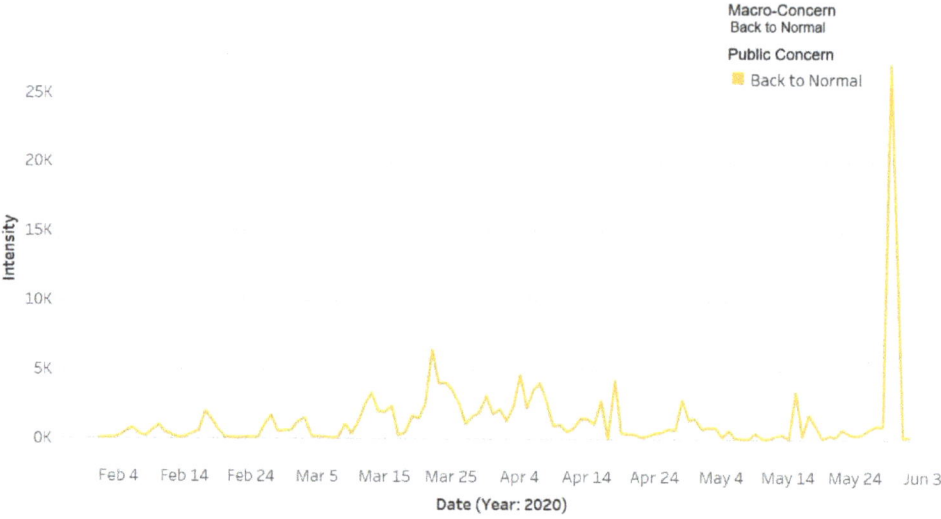

Figure 9. Daily Twitter activity for a public macro-concern (back to normal).

This tweet was posted by the end of the nationwide coronavirus curfew. The Ministry of Health considered it the first stage to return to normal and started a new awareness campaign under the slogan "العودة بحذر" (returning with caution). The interaction of people with this announcement as well as the use of the hashtag "#بحذر_العودة" explain the increase in the tweet intensity on that day.

Figure 10 plots the intensity of the tweets for the public macro-concern **Daily Matters** that includes three public concerns: **Five Daily Prayers (Salah)**, **Supplications**, and **Mobility**. Note in the figure that the intensity of the tweets about **Supplications** (see camel color) increased with the spreading of the virus and the increased number of cases. People in Saudi Arabia increased their supplications in response to the COVID-19 crisis. They ask God to protect them and their families from the virus, as well as asking for an end to the pandemic. The light blue color represents the **Salah** concern. The highest peak is on 26 May. Looking in the news media, we found that on that day an official source in the Ministry of Interior announced that, starting from Sunday 8 Shawwal (31 May) until Saturday 28 Shawwal (20 June), they will allow prayers to be held in all mosques of the Kingdom (except the mosques in the Makkah city) [72]. This explains the sharp increase in the tweet intensity on that day, because people were very happy with this news since praying at the mosque is critical for Muslims. The orange color represents the intensity of tweets about the **Mobility** concern. Note in the figure that the highest peak is on 24 March, which is two days after the curfew was implemented in Saudi Arabia. This Twitter activity was in response to how the roads appeared (empty) on the first day of the curfew. We verified this through online articles (see, e.g., [73]). The users of social media shared videos and photos showing the main streets empty due to the coronavirus curfew.

Figure 11 shows the intensity of the tweets for the public macro-concern **Social Sustainability**, which includes one public concern, **Hospital Treatment**. There was an increase over time in the Twitter activity on this concern during the pandemic, particularly during the later part of March up until mid-April. This was due to the difficulties related to the difficulties in getting treatment at hospitals and other related matters. Particularly, we found several articles in the local newspaper (Okaz) [74,75] encouraging people to donate blood because the blood bank supplies became low due to the COVID-19 situation. Additionally, we found in the collected dataset several tweets about the need for blood donation where they shared the patient files numbers in different hospitals in different cities. Furthermore, the Saudi Twitter hashtags account (@HashKSA) posted the following tweet on 12 April:

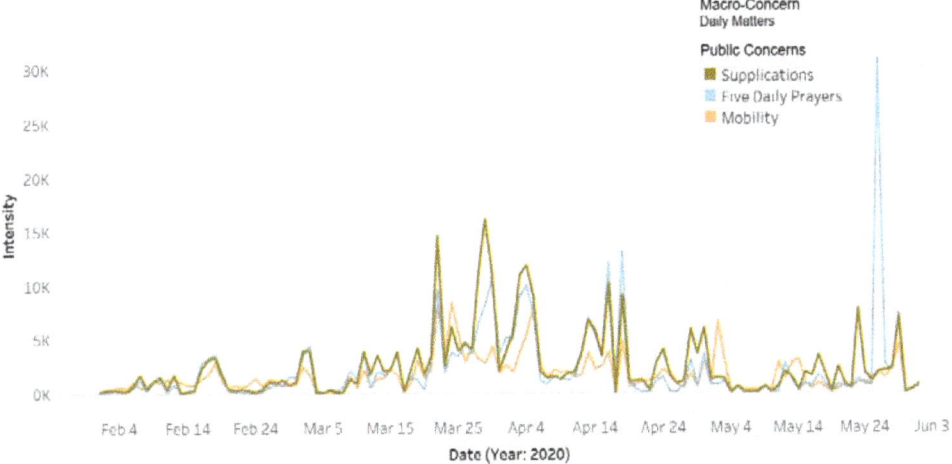

Figure 10. Daily Twitter activity for a public macro-concern (impact on daily life).

بنوك الدم تشكو قلة المتبرعين بعد جائحة #كورونا
مديرة بنك الدم في التخصصي "د. الحميدان" تؤكد شدة الحاجة وتحث على التبرع بالدم والصفائح خصوصاً لمرضى #الأورام و #زراعة_الأعضاء

Blood banks complain about the lack of donors after the Corona pandemic. The director of the blood bank in Specialist Hospital, Dr. Al-Humaidan, emphasizes the need and urges to donate blood and platelets, especially for the patients of #oncology and #organ_transplants.

Figure 12 depicts the Twitter activity related to the macro-concern economic sustainability, which includes the public concerns **Prize Draw**, **Salary**, **Loan**, and **Offers**. The blue color represents the **Prize Draw** concern. A well-known Twitter activity is about some Twitter users who post about a prize and then pick randomly from users who retweeted their tweet about the prize. One of the reasons for them to do this is to get more followers and become famous, and then this is one of the ways to earn income. This activity helps both the person who wins the prize and the one who announced it. It can be noticed in the graph that, during the pandemic, the intensity of the tweets related to this concern was on the rise. We think that having more free time due to staying at home could be a reason for the increase in such activities on social media. Besides this, the financial difficulties that have become a concern for many people due to the pandemic perhaps have led the people to find other ways to earn income. The green color represents activity for the concern **Offers**. Note in the figure that the intensity of the tweets began to increase around the end of March. The timeline coincides with the timeline of curfew enforcement and shop closures. This, we believe, led business owners to increase sale offers on their products to attract customers to keep shopping from their online stores. Our personal experience in Saudi Arabia in the last few months is that many businesses have gone online or have increased their online sales activities. Social media is one of the free and powerful ways for marketing, and the trend of online shopping and sales offers can be witnessed here.

The public concern **Salary** in Figure 12 is represented by the magenta color plot in the figure. We found that on 3 April King Salman of Saudi Arabia ordered the government to contribute towards 60% of the salaries of Saudi private-sector employees with a financial incentive of 9 billion Riyals in total [21]. This explains the dramatic rise in the intensity of tweets on that day. The brown color represents the **Loan** concern; its highest peak was on 22 March. We found that on that day the Saudi Arabian Monetary Agency (SAMA) announced that Saudi local banks will postpone the 3-month mortgage installments of all public and private health workers starting from April 2020 [20].

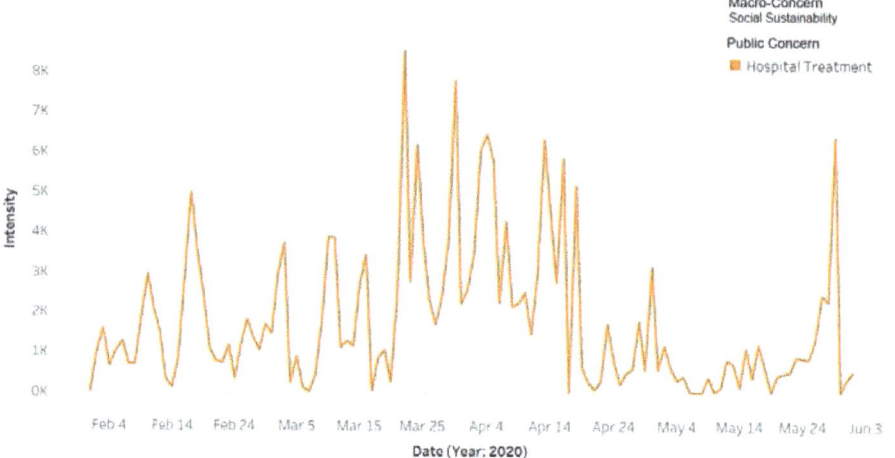

Figure 11. Daily Twitter activity for a public macro-concern (social sustainability).

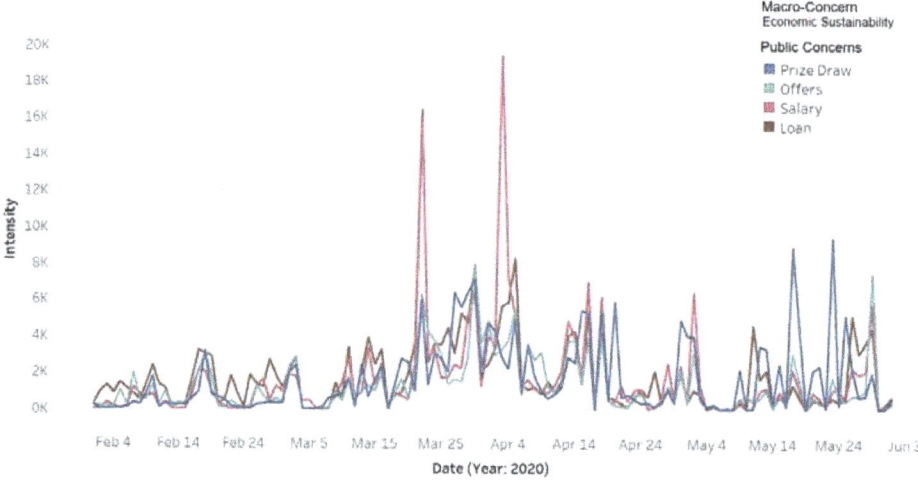

Figure 12. Daily Twitter activity for a public macro-concern (economic sustainability).

4.3. Spatio-Temporal Analysis

We investigate in this section the spatio-temporal behavior of selected public concerns during the pandemic. We overlay the location of the specific detected concerns on top of the map of Saudi Arabia. We plot only the tweets that include location information. The size of the circle represents the intensity of the relevant tweets.

Figure 13 depicts the location of tweets about the public concern **Curfew** posted on 2 April 2020. For governance purposes, Saudi Arabia is divided into 13 provinces. Their names are listed on the left of the figure. We have selected the spatial behavior of the concern curfew on this date because the temporal analysis we presented earlier (see Section 4.2, Figure 7) revealed that on that day a 24 h curfew was enforced in the

Makkah and Madinah cities. Note in the figure that the largest circle is over Makkah, and this validates the information we already have. We were expecting to find another large circle over Madinah city, but we did not. The official name of Madinah city in Arabic is "المدينة المنورة", transliterated as "Al-Madinah Al-Munawwarah". The Arabic word "المدينة" (Al-Madinah) can also mean "the city", referring to a city that is being referred to in a context, implicitly or explicitly—that is, people may refer to a city as "the city" that is being mentioned in the same tweet or the name of the city may be known from the context of the tweet. The choice we have made in designing the location extractor is that the word "Al-Madinah" if appearing without "Al-Munawwarah" is not considered as a location. We consider the tweet to be about the Madinah city only if the city name is mentioned in full (Al-Madinah Al-Munawwarah). Note in Figure 13 that the activities related to the concern curfew can also be seen in other cities around the kingdom, with some circles (Riyadh) larger than the others. This is because prayers in the main mosques of Makkah (Mecca) and Medina are important for people all around the world.

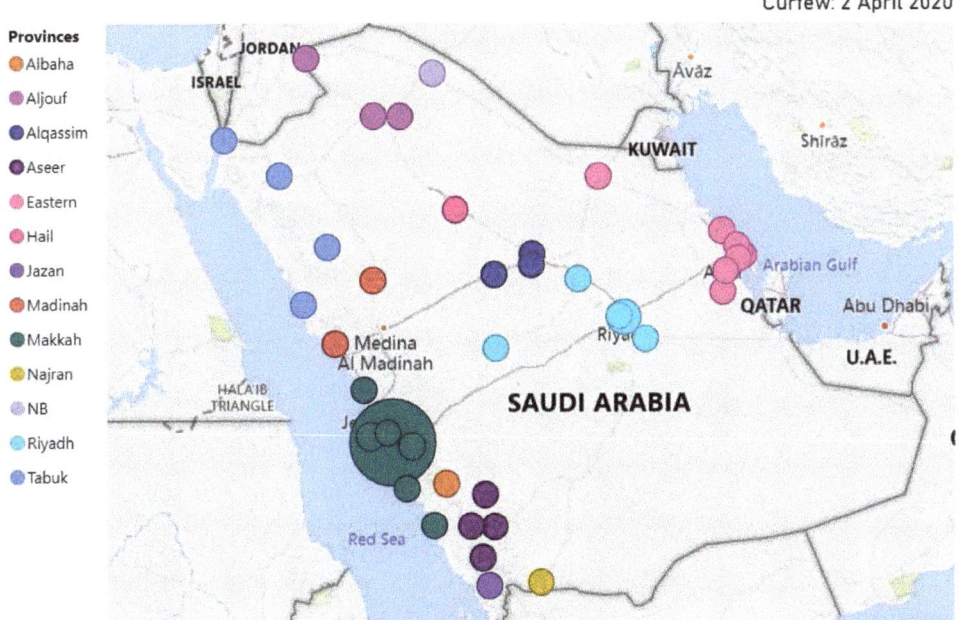

Figure 13. Spatio-temporal behavior of public concern (curfew: 2 April 2020).

Figures 14 and 15 illustrate the location of the tweets about the public concern **COVID-19 Cases** on 22 March and 30 March, respectively. These two dates are selected for the concern **COVID-19 Cases** because the temporal analysis we presented earlier (see Section 4.2, Figure 8) has revealed that the two top peak intensities for the concern happened on these two dates. A total of 119 cases were reported on 22 March, 72 of these in Makkah, 43 in Riyadh, 15 in Eastern Province (4 in Dammam, 4 in Qatif, 3 in Alhasa, 3 in Alkhobar, and one in Dhahran), and one in Alqassim [76]. This explains many circles in the eastern province in Figure 14. Each circle represents a city and the size reflects the tweets' intensity. Note the large light blue circle over Riyadh city and large green circles around Jeddah and Makkah (Jeddah is in Makkah province). We also know that people all around the country were interested in the situation, so they posted about the virus spread and the number of infected people. This explains the presence of circles in different cities around the kingdom.

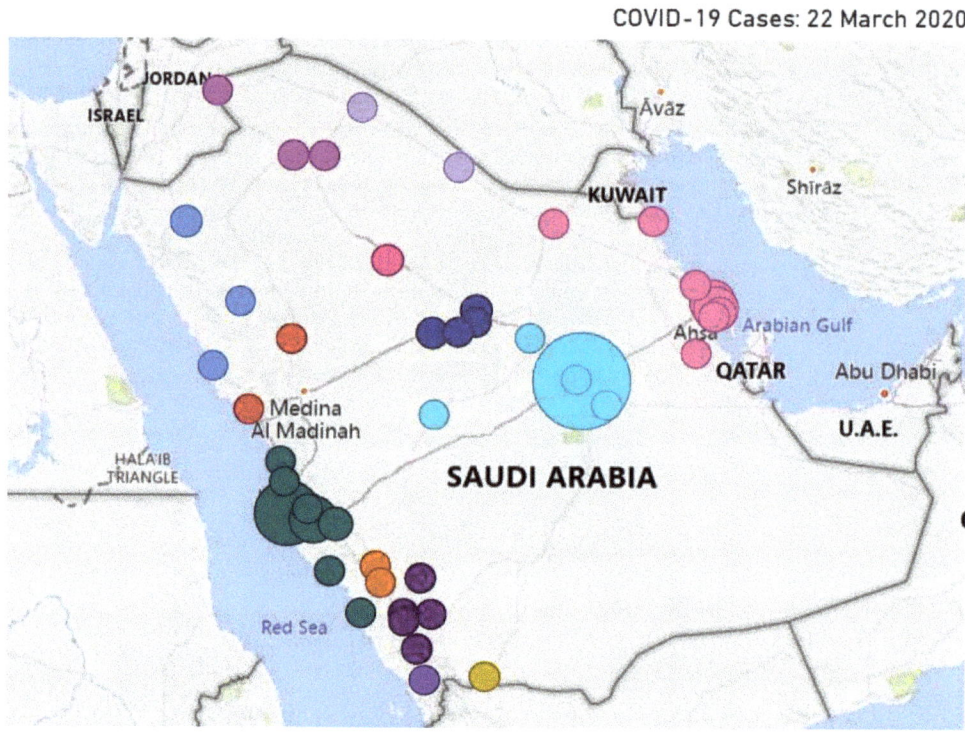

Figure 14. Spatio-temporal behavior of public concern (COVID-19 cases: 22 March 2020).

Figure 15 depicts the spatial information for 30 March. A total of 154 cases were reported on the day with the following distribution: Makkah (40), Dammam (34), Riyadh (22), Madinah (22), Jeddah (9), Haffof (6), Alkhobar (6), Qatif (5), Taif (2), and one in each of the following cities: Yanbu, Buraydah, Alras, Khamis Mushait, Alduwadimi, Dhahran, Samta, Tabuk [77]. To help to understand the map, note that Dammam, Haffof, Alkhobar, Dhahran, and Qatif are in the Eastern Province, whereas the Makkah, Jeddah, and Taif cities are in Makkah Province. Comparing Figure 15 with Figure 14, note that there are some additional circles in Figure 15, implying that the discussion about the public concern had spread to other cities. Moreover, the discussions on the public concern increased in Makkah (dark green circles), perhaps mostly due to the concern becoming a bigger issue over time during March 2020.

4.4. Execution Time Analysis

We explained earlier that our tool is designed as a distributed computing tool to address scalability in terms of big data and compute-intensive analytics applications. The tool was developed using the distributed computing platform Apache Spark and was executed on the Aziz supercomputer (see Section 3.1). LDA clustering is RAM-intensive. We have used multiple nodes with 256 GB RAM each.

Figure 16 plots the execution times of the LDA algorithm with five iterations against a varying number of cores (24, 48, 72, 96, 120, 144, and 168). The number of features, in this case, was not limited (compare with Figure 17). The results show that parallelizing the LDA algorithm on a higher number of cores (up to a certain extent) reduces the execution time. The LDA algorithm took 163.9 h (6 days) on 24 cores. We were able to reduce this time to the minimum time of 23.6 h using 168 cores. Increasing the number of cores beyond 120 (to 144 and 168) did not help much and only managed to reduce the execution time of the LDA algorithm a little. This behavior where the execution time of a parallel algorithm does not decrease with an increase in the number of computing cores or nodes is a normal behavior in parallel or distributed computing and happens when the task size is small relative to the number of cores. This is caused by the overhead of parallelizing or distributing a task. Usually, once the parallelization reaches a saturation point where an increase in the number of cores does not decrease the execution time, the execution time may even begin increasing with an increase in the number of cores (see Figure 17).

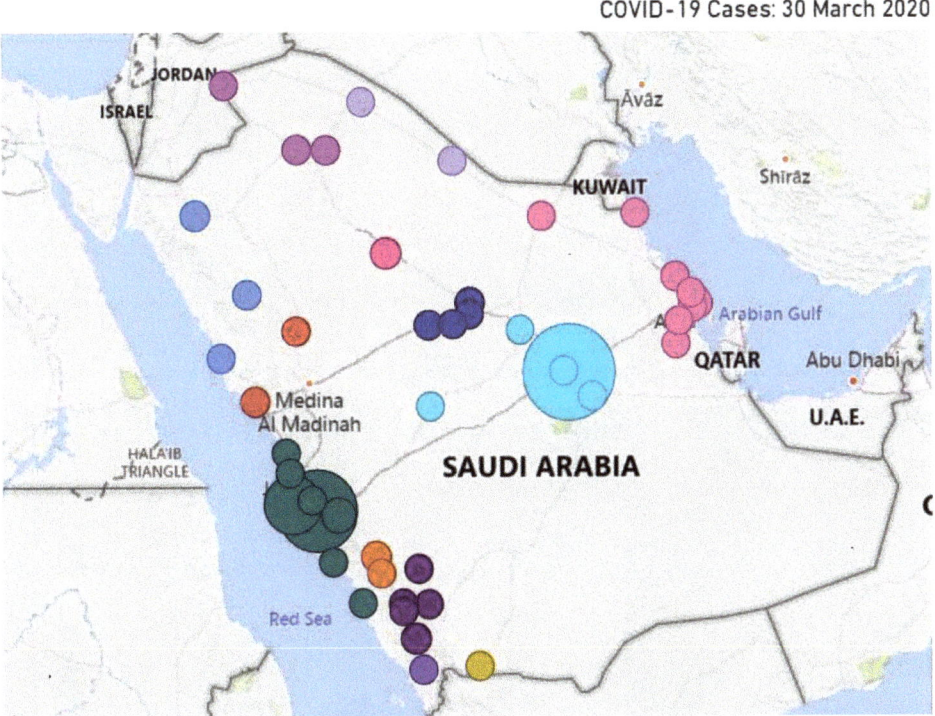

Figure 15. Spatio-temporal behavior of public concern (COVID-19 cases: 30 March 2020).

Figure 17 plots the execution times against the number of cores (24, 48, and 72) for a varying number of LDA iterations (5, 10, 50, 100, 250, 500, 1000) using 10,000 features/keywords (we have limited the number of features to reduce execution times). For the LDA algorithm with 1000 iterations, we are able to reduce the execution time by more than half, from 16.8 h on 24 cores to 7.4 h on 48 cores, benefitting from an increase in the number of cores. The LDA algorithms with the lower number of iterations (5, 10, 50, . . . , 500) have also benefited by their execution on a higher number of cores. However, a further increase in the number of cores (72 from 48) does not improve execution speed and rather increases the execution time. As explained earlier, this is a normal behavior in parallel computing due to the parallelization reaching the saturation point.

Generally speaking, a higher number of iterations is expected to produce better clusters. Our experiences in this work suggest that the clusters (public concerns) obtained from 100 iterations were better than the other configurations in terms of the relationship between the keywords of a cluster, etc., enabling us to better label the clusters with appropriate public concern names. Based on the results, the best choice was to execute LDA with 100 iterations on 72 cores. The results reported in this paper are based on this configuration (LDA with 100 iterations and 10,000 features).

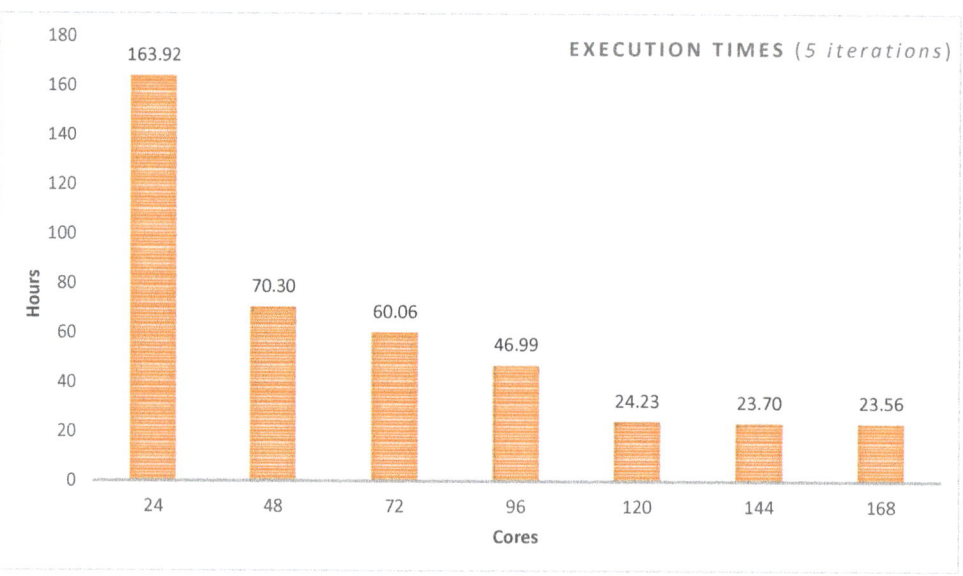

Figure 16. Execution time vs. number of cores for varying number of LDA iterations (no limit on the number of features).

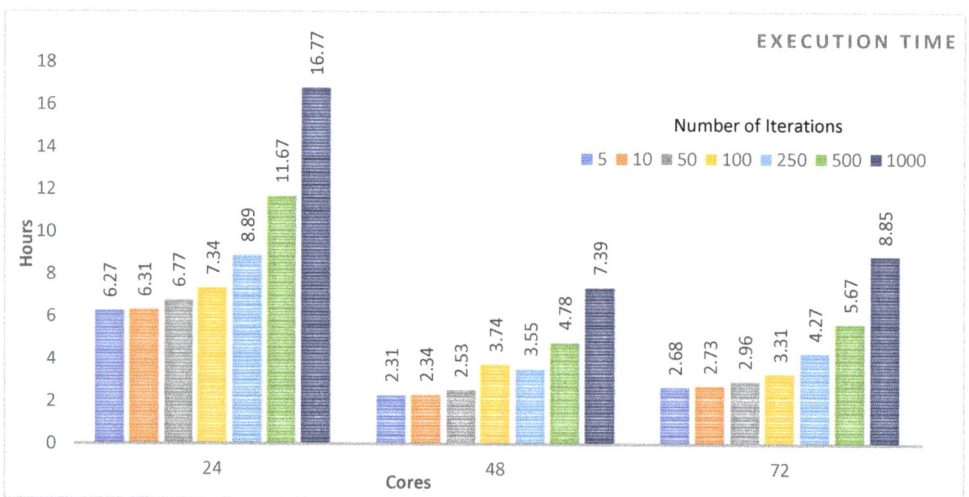

Figure 17. Execution time vs. number of cores for various numbers of LDA iterations (a limited number of features—10,000 keywords).

It may appear that the total savings one would obtain by using our tool on Apache Spark would be 4 h (7.34–3.31 h, for the LDA algorithm with 100 iterations). The process of LDA clustering such as presented in this paper may require running the LDA algorithm many times on large volumes of data with different numbers of iterations and features. In our case, we executed the LDA algorithm with various configurations between 30 to 40 times. For this, using the LDA algorithm with 5 to 1000 iterations would easily require over a month of computing time. The ability of the tool to execute in parallel could save a month of computing time in this case and speed up the development process. For larger datasets, executing sequential codes may not even be possible, or distributed computing could save years of development time. How to select the number of cores for a given job that could save experimental time and energy itself is a challenge and has been addressed in our other works [78,79].

4.5. Pandemic Measures, and Public Concerns, and Their Interrelationship

Table 1 lists the fifteen major pandemic measures and public concerns discussed by the public on Twitter during the COVID-19 pandemic. The pandemic measures are quarantine, stay home, prevention (COVID-19), cleaning services, curfew, loan, salary, and back to normal. The measures taken by the public and industry to address the economic difficulties caused due to the COVID-19 pandemic are offers and prize draw. The public concerns are COVID-19 cases, supplications, Five Daily Prayers (Salah), mobility, hospital treatment. Some measures, in a way, could also be concerns. For example, quarantine, stay home, prevention (COVID-19), curfew, loan, salary, and back to normal are both measures and concerns.

The interrelationship or impact of public, industry, or government measures on public concerns can be evidenced in our analysis presented in this section. For example, the events related to loans were being discussed by the public, but were the highest peak was detected on 22 March, the day when the Saudi Arabian Monetary Agency (SAMA) announced it in the media (see [20]). Another example is the "No Mobility" event (empty roads) that was vigorously discussed on 24 March, two days after the curfew measure was announced. The impact of the quarantine and curfew measures was also seen in a reduction in blood donations and blood supplies, leading to increased Twitter activity (concern) on this topic requesting blood donations from late March to mid-April. This concern can also be seen as a measure by the hospital authorities to announce the blood shortage and request action from the public.

5. Conclusions

The level of digital and physical connectedness of today's societies has never been seen before. We travel a lot to distant lands and frequently share gifts and viruses with each other. Unfortunately, the COVID-19 pandemic has exposed the vulnerabilities of this unprecedentedly connected world. The COVID-19 pandemic is rapidly growing across the world. Many countries have been affected and the number of cases has greatly increased. World Health Organization (WHO) declared it a pandemic on 11 March 2020. Currently, medical specialists can only treat the symptoms of the disease, since there are no cures for this disease, and developing a new vaccine with low risks and a high success rate will take time. Therefore, it is a serious global health issue.

Social networking platforms such as Twitter streams hundreds of millions of posts daily. They can be treated as a useful medium for the dissemination of information about diseases. This provides us a great opportunity to study and capture the dynamics of real-world events and understand the various public measures being undertaken by governments, as well as the changes in the daily activities of people during such outbreaks.

In this paper, we proposed a software tool that aims to detect government pandemic measures and public concerns during the COVID-19 pandemic. The methods used in the tool include an unsupervised Latent Dirichlet Allocation (LDA) topic modeling algorithm, natural language processing (NLP), correlation analysis, and other spatio-temporal information extraction and visualization methods. The tool is built using a range of technologies, including MongoDB, Parquet, Apache Spark, Spark SQL, and Spark ML. The tool, its architecture, five software components, and its algorithms are described in detail. Using the tool, we collected a dataset comprising 14 million tweets from the Kingdom of Saudi Arabia (KSA) for the period 1 February 2020 to 1 June 2020. We formulated and analyzed the findings of this paper from three relationship perspectives: information-structural, temporal, and spatio-temporal.

Concerning the information-structural or subject matter perspective, we have detected 15 government pandemic measures and public concerns and have grouped them into six macro-concerns. For the **pandemic measures** implemented by the Saudi government concerning the COVID-19 pandemic, we detected curfew and restrictions on mobility in the country, quarantine and fines, restrictions on praying in the mosques, campaigns to stay home, COVID-19 prevention, and cleaning services provided to curb the coronavirus spread. For **economic sustainability**, we detected that the government provided financial incentives including loans and private-sector salaries. Businesses increased offers to increase their sales. People moved to or increased in their online economic activities, such as activities related to prize draws for income earnings. For health, well-being, and **social sustainability**, we detected that blood donation and treatment at hospitals have been a major cause of concern. People also actively talked about the new number of cases. The **daily livelihood** issues in Saudi Arabia include the five daily congregational prayers at the mosques that were suspended by the government. People also increased in supplications for the safety of people. A significant reduction in mobility was noted across the country that was related to **environmental sustainability**, health, and well-being due to the reduction in traffic congestion and air pollution. As regards the temporal perspective, we were able to detect the timewise progression of events from the public discussions on COVID-19 cases in mid-March to the first curfew on 22 March, financial loan incentives on 22 March, the increased quarantine discussions during March–April, the discussions on the reduced mobility levels from 24 March onwards, the blood donation shortfall from late March onwards, the government's 9 billion SAR salary incentives on 3 April, lifting the ban on five daily prayers in mosques on 26 May, and finally the return to normal government measures on 29 May 2020. For the **spatio-temporal** perspective, we extracted location information using different approaches including tweet text and hashtags, geo-coordinate attributes, and user profiles. We were able to detect important events in over 50 cities around the kingdom, with major activities related to COVID-19 cases, curfew, etc., in the Makkah, Riyadh, and Eastern provinces. We validated the detected government measures and public concerns and their spatial and temporal nature through external validation by searching online news media or internal validation by checking tweets.

The detected events in KSA are also aligned with **international concerns,** such as various lockdown measures [14], reduced mobility [15], reduction in blood donations [16], financial difficulties and related government incentives [17,18], and worries related to returning to normal times [19]. Saudi Arabia has followed different strategies to fight the outbreak, instill a sense of responsibility, and raise awareness among people about the importance of their role in the fight against coronavirus. The government undertook early actions to prevent the spread of the virus. KSA reported its first case of the COVID-19 on 2 March. One week later, they closed the schools. On 16 March, they suspended all international and national flights, closed shopping malls, and suspended all sports activities. On 18 March, the attendance of employees at their workplaces in government agencies and the private sector was suspended. Furthermore, the king ordered free treatment for all citizens and residents, even for the violators of the residency system. The KSA government also provided financial incentives in terms of private-sector salaries and the temporary postponement of loan payments.

The research reported in this paper is different from the existing works on social media analytics for COVID-19-related studies in several respects, as has been discussed in detail in Section 2. None of the existing works have reported a similar COVID-19 analysis of Twitter data in the Arabic language in terms of the modelling methods used and the depth of the analysis. The software developed for this work is part of the tool Iktishaf [6–9] that we have been developing for the last few years. The ability of the tool to execute in parallel could save a month of computing time for the specific dataset size and the problem addressed in this paper and speed up the development process. For larger datasets, executing sequential codes may not even be possible, or distributed computing could save years of development time.

The findings presented in this paper show the effectiveness of the Twitter media in detecting important events, government measures, public concerns, and other information in time, space, and information-structure with no earlier knowledge about them. The utilization possibilities of such tools are unlimited. For example, governments could learn about the various public concerns in pandemic and normal times and develop policies and measures to address these concerns. The public could raise their concerns and give feedback on government policies. The public could learn about various public and industry activities (such as economic activities detected by our tool) and get involved in these to address financial, social, and other difficulties. The standardization and adoption of such tools could lead to real-time surveillance and the detection of disease outbreaks (and other potentially dangerous phenomena) across the globe and allow governments to take timely actions to prevent the spread of diseases and other disasters. The international standardization of such tools could allow governments to learn about the impact of policies of various countries and develop best practices for national and international response.

While we have shown good evidence of the use of LDA, NLP, and other methods, more work is needed to improve the breadth and depth of the work with regard to what can be detected, the diversity of data and machine and deep learning methods, the accuracy of detection in space and time, and the real-time analysis of the tweets.

Our focus in this work is on Saudi Arabia. The tool hence currently works with tweets only in the Arabic language. The tool can be used in other Arabic language-speaking countries, such as Egypt, Kuwait, Bahrain, and UAE. The system methodology and design of the tool developed in this paper are generic, and therefore the tool can be extended to other countries globally. This will require the adaptation of the tool with additional languages, such as English, Spanish, or Chinese, by additional modules in the pre-processing and clustering modules.

Author Contributions: Conceptualization, E.A. and R.M.; methodology, E.A. and R.M.; software, E.A.; validation, E.A. and R.M.; formal analysis, E.A. and R.M.; investigation, E.A. and R.M.; resources, R.M., I.K., and A.A.; data curation, E.A.; writing—original draft preparation, E.A. and R.M.; writing—review and editing, R.M., A.A., and I.K; visualization, E.A.; supervision, R.M.; project administration, R.M., I.K., and A.A.; funding acquisition, R.M., A.A., and I.K. All authors have read and agreed to the published version of the manuscript.

Funding: This project was funded by the Deanship of Scientific Research (DSR) at King Abdulaziz University, Jeddah, under grant number RG-6-611-40. The authors, therefore, acknowledge with thanks the DSR for their technical and financial support.

Institutional Review Board Statement: Not applicable.

Informed Consent Statement: Not applicable.

Data Availability Statement: Data was obtained from Twitter. Restrictions apply to the availability of these data.

Acknowledgments: The experiments reported in this paper were performed on the Aziz supercomputer at King Abdulaziz University.

Conflicts of Interest: The authors declare no conflict of interest.

References

1. Johns Hopkins University. *Coronavirus COVID-19 Global Cases by the Center for Systems Science and Engineering (CSSE) at Johns Hopkins University (JHU)*; Johns Hopkins University: Baltimore, MD, USA, 2020.
2. Agarwal, S.; Mittal, N.; Sureka, A. Potholes and Bad Road Conditions- Mining Twitter to Extract Information on Killer Roads. In Proceedings of the ACM India Joint International Conference on Data Science and Management of Data, Dona Paula, India, 11–13 January 2018.
3. Klaithin, S.; Haruechaiyasak, C. Traffic Information Extraction and Classification from Thai Twitter. In Proceedings of the 13th International Joint Conference on Computer Science and Software Engineering (JCSSE), Khon Kaen, Thailand, 13–15 July 2016; pp. 1–6. [CrossRef]
4. D'Andrea, E.; Ducange, P.; Lazzerini, B.; Marcelloni, F. Real-Time Detection of Traffic from Twitter Stream Analysis. *IEEE Trans. Intell. Transp. Syst.* **2015**, *16*, 2269–2283. [CrossRef]
5. Kurniawan, D.A.; Wibirama, S.; Setiawan, N.A. Real-time Traffic Classification with Twitter Data Mining. In Proceedings of the 2016 8th International Conference on Information Technology and Electrical Engineering (ICITEE), Yogyakarta, Indonesia, 5–6 October 2016; [CrossRef]

6. Alomari, E.; Katib, I.; Mehmood, R. Iktishaf: A Big Data Road-Traffic Event Detection Tool Using Twitter and Spark Machine Learning. *Mob. Netw. Appl.* **2020**. [CrossRef]
7. Alomari, E.; Mehmood, R.; Katib, I. Sentiment Analysis of Arabic Tweets for Road Traffic Congestion and Event Detection. In *Smart Infrastructure and Applications: Foundations for Smarter Cities and Societies*; Springer International Publishing: Cham, Switzerland, 2020; pp. 37–54.
8. Alomari, E.; Mehmood, R. Analysis of tweets in Arabic language for detection of road traffic conditions. In *Lecture Notes of the Institute for Computer Sciences, Social-Informatics and Telecommunications Engineering*; Springer: Cham, Switzerland, 2018; Volume 224, pp. 98–110. [CrossRef]
9. Alomari, E.; Mehmood, R.; Katib, I. Road Traffic Event Detection Using Twitter Data, Machine Learning, and Apache Spark. In Proceedings of the 2019 IEEE SmartWorld, Ubiquitous Intelligence & Computing, Advanced & Trusted Computing, Scalable Computing & Communications, Cloud & Big Data Computing, Internet of People and Smart City Innovation (SmartWorld/SCALCOM/UIC/ATC/CBDCom/IOP/SCI), Leicester, UK, 19–23 August 2019; pp. 1888–1895. [CrossRef]
10. Alotaibi, S.; Mehmood, R.; Katib, I.; Rana, O.; Albeshri, A. Sehaa: A Big Data Analytics Tool for Healthcare Symptoms and Diseases Detection Using Twitter, Apache Spark, and Machine Learning. *Appl. Sci.* **2020**, *10*, 1398. [CrossRef]
11. Suma, S.; Mehmood, R.; Albeshri, A. Automatic Detection and Validation of Smart City Events Using HPC and Apache Spark Platforms. In *Smart Infrastructure and Applications: Foundations for Smarter Cities and Societies*; Springer: Cham, Switzerland, 2020; pp. 55–78.
12. Suma, S.; Mehmood, R.; Albugami, N.; Katib, I.; Albeshri, A. Enabling Next Generation Logistics and Planning for Smarter Societies. *Procedia Comput. Sci.* **2017**, *109*, 1122–1127. [CrossRef]
13. Alsulami, M.; Mehmood, R. Sentiment Analysis Model for Arabic Tweets to Detect Users' Opinions about Government Services in Saudi Arabia: Ministry of Education as a case study. In Proceedings of the Al Yamamah Information and Communication Technology Forum, Riyadh, Saudi Arabia, 4 March 2018.
14. The Best Global Responses to COVID-19 Pandemic | Time. Available online: https://time.com/5851633/best-global-responses-covid-19/ (accessed on 26 July 2020).
15. Jeremy, S.; Monschauer, Y. Changes in Transport Behaviour during the Covid-19 Crisis. IEA. Available online: https://www.iea.org/articles/changes-in-transport-behaviour-during-the-covid-19-crisis (accessed on 1 January 2021).
16. Marks, P. Coronavirus (COVID-19) Update: Blood Donations FDA. 2020. Available online: https://www.fda.gov/news-events/press-announcements/coronavirus-covid-19-update-blood-donations (accessed on 1 January 2021).
17. Covid-19 Coronavirus: Finance Minister Says Government Has More Fiscal Firepower to Fight Virus—NZ Herald. Available online: https://www.nzherald.co.nz/nz/news/article.cfm?c_id=1&objectid=12319300 (accessed on 26 July 2020).
18. FACTBOX-Global Economic Policy Response to the Coronavirus Crisis—Reuters. Available online: https://www.reuters.com/article/health-coronavirus-economy/factbox-global-economic-policy-response-to-the-coronavirus-crisis-idUSL3N2C11C3 (accessed on 26 July 2020).
19. How is WHO responding to COVID-19? Available online: https://www.who.int/emergencies/diseases/novel-coronavirus-2019/who-response-in-countries (accessed on 26 July 2020).
20. 4 'SAMA' Initiatives to Mitigate Corona's Economic Impacts. Available online: https://ajel.sa/9JRdyv/ (accessed on 1 January 2021).
21. By Order of the King . . . the State Bears 60% of the Salaries of Saudis in the 'Private Sector'. Available online: https://www.okaz.com.sa/news/local/2018078 (accessed on 1 January 2021).
22. Mehmood, R.; See, S.; Katib, I.; Chlamtac, I. (Eds.) *Smart Infrastructure and Applications: Foundations for Smarter Cities and Societies*; EAI/Springer Innovations in Communication and Computing, Springer International Publishing: Cham, Switzerland, 2020; p. 692.
23. Mehmood, R.; Bhaduri, B.; Katib, I.; Chlamtac, I. (Eds.) *Smart Societies, Infrastructure, Technologies and Applications*; Lecture Notes of the Institute for Computer Sciences, Social Informatics and Telecommunications Engineering (LNICST); Springer: Cham, Switzerland, 2018; Volume 224, p. 367.
24. Janbi, N.; Katib, I.; Albeshri, A.; Mehmood, R. Distributed Artificial Intelligence-as-a-Service (DAIaaS) for Smarter IoE and 6G Environments. *Sensors* **2020**, *20*, 5796. [CrossRef]
25. Yigitcanlar, T.; Butler, L.; Windle, E.; Desouza, K.C.; Mehmood, R.; Corchado, J.M. Can Building 'Artificially Intelligent Cities' Safeguard Humanity from Natural Disasters, Pandemics, and Other Catastrophes? An Urban Scholar's Perspective. *Sensors* **2020**, *20*, 2988. [CrossRef]
26. Mohammed, T.; Albeshri, A.; Katib, I.; Mehmood, R. UbiPriSEQ—Deep reinforcement learning to manage privacy, security, energy, and QoS in 5G IoT hetnets. *Appl. Sci.* **2020**, *10*, 7120. [CrossRef]
27. Kemp, S. Digital Trends 2019: Every Single Stat you Need to Know about the Internet, *thenextweb.com*. 2019. Available online: https://thenextweb.com/contributors/2019/01/30/digital-trends-2019-every-single-stat-you-need-to-know-about-the-internet/ (accessed on 10 January 2020).
28. Liu, B. Sentiment Analysis and Opinion Mining. *Synth. Lect. Hum. Lang. Technol.* **2012**, *5*, 1–167. [CrossRef]
29. Yigitcanlar, T.; Kankanamge, N.; Vella, K. How Are Smart City Concepts and Technologies Perceived and Utilized? A Systematic Geo-Twitter Analysis of Smart Cities in Australia. *J. Urban Technol.* **2020**. [CrossRef]

30. Amaxilatis, D.; Mylonas, G.; Theodoridis, E.; Diez, L.; Deligiannidou, K. Learningcity: Knowledge generation for smart cities. In *EAI/Springer Innovations in Communication and Computing*; Springer Science and Business Media Deutschland GmbH: Berlin, Germany, 2020; pp. 17–41.
31. Yigitcanlar, T.; Kankanamge, N.; Regona, M.; Maldonado, A.; Rowan, B.; Ryu, A.; Desouza, K.C.; Corchado, J.M.; Mehmood, R.; Li, R.Y.M. Artificial Intelligence Technologies and Related Urban Planning and Development Concepts: How Are They Perceived and Utilized in Australia? *J. Open Innov. Technol. Mark. Complex.* **2020**, *6*, 187. [CrossRef]
32. Bello, J.P.; Silva, C.; Nov, O.; DuBois, R.L.; Arora, A.; Salamon, J.; Mydlarz, C.; Doraiswamy, H. SONYC: A System for Monitoring, Analyzing, and Mitigating Urban Noise Pollution. *Commun. ACM* **2019**, *62*, 68–77. [CrossRef]
33. Pandhare, K.R.; Shah, M.A. Real Time Road Traffic Event Detection Using Twitter and Spark. Available online: https://ieeexplore.ieee.org/document/7975237 (accessed on 1 January 2021).
34. Salas, A.; Georgakis, P.; Nwagboso, C.; Ammari, A.; Petalas, I. Traffic event detection framework using social media. In Proceedings of the 2017 IEEE International Conference on Smart Grid and Smart Cities (ICSGSC), Singapore, 23–26 July 2017; pp. 303–307. [CrossRef]
35. Lau, R.Y.K. Toward a social sensor based framework for intelligent transportation. In Proceedings of the 2017 IEEE 18th International Symposium on A World of Wireless, Mobile and Multimedia Networks (WoWMoM), Macau, 12–15 June 2017; pp. 1–6. [CrossRef]
36. Parker, J.; Yates, A.; Goharian, N.; Frieder, O. Health-related hypothesis generation using social media data. *Soc. Netw. Anal. Min.* **2015**, *5*, 1–15. [CrossRef]
37. Bian, J.; Topaloglu, U.; Yu, F. Towards large-scale twitter mining for drug-related adverse events. In Proceedings of the 2012 International Workshop on Smart Health and Wellbeing—SHB '12, Maui, HI, USA, 29 October 2012; p. 25. [CrossRef]
38. Lamb, A.; Paul, M.J.; Dredze, M. Separating fact from fear: Tracking flu infections on Twitter. In Proceedings of the 2013 Conference of the North American Chapter of the Association for Computational Linguistics: Human Language Technologies, Atlanta, GA, USA, 9–14 June 2013; pp. 789–795.
39. Aramaki, E. Twitter Catches The Flu: Detecting Influenza Epidemics using Twitter. In Proceedings of the 2011 Conference on Empirical Methods in Natural Language Processing, EMNLP 2011, Edinburgh, UK, 27–31 July 2011.
40. Wakamiya, S.; Kawai, Y.; Aramaki, E. Twitter-based influenza detection after flu peak via tweets with indirect information: Text mining study. *J. Med. Internet Res.* **2018**, *20*. [CrossRef] [PubMed]
41. Wakamiya, S.; Morita, M.; Kano, Y.; Ohkuma, T.; Aramaki, E. Tweet Classification Toward Twitter-Based Disease Surveillance: New Data, Methods, and Evaluations. *J. Med. Internet Res.* **2019**, *21*, e12783. [CrossRef] [PubMed]
42. Singh, L.; Bansal, S.; Bode, L.; Budak, C.; Chi, G.; Kawintiranon, K.; Padden, C.; Vanarsdall, R.; Vraga, E.; Wang, Y. A first look at COVID-19 information and misinformation sharing on Twitter. *arXiv* **2020**, arXiv:2003.13907.
43. Gencoglu, O. Large-scale, Language-agnostic Discourse Classification of Tweets During COVID-19. *Learn. Knowl. Extr.* **2020**, *2*, 603–616. [CrossRef]
44. Li, X.; Zhou, M.; Wu, J.; Yuan, A.; Wu, F.; Li, J. Analyzing COVID-19 on Online Social Media: Trends, Sentiments and Emotions. *arXiv* **2020**, arXiv:2005.14464.
45. Sri, V.; Venigalla, M.; Vagavolu, D.; Chimalakonda, S. Mood of India During Covid-19—An Interactive Web Portal Based on Emotion Analysis of Twitter Data. *arXiv* **2020**, arXiv:2005.02955.
46. Ziems, C.; He, B.; Soni, S.; Kumar, S. Racism is a Virus: Anti-Asian Hate and Counterhate in Social Media during the COVID-19 Crisis. *arXiv* **2020**, arXiv:2005.12423.
47. Marli, F.; de Andrade, R.; Lu, Y. Twitter in Brazil: Discourses on China in Times of Coronavirus. Available online: https://ssrn.com/abstract=3608566 (accessed on 1 January 2021).
48. Medford, R.J.; Saleh, S.N.; Sumarsono, A.; Perl, T.M.; Lehmann, C.U. An 'Infodemic': Leveraging High-Volume Twitter Data to Understand Public Sentiment for the COVID-19 Outbreak. Available online: https://www.medrxiv.org/content/10.1101/2020.04.03.20052936v1 (accessed on 1 January 2021).
49. Kouzy, R.; Abi Jaoude, J.; Kraitem, A.; El Alam, M.B.; Karam, B.; Adib, E.; Zarka, J.; Traboulsi, C.; Akl, E.W.; Baddour, K. Coronavirus Goes Viral: Quantifying the COVID-19 Misinformation Epidemic on Twitter Data collection. *Cureus* **2020**, *12*. [CrossRef]
50. Yang, K.; Torres-lugo, C.; Menczer, F. Prevalence of Low-Credibility Information on Twitter During the COVID-19 Outbreak. *arXiv* **2020**, arXiv:2004.14484.
51. Memon, S.A.; Carley, K.M. Characterizing COVID-19 Misinformation Communities Using a Novel Twitter Dataset. 2020. Available online: https://arxiv.org/abs/2008.00791 (accessed on 1 January 2021).
52. Ferrara, E. What Types of COVID-19 Conspiracies are Populated by Twitter Bots? 2020. Available online: https://arxiv.org/abs/2004.09531 (accessed on 1 January 2021).
53. Gencoglu, O.; Gruber, M. Causal Modeling of Twitter Activity During COVID-19. *arXiv* **2020**, arXiv:2005.07952.
54. Budhwani, H.; Sun, R. Creating COVID-19 Stigma by Referencing the Novel Coronavirus as the 'Chinese virus' on Twitter: Quantitative Analysis of Social Media Data Corresponding Author. *J. Med. Internet Res.* **2020**, *22*, 1–7. [CrossRef] [PubMed]
55. Liu, Q.; Zheng, Z.; Zheng, J.; Chen, Q.; Liu, G. Health Communication Through News Media During the Early Stage of the COVID-19 Outbreak in China: Digital Topic Modeling Approach Corresponding Author. *J. Med. Internet Res.* **2020**, *22*, 1–12. [CrossRef]

56. Prabhakar Kaila, D.; Prasad, D.A. Informational Flow on Twitter—Corona Virus Outbreak—Topic. *Int. J. Adv. Res. Eng. Technol.* **2020**, *11*, 128–134.
57. Abd-alrazaq, A.; Alhuwail, D.; Househ, M.; Hamdi, M.; Shah, Z. Top Concerns of Tweeters During the COVID-19 Pandemic: Infoveillance Study Corresponding Author. *J. Med. Internet Res.* **2020**, *22*, 1–9. [CrossRef] [PubMed]
58. Med, J.G.I. Public Priorities and Concerns Regarding COVID-19 in an Online Discussion Forum: Longitudinal Topic Modeling. *J. Gen. Intern. Med.* **2020**. [CrossRef]
59. Ordun, C.; Hamilton, B.A.; Raff, E.; Hamilton, B.A. Exploratory Analysis of Covid-19 Tweets using Topic Modeling, UMAP, and DiGraphs. *arXiv* **2020**, arXiv:2005.03082.
60. Mackey, T.; Purushothaman, V.; Li, J.; Shah, N.; Nali, M.; Bardier, C.; Liang, B.; Cai, M.; Cuomo, R. Machine Learning to Detect Self-Reporting of Symptoms, Testing Access, and Recovery Associated With COVID-19 on Twitter: Retrospective Big Data Infoveillance Study. *JMIR Public Health Surveill.* **2020**, *6*, e19509. [CrossRef]
61. Li, D.; Chaudhary, H.; Zhang, Z. Modeling spatiotemporal pattern of depressive symptoms caused by COVID-19 using social media data mining. *Int. J. Environ. Res. Public Health* **2020**, *17*, 4988. [CrossRef]
62. Alam, F.; Shaar, S.; Nikolov, A.; Mubarak, H.; Martino, G.D.S.; Abdelali, A.; Dalvi, F.; Durrani, N.; Sajjad, H.; Darwish, K. Fighting the COVID-19 Infodemic: Modeling the Perspective of Journalists, Fact-Checkers, Social Media Platforms, Policy Makers, and the Society. *arXiv* **2020**, arXiv:2005.00033.
63. Alshaabi, T.; Minot, J.R.; Arnold, M.V.; Adams, J.L.; Dewhurst, D.R.; Reagan, A.J.; Muhamad, R.; Danforth, C.M.; Dodds, P.S. How the world's collective attention is being paid to a pandemic: COVID-19 related 1-gram time series for 24 languages on Twitter. *arXiv* **2020**, arXiv:2003.12614.
64. Alsudias, L.; Rayson, P. COVID-19 and Arabic Twitter: How can Arab World Governments and Public Health Organizations Learn from Social Media? In Proceedings of the 1st Workshop on NLP for COVID-19 at ACL 2020, Seattle, WA, USA, 9–10 July 2020.
65. Diab, M.; Ghoneim, M.; Habash, N. Arabic Diacritization in the Context of Statistical Machine Translation. In Proceedings of the Eleventh Machine Translation Summit (MT-Summit XI), Copenhagen, Denmark, 10–14 September 2007.
66. Blei, D.M.; Edu, B.B.; Ng, A.Y.; Edu, A.S.; Jordan, M.I.; Edu, J.B. Latent Dirichlet Allocation. *J. Mach. Learn. Res.* **2003**, *3*, 993–1022. [CrossRef]
67. Tweet Objects. Available online: https://developer.twitter.com/en/docs/tweets/data-dictionary/overview/intro-to-tweet-json (accessed on 1 January 2021).
68. 24-Hour Curfew in Mecca and Medina. Available online: https://www.skynewsarabia.com/middle-east/1333463-%D9%85%D9%86%D8%B9-%D8%A7%D9%84%D8%AA%D8%AC%D9%88%D9%84-%20%D9%85%D9%83%D8%A9-%D9%88%D8%A7%D9%84%D9%85%D8%AF%D9%8A%D9%86%D8%A9-%D9%85%D8%AF%D8%A7%D8%B1-24-%D8%B3%D8%A7%D8%B9%D8%A9 (accessed on 1 January 2021).
69. Althumairi, A. 'Governmental Communication' Launches the Visual Identity of the 'We are All Responsible' Initiative to Confront 'Covid 19'. Available online: https://www.aleqt.com/2020/03/21/article_1785661.html (accessed on 1 January 2021).
70. WAS, S.P.A. General/Custodian of the Two Holy Mosques Issues a Curfew Order to Limit the Spread of the New Corona Virus Starting from 7 pm until Six in the Morning for 21 days from the Evening of Monday 28 Rajab 23 March. Available online: https://www.spa.gov.sa/2050399 (accessed on 1 January 2021).
71. The Minister of Health: The Custodian of the Two Holy Mosques Orders the Treatment of all (Corona) Patients Free of Charge. Ministry of Health. Available online: https://www.moh.gov.sa/Ministry/MediaCenter/News/Pages/News-2020-03-30-005.aspx (accessed on 1 January 2021).
72. Allow Prayer to be Held in Mosques. «Interior»: The Return of Normal Life in all Regions Except Mecca. Available online: https://www.okaz.com.sa/news/local/2025741 (accessed on 1 January 2021).
73. Corona . . . This is How the Streets of Saudi Arabia Appeared in the First Days of the Curfew. Available online: https://www.aljazeera.net/news/politics/2020/3/24/%D8%A7%D9%84%D8%B3%D8%B9%D9%88%D8%AF%D9%8A%D8%A9-%D8%AD%D8%B8%D8%B1-%D8%A7%D9%84%D8%AA%D8%AC%D9%88%D9%84-%D9%83%D9%88%D8%B1%D9%88%D9%86%D8%A7-%D8%A7%D9%84%D8%AD%D8%B1%D8%B3 (accessed on 1 January 2021).
74. Alnajar, S. Umloj Blood Bank: Corona Reduced the Number of Donors. Available online: https://www.okaz.com.sa/news/local/2018263 (accessed on 1 January 2021).
75. Alqarni, A. 'Iradat Riyadh' Donates Blood to 'Specialist' Patients. Available online: https://www.okaz.com.sa/news/local/2018828 (accessed on 1 January 2021).
76. Alsaeid, A. 'Health': 119 New Cases of 'Corona Case' . . . and the Total is 511. 2020. Available online: https://www.okaz.com.sa/news/local/2016269 (accessed on 1 January 2021).
77. COVID-19 Cases on 30 March 2020. Available online: https://twitter.com/SaudiMOH/status/1244609485563461633 (accessed on 1 January 2021).
78. Usman, S.; Mehmood, R.; Katib, I.; Albeshri, A.; Altowaijri, S.M. ZAKI: A Smart Method and Tool for Automatic Performance Optimization of Parallel SpMV Computations on Distributed Memory Machines. *Mob. Netw. Appl.* **2019**. [CrossRef]
79. Usman, S.; Mehmood, R.; Katib, I.; Albeshri, A. ZAKI+: A Machine Learning Based Process Mapping Tool for SpMV Computations on Distributed Memory Architectures. *IEEE Access* **2019**, *7*, 81279–81296. [CrossRef]

Article

Enhanced Sentinel Surveillance System for COVID-19 Outbreak Prediction in a Large European Dialysis Clinics Network

Francesco Bellocchio [1], Paola Carioni [1], Caterina Lonati [2], Mario Garbelli [1], Francisco Martínez-Martínez [3], Stefano Stuard [4] and Luca Neri [1,*,†]

[1] Fresenius Medical Care Italia SpA, Palazzo Pignano, 26020 Lombardia, Italy; francesco.bellocchio@fmc-ag.com (F.B.); paola.carioni@fmc-ag.com (P.C.); mario.garbelli@fmc-ag.com (M.G.)
[2] Center for Preclinical Research, Fondazione IRCCS Ca' Granda Ospedale Maggiore Policlinico, 20122 Milan, Italy; caterina.lonati@gmail.com
[3] Santa Barbara Smart Health S. L., Parc Cientific Universitat id Valencia, Carrer del Catedràtic Agustín Escardino Benlloch, 9, 46980 Paterna, Spain; francisco.martinezmartinez@fmc-ag.com
[4] Fresenius Medical Care Deutschland GmbH, 61352 Bad Homburg, Germany; Stefano.stuard@fmc-ag.com
* Correspondence: luca.neri@fmc-ag.com; Tel.: +39-037-327-7579 or +39-345-391-5542
† Current address: Clinical & Data Intelligence Systems—Advanced Analytics, Fresenius Medical Care Deutschland GmbH, Via Papa Giovanni Paolo II, 41, 26020 Vaiano Cremasco, Italy.

Abstract: Accurate predictions of COVID-19 epidemic dynamics may enable timely organizational interventions in high-risk regions. We exploited the interconnection of the Fresenius Medical Care (FMC) European dialysis clinic network to develop a sentinel surveillance system for outbreak prediction. We developed an artificial intelligence-based model considering the information related to all clinics belonging to the European Nephrocare Network. The prediction tool provides risk scores of the occurrence of a COVID-19 outbreak in each dialysis center within a 2-week forecasting horizon. The model input variables include information related to the epidemic status and trends in clinical practice patterns of the target clinic, regional epidemic metrics, and the distance-weighted risk estimates of adjacent dialysis units. On the validation dates, there were 30 (5.09%), 39 (6.52%), and 218 (36.03%) clinics with two or more patients with COVID-19 infection during the 2-week prediction window. The performance of the model was suitable in all testing windows: AUC = 0.77, 0.80, and 0.81, respectively. The occurrence of new cases in a clinic propagates distance-weighted risk estimates to proximal dialysis units. Our machine learning sentinel surveillance system may allow for a prompt risk assessment and timely response to COVID-19 surges throughout networked European clinics.

Keywords: SARS-CoV-2; COVID-19; sentinel surveillance system; outbreak prediction; machine learning; artificial intelligence

1. Introduction

Due to its unique characteristics, the Severe Acute Respiratory Syndrome Coronavirus 2 (SARS-CoV-2) pandemic has posed unprecedented challenges to clinics providing life-saving services to patients suffering from chronic illnesses, including chronic kidney disease (CKD). In fact, non-specific clinical manifestations of Coronavirus disease 2019 (COVID-19) [1] as well as the viral transmission from asymptomatic or pre-symptomatic individuals [2–4] make the early recognition of newly infected cases extremely difficult. Moreover, the occurrence of superspreading events (SSEV), during which few individuals are able to infect many people [5], hampers infection control measures [6,7].

Social distancing, preventive quarantine, and the isolation of infected subjects still represents the most effective means to reduce the risk of SARS-CoV-2 human-to-human transmission [8,9]. However, patients with end-stage kidney disease (ESKD) need to undergo in-center dialysis three times per week for 4 h per session, which makes physical distancing more difficult to achieve due to repeated, prolonged interactions with other patients and healthcare staff [10–13]. Unfortunately, ESKD individuals also show a higher risk of complications following SARS-CoV-2 infection due to weakened immune response [14–17] and to the occurrence of many of the risk factors commonly associated with development of severe COVID-19 [18,19], including older age and comorbidities [20,21]. Moreover, because of compromised host immunity, a vaccine may not exhibit the same efficacy on hemodialysis patients as it does in immunocompetent individuals [13].

Therefore, the reduction of the contagion risk within dialysis clinics while preserving clinical operations is a key challenge for healthcare systems during this pandemic. To help anticipate local epidemic dynamics and adjust non-pharmacological interventions to the changing background of infection risk, we sought to develop an advanced sentinel surveillance system supported by a machine learning (ML) prediction model, where the occurrence of COVID-19 cases in a clinic propagates distance-weighted risk estimates to adjacent dialysis units. The present study describes the derivation and validation of the prediction model, as well as the strategies adopted to monitor its performance throughout the pandemic period.

2. Materials and Methods

2.1. Design and Setting

All dialysis clinics belonging to the Fresenius Medical Care (FMC) European Nephrocare Network confer clinical data to a centralized data-repository, namely the European Clinical Database (EuCliD®, Fresenius Medical Care, Deutschland GmbH, Vaiano Cremasco, Italy) [22,23]. Since April 2020, all SARS-CoV-2 infections (suspected and confirmed cases as well as initial symptoms), diagnostic procedures, and clinical endpoints are reported in the treatment incident report (TIR) module in EuCliD®. We used aggregated data abstracted from the TIR, open source data describing epidemic dynamics in European countries, as well as aggregated data on biochemical assays prescriptions and results to estimate outbreak risk in dialysis clinics belonging to the FMC European Nephrocare Network.

2.2. Outcome Variable

The model forecasts the risk of a COVID-19 outbreak in each dialysis clinic in a 2-week horizon. Clinic outbreak is defined as the occurrence of two or more COVID-19-confirmed cases in a given clinic. Therefore, for each clinic registered in the Nephrocare network, the model estimates the probability of COVID-19 outbreak (2 or more PCR confirmed cases within a 2-week horizon) as a function of a vector of input variables. Study design is represented in Figure 1.

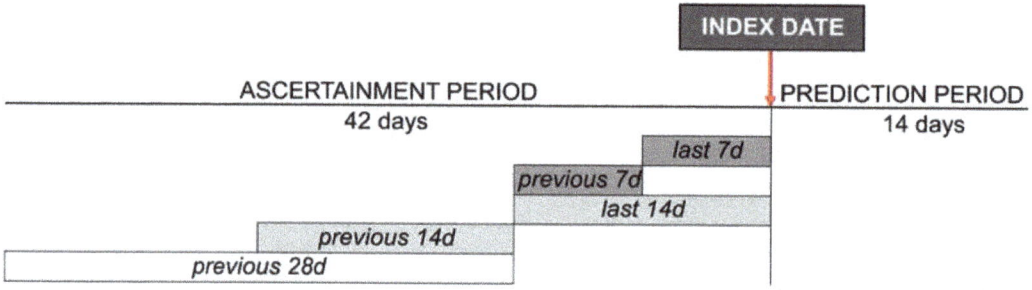

Figure 1. Study design: Reference timeframe for data collection/calculation is shown.

For illustrative purposes, we established 3 risk categories: (1) low (L), when outbreak risk is less than or equal to 1.5%; (2) medium (M), risk greater than 1.5% and less than or equal to 12.5%; (3) high (H), if risk is greater than 12.5%. For this purpose, the action threshold defining the low risk class has been chosen to select a subpopulation of clinics where the risk of outbreak is very small so that non-pharmacological interventions to prevent the spread of COVID-19 can be temporarily and partially mitigated. In this context, a costly error would be to assign to the Low Risk class a clinic which will experience an outbreak in the following two weeks. Such threshold would be useful when a sufficiently large share of clinics (i.e., P(Class = L)) could be found, so that P(Class = L | Outbreak = No) is high and P(Outbreak = Yes | Class = L) is, conversely, very small. On the other hand of the spectrum, we selected a more specific action threshold, which defines a High-Risk Class of clinics. In this risk group, additional non-pharmacological intervention should be initiated including, for example, the formal testing of temperature and thorough physical examination administered to each patient before entering the clinic or even periodical screening test (i.e., once-weekly). Since the intervention would require intensive resources, may be constraint by procurement difficulties, and would unduly overburden patients with unnecessary testing, the High Risk threshold should ideally define a group where P(Outbreak = Yes | Class = H) is high and both P(Class = H | Outbreak = No) and P(Outbreak = Yes | Class $\neq$ H) are low. It is important to remark that the choice and number of the action thresholds depends on the intended use of the risk score, the set of interventions available to the organization, the price cost of each intervention, and ultimately by the value function ranking the desirability/undesirability of different health outcomes. Therefore, the thresholds presented in this paper should not be considered generalizable per se: different institutions may choose different thresholds (or no thresholds at all) depending on the availability, cost, and expected outcomes of COVID-19-related interventions (i.e., email alerts to medical directors, shipments of medical equipment such as face masks or diagnostics kits, delivery of health education modules, PCR screening, etc.,). Therefore, the problem is not diagnostic in nature, yet reduces to optimal ranking (and longitudinal stability of such ranking of risk) in order to efficiently allocate limited resources and minimize risk for the patients throughout a continuously changing epidemic landscape.

2.3. Input Variables

The model is computed using aggregated data provided by all the dialysis centers (min: 545; max: 611) located in one of the 23 countries of the FMC European Nephrocare Network. The final model incorporates 74 variables belonging to one of the following categories (Appendix A):

1. Open Source Data [24];
2. Epidemic status in the clinical country/region (prefix: RG): 15 parameters;
3. Aggregated Data abstracted from EuCLiD®:
   a. Epidemic status in the target clinic (prefix: CL): 5 variables;
   b. Distance-weighted information of the adjacent clinics (prefix: CLS); 5 variables. Adjacent clinics were defined as the 3 centers with shorter distance in terms of both latitude and longitude to the target clinic. Measures of the adjacent clinics, including cases and trends, were computed as the average value weighted for the inverse of the distance to the target clinic;
   c. Other parameters related to the target clinic (prefix: CL): 49 parameters.

As detailed in Appendix A, each variable can be calculated/collected over different timeframes of the ascertainment period, i.e., the last 7 days (d), previous 7 d, last 14 d, previous 14 d, and previous 28 d.

2.4. Statistical Analysis

2.4.1. Model Derivation

We used XG Boost, a scalable ML system for tree boosting [25]. We used the available open source package [26] for Python, Version 3.7.4 (Python Software Foundation, Delaware, DE, United States) [27].

The first release of the model was trained using data related to 1st April 2020 (training dataset index date), while the second and the third versions were derived using data related to 15th July 2020 and 1st November 2020, respectively. We considered all the clinics delivering services to at least one patient on the index date as well as over the week before index date.

2.4.2. Model Accuracy and Feature Importance

Prediction accuracy of each release was tested every first and fifteenth day (validation dataset index dates). Therefore, development and validation datasets can include the same set of clinics/patients every two weeks.

To evaluate model performance, we measured the area under the curve (AUC) of the receiver operating characteristics (ROC) curve in the testing datasets [28] using Python, Version 3.7.4 (Python Software Foundation, Delaware, DE, United States) [27]. The AUC provides an aggregate measure of performance as the ROC curve plots the true positive rate (TPR) against the false positive rate (FPR) at all classification thresholds. Model discrimination ability over time was monitored by visual inspection of AUC trends. For illustrative purposes, we also reported the classification performance in terms of P(Outbreak | Class) (i.e., probability of outbreak (Yes/No) given the assigned risk class (L/M/H)) and P(Class | Outbreak) (i.e., probability of the assigned risk class given the outbreak) for the two action-thresholds chosen (0.015 and 0.125). In order to calculate P(Outbreak | Class) and P(Class | Outbreak) we artificially treated our problem as a binary decision for each threshold. We computed average probability values across the whole study period.

Feature importance was computed using the SHapley Additive exPlanations (SHAP) method [29]. This analysis enables intuitive model explainability via an accurate and efficient estimation of the contribution to risk of each input variable.

2.4.3. Descriptive Statistics

For both the training and validation datasets, we analyzed the number of active clinics, frequency and incidence of a COVID-19 outbreak, the distribution of clinics in each prediction level of risk (low, medium, high), as well as the relative risk compared to clinics in low-risk groups with Python, Version 3.7.4.

3. Results

3.1. Dialysis Clinic Characteristics

Model version 1, 2, and 3 were trained using a dataset related to 1st April 2020, 15th July 2020, and 1st November 2020, respectively. On these dates, active clinics were 589, 597, 603, while 34 (5.77%), 44 (7.37%), and 233 (38.64%) clinics had two or more patients with COVID-19 infection in the fortnight after the index date.

The surveillance system stratifies clinics by their risk of new local outbreak within two weeks. To facilitate the interpretation of the results, we established three risk categories: (1) Low, when outbreak risk is less than or equal to 1.5%; (2) Medium, risk greater than 1.5% and less than or equal to 12.5%; (3) High, if risk is greater than 12.5%. Risk thresholds depend both on the incidence of pandemic and on the ability of any given clinic to implement containment measures. Figure 2 reports the share of active dialysis clinics in different risk classes at each testing date.

The actual outbreak incidence in the dialysis clinics during the validation period is reported in Figure 3.

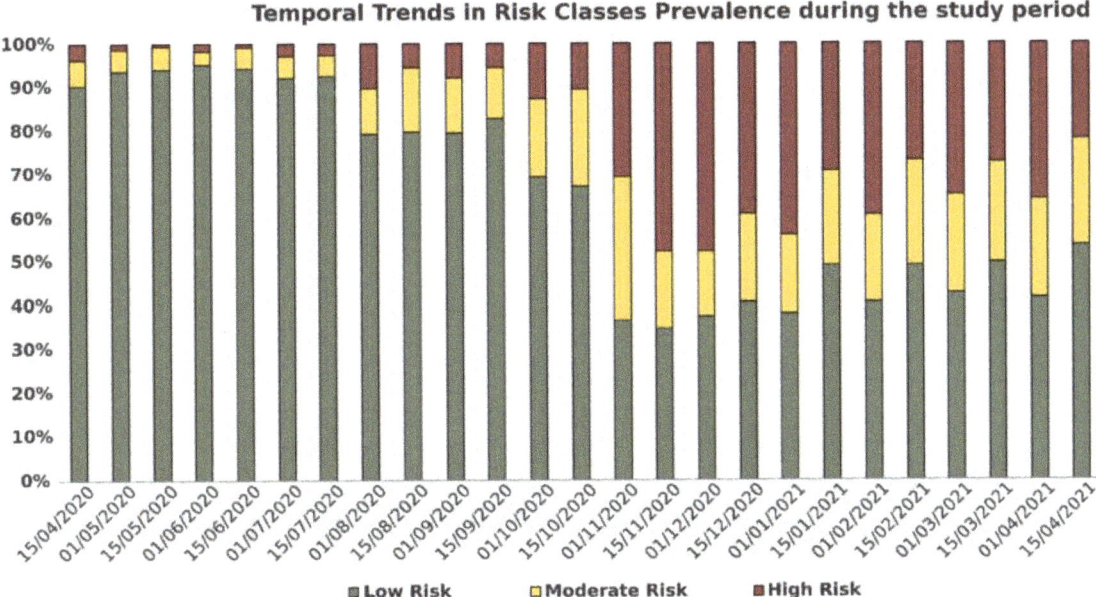

Figure 2. Number of dialysis clinics at the validation dates. Colors denote risk categories: Red, high > 12.5%; Yellow, medium 1.5% < x ≤ 12.5%; Green, low ≤ 1.5%.

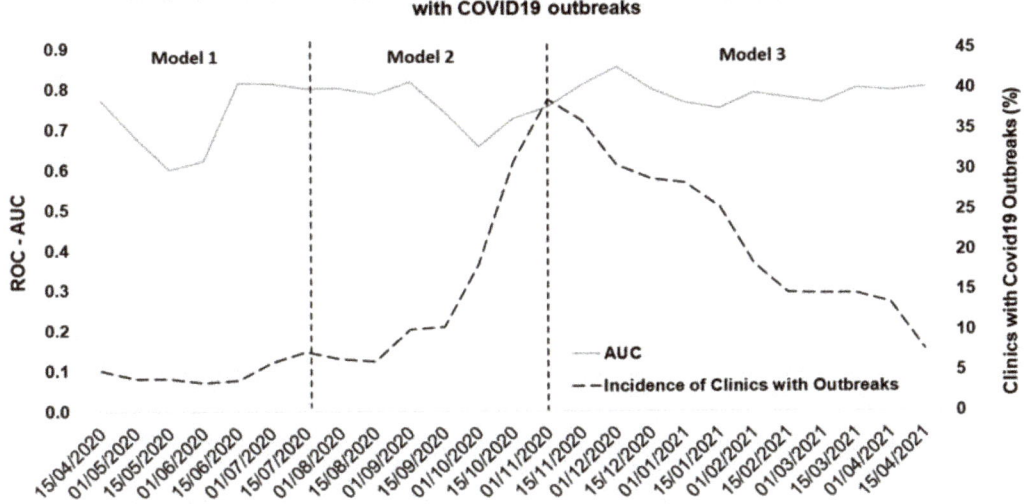

Figure 3. Model Performance and Incidence of Clinics with Outbreaks: the plot reports data related to the 1 year observation period.

3.2. Model Performance

All versions of the model showed a good performance over the validation period. Figure 3 shows trends in AUC values of the three model versions over a 1-year observation period. Variability in prediction accuracy decreased as retraining was applied: version 1's average AUC was 0.73 (95% CI 0.55–0.91), AUC of version 2 was 0.75 (95% CI 0.65–0.86), while version 3 had a more stable performance with an average AUC of 0.79 (0.74–0.85). The ROC-AUC diagram for the three model versions have been reported in Figure 4.

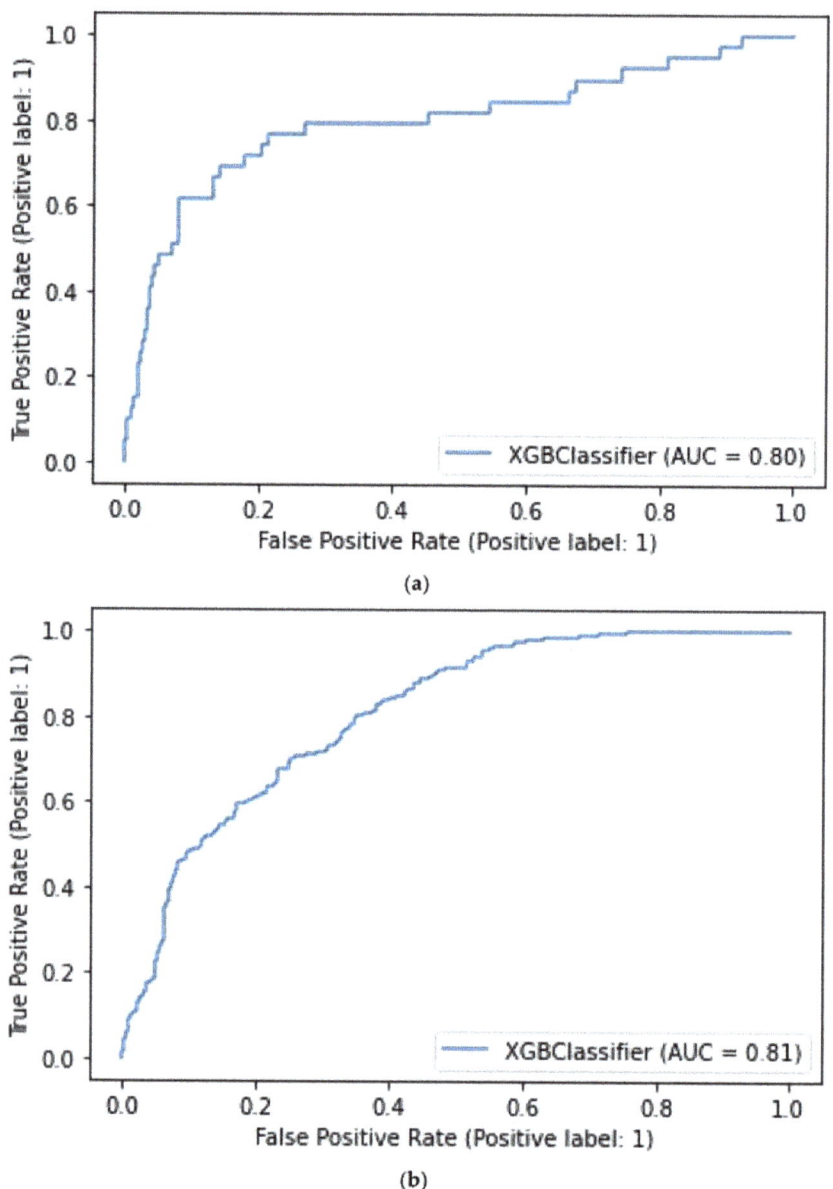

Figure 4. Cont.

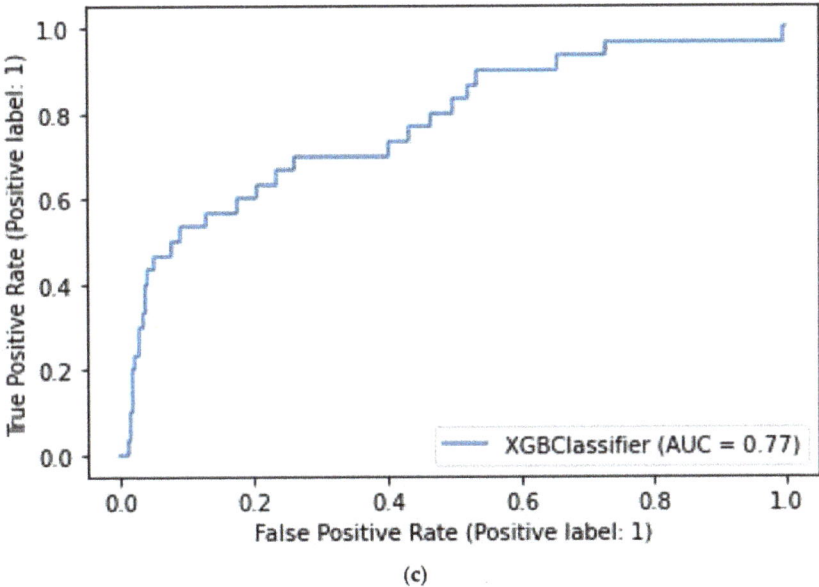

(c)

Figure 4. Panel (**a**–**c**) respectively contain the ROC-AUC plot related to Model 1, Model 2, and Model 3 evaluated on the following dates: 15 April 2020, 1 August 2020, and 15 November 2020.

In order to demonstrate the potential use of the model, we geographically mapped the risk on a few exemplary dates, i.e., the 2 August 2020, 4 October 2020, 1 November 2020, and 3 January 2020 (Figure 5). The graphical representation visually highlights clinic clusters according to the risk of a COVID-19 outbreak occurrence within 2 weeks (Figure 5, left panels, colored circles denote the low, medium, and high-risk categories). There was substantial correlation between the predicted risk (Figure 5, left panels) and the actual outcome (Figure 5, right panels) on all of the validation dates.

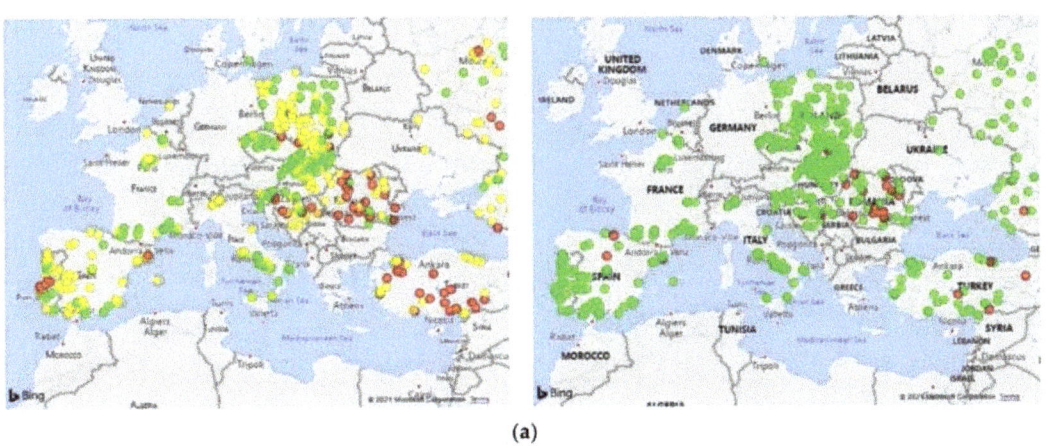

(a)

Figure 5. *Cont.*

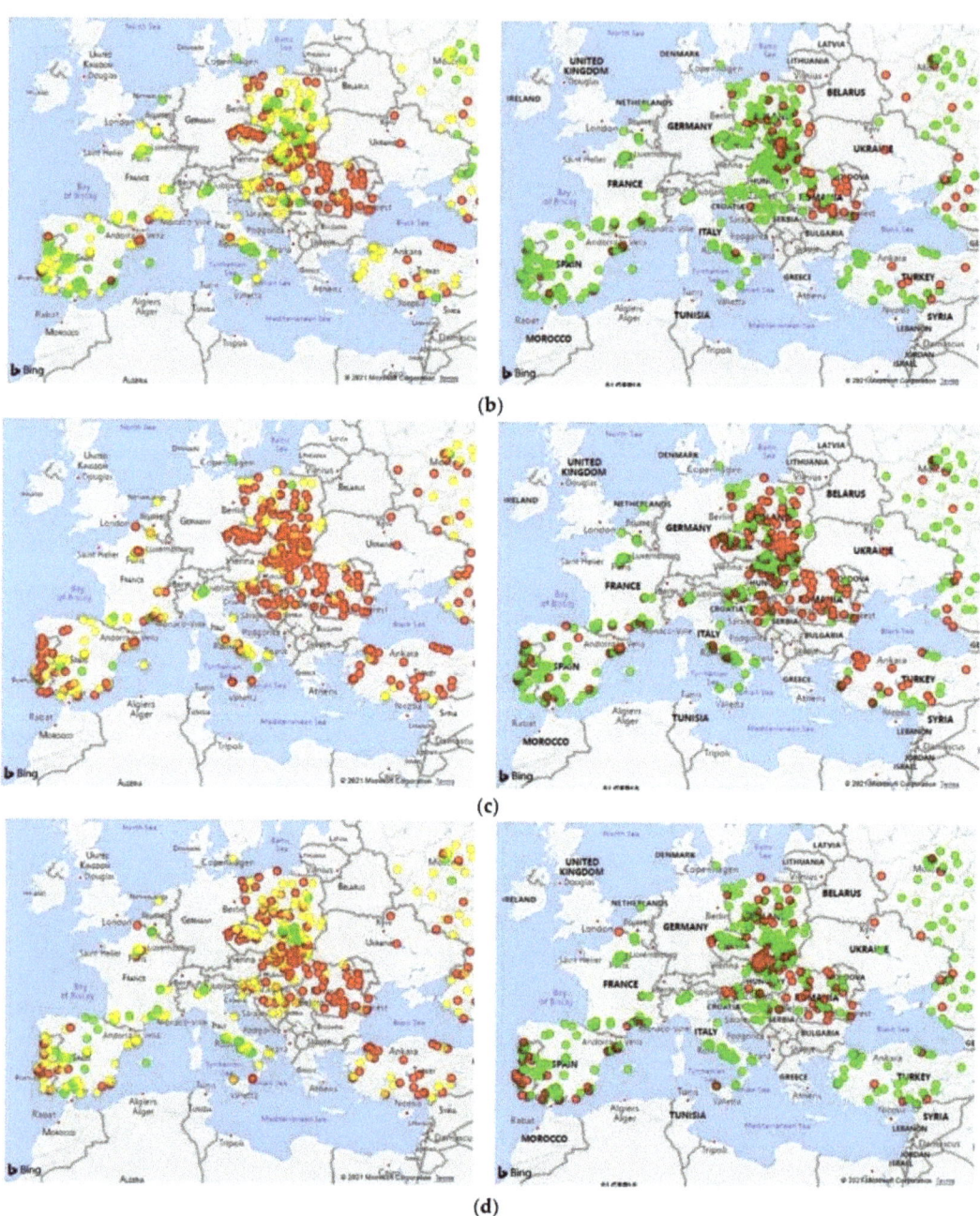

Figure 5. COVID-19 outbreak risk mapping in European clinics of the Nephrocare network. Geographical risk maps were built considering epidemic data related to the following exemplary dates: (**a**) 2 August 2020, (**b**) 4 October 2020, (**c**) 1 November 2020, and (**d**) 3 January 2020. Panels on the left show clinic clusters according to the risk of a COVID-19 outbreak occurrence within 2 weeks: Red circles: risk > 12.5%; Yellow, 1.5% < risk ≤ 12.5%; Green, risk ≤ 1.5%. Panels on the right report the actual incidence of COVID-19 outbreaks in the forecasting period.

Tables 1 and 2 report the classification performance in terms of P(Outbreak | Class) (i.e., probability of outbreak (Yes/No) given the assigned risk class (L/M/H)) and P(Class | Outbreak) (i.e., probability of the assigned risk class given the outbreak) for the two action-thresholds chosen (0.015 and 0.125). In order to calculate P(Outbreak | Class) and P(Class | Outbreak), we artificially treated our problem as a binary decision for each threshold. We computed average probability values across the whole study period.

Table 1. Average classification performance in terms of P(Outbreak | Class) (i.e., probability of outbreak (Yes/No) given the assigned risk class, L) and P(Class | Outbreak) (i.e., probability of the assigned risk class given the outbreak) at the low action-thresholds (predicted risk = 0.015).

Low Risk Group. P(Class = L) = 0.648			
P(Class = L | Outbreak = Yes) 0.23	P(Class ≠ L | Outbreak = Yes) 0.77	P(Class = L | Outbreak = No) 0.73	P(Class ≠ L | Outbreak = No) 0.27
P(Outbreak = Yes | Class = L) 0.06	P(Outbreak = No | Class = L) 0.94	P(Outbreak = Yes | Class ≠ L) 0.37	P(Outbreak = No | Class ≠ L) 0.63

Table 2. Average classification performance in terms of P(Outbreak | Class) (i.e., probability of outbreak (Yes/No) given the assigned risk class, H) and P(Class | Outbreak) (i.e., probability of the assigned risk class given the outbreak) at the high action-thresholds (predicted risk = 0.125).

High Risk Group P(Class = H) = 0.197			
P(Class = H | Outbreak = Yes) 0.51	P(Class ≠ H | Outbreak = Yes) 0.49	P(Class = H | Outbreak = No) 0.14	P(Class ≠ H | Outbreak = No) 0.86
P(Outbreak = Yes | Class = H) 0.40	P(Outbreak = No | Class = H) 0.60	P(Outbreak = Yes | Class ≠ H) 0.09	P(Outbreak = No | Class ≠ H) 0.91

Overall, the risk score was strongly associated with the likelihood of COVID-19 outbreak, as demonstrated by the relative risk of outcome occurrence in the three risk classes over the study period (Table 3).

Table 3. Average classification performance in terms of relative risk of COVID-19 outbreak by risk class. The relative risk is calculated as $RR = \frac{P(Outbreak=Yes|Class)}{P(Outbreak=Yes|Class=L)}$.

Risk Class	RR
L	−ref
M	3.45
H	5.95

3.3. Model Feature Importance

Feature analysis investigated the impact of each variable on model output (Figure 6). Although there are some differences among the model versions, overall, the most important variables are related to the epidemic dynamics in the clinic in the period immediately preceding the index date for risk evaluation. Regional data on the number of COVID-19 cases and deaths were likewise ranked high. The number of COVID-19 cases in adjacent clinics resulted in the top predictor list of all three model versions. Of note, variables routinely measured in clinical practice, including changes in CRP and blood white cell count over the observation period, were also strongly associated with outbreak risk.

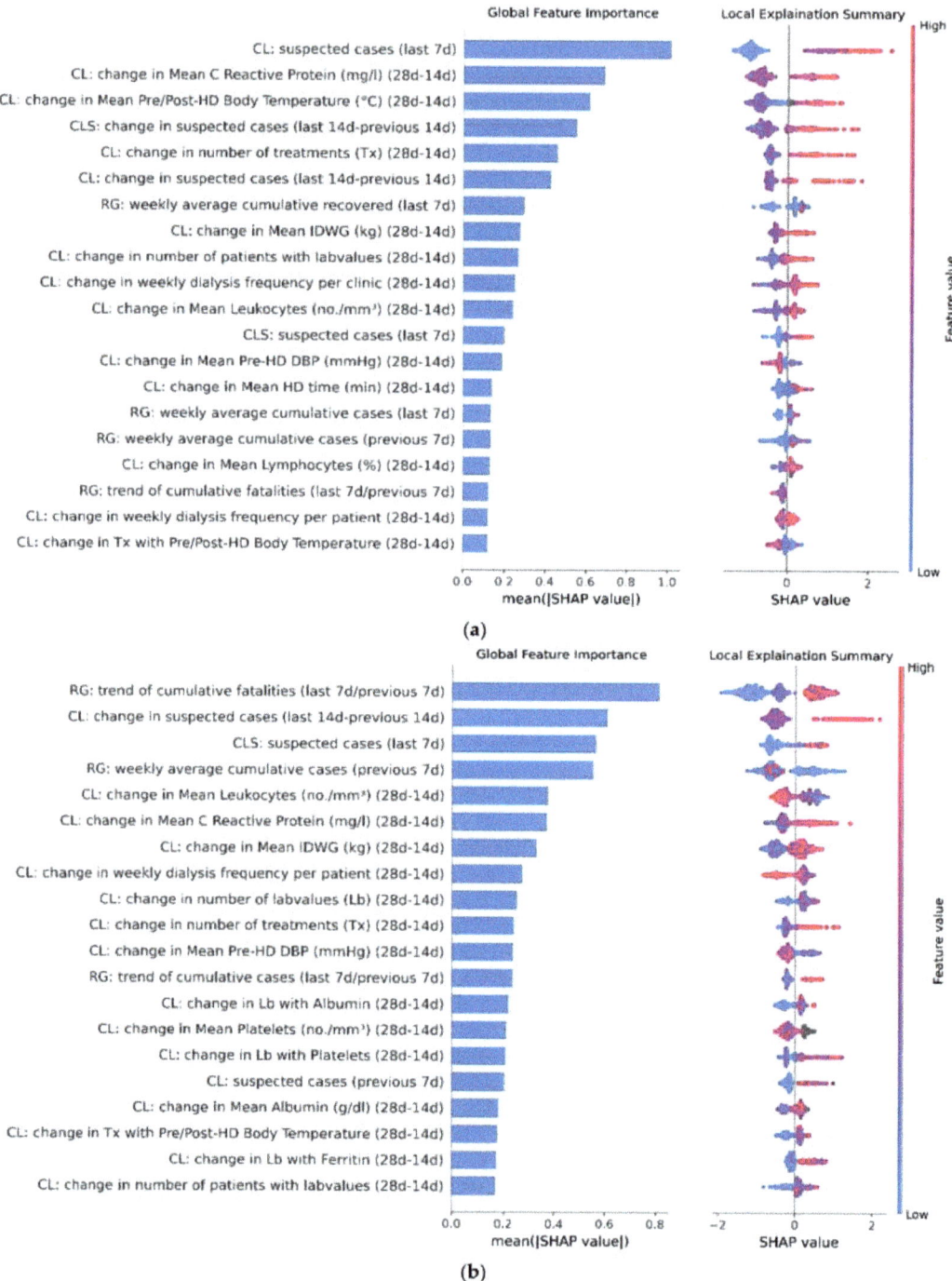

Figure 6. *Cont.*

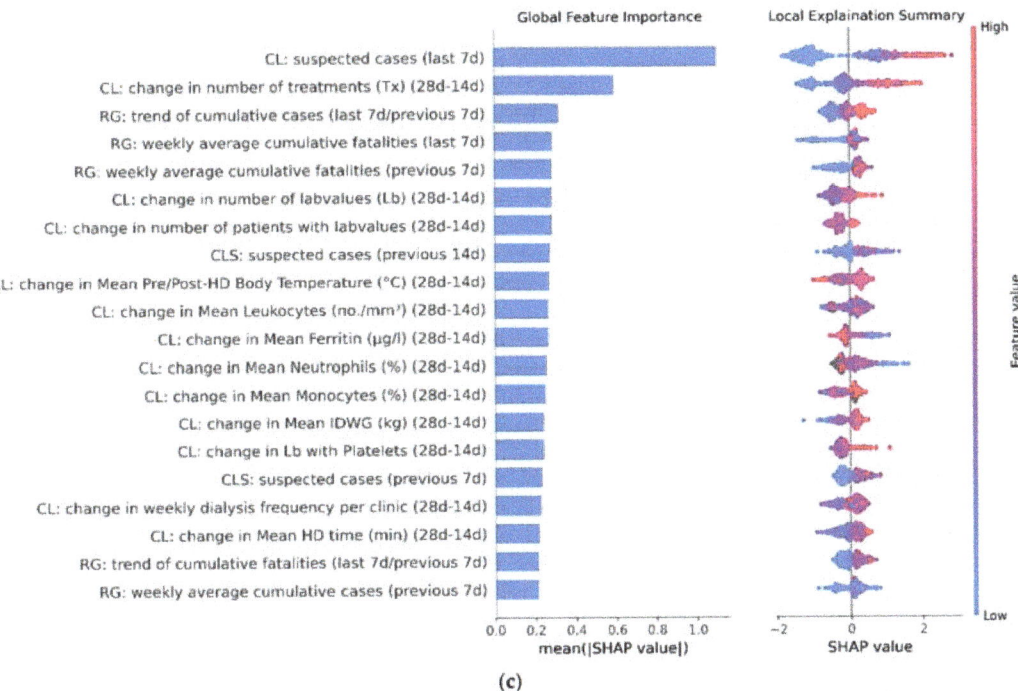

(c)

Figure 6. Panel (a–c) respectively contain the Shapley additive explanations (SHAP) related to Model 1, Model 2, and Model 3 evaluated on the following dates: 15 April 2020, 1 August 2020, and 15 November 2020. SHAP plots show relative feature importance. The blue bar represents overall SHAP values for each variable and are interpreted as relative importance of each variable to risk estimates. On the right side, SHAP values show the direction of association between predictor and risk estimates. Each dot represents one individual clinic from the test dataset. Higher values of the predictors are represented in red color; lower values of the predictors are represented in blue color. The X axis represents the impact of variables on risk in terms of SHAP values. Red color in correspondence with positive values suggests direct correlations between risk factors and the occurrence of COVID-19 outbreak, while red color in the region of negative SHAP values suggests inverse correlation.

4. Discussion

The present study describes the development and validation of a novel sentinel surveillance system allowing for the prompt risk assessment of a COVID-19 outbreak in a large European network of dialysis clinics over a 2-week forecasting horizon. The model had a stable accuracy over time and was able to consistently discriminate outbreak risk in dialysis units across all European countries at every stage of the current pandemic, i.e., during epidemic growth and decay phases. The design of our ML prediction model enables administrators and developers to quickly retrain this tool in case the visual inspection of AUC values over time suggests a trend toward a decrease in its discrimination ability.

Nosocomial transmission has greatly contributed to an increase in the global burden of COVID-19 pandemic by extremely affecting the capacity of the health system, not only to provide medical support to patients, but also to protect healthcare professionals [30,31]. Dialysis centers are particularly vulnerable to outbreak development [11,12,32] in that mitigation strategies are not entirely feasible due to the necessity of in-person encounters to provide a life-saving treatment such as hemodialysis [11]. Considering the peculiar frailty of ESKD patients, all scientific nephrology societies have provided guidance on COVID-19 transmission prevention in dialysis facilities [33–35]. In this regard, surveillance and early contagion detection are essential to reduce the risk of local outbreaks developing into epidemics.

Clinics of the FMC European Nephrocare Network have implemented multiple non-pharmacological interventions to limit viral spreading among the CKD community, including stringent hygiene procedures, social distancing, and the identification and isolation of suspected cases. In addition, dialysis facilities have established recording pathways to report any infection event in the EuCliD® TIR System. Such data are used to monitor the effectiveness of non-pharmacological intervention and to detect high-risk patients needing special attention [36–38].

One important feature of our modeling strategy entailed the combined use of open source and clinical data collected in standard clinical practice. In fact, we exploited the interconnection of the European Nephrocare clinics to augment background epidemic data with a surveillance system based on incident reports and practice pattern variation at each dialysis unit. Information about local epidemic status in a given clinic was then propagated through distance-weighting metrics to the surrounding facilities. An ML method was used to integrate all information into a summary score metric. Remarkably, variables related to the epidemic dynamics in the clinic and to the regional epidemic status, as well as to the risk proxies propagated from adjacent clinics, were all important predictors of outbreak occurrence. Such an approach is particularly relevant because it enabled us to capture local disease spread beyond the registry data compiled for the general population, which does not capture the heterogeneity of viral transmission in a setting where frequent and multiple human interactions necessarily occur. Indeed, as the basic reproduction index (R0) is a function of both the transmissibility of a disease and the contact patterns that underlie transmission [39], the regional/provincial R0 cannot be translated in dialysis facilities in that ESKD patients' biological and socio-behavioral factors significantly differ from those of the general population [40]. The occurrence of SSEVs further complicates the picture, making generalizations of regional epidemic trends that are not entirely appropriate for the reliable prediction of viral spreading in healthcare settings [41,42].

The interconnection of the FMC network allows for the collection and subsequent central integration of a bulk of information provided by facilities distributed throughout European countries. This particular setting offers the advantage to perform the real-time monitoring of sentinel sensors that are likely to provide timely and accurate indications of epidemic activity [43], while considering the heterogeneity underlying transmission dynamics. Sentinel surveillance in outpatient settings was previously shown to provide a robust approach to oversee SARS-CoV-2 spreading [44]. In general, the monitoring of community transmission in nodes distributed across different regions was reported to ensure efficient disease detection in networked populations [45]. It is important to highlight that the analytic strategy adopted in this study is general and can be applied to any epidemic communicable disease, as all naturally occurring, clustering units where social promiscuity, density, and duration of interactions are substantially different compared to the general population. Henceforth, this method may be applied to social contexts with a high risk of outbreak generation, including schools, hospitals, and workplaces from which the provided infection data are promptly captured and conferred to a central database, even in aggregated form. Monitoring of the pandemic situation within the network allows for the timely implementation of infection control procedures in the adjacent networked unit and efficiently anticipates resource needs.

Finally, variable importance analysis has indicated that trends in clinical practice patterns are among the top predictors. This observation indicates that the tracking of physicians' prescription behavior can provide valuable information to assess epidemic dynamics also during explosive growth, when surveillance and laboratory resources are limited and COVID-19 cases may be recorded with some delay due to the emergency situation [46].

5. Conclusions

Our sentinel surveillance system allows for a prompt risk assessment and timely response to the challenges posed by the COVID-19 epidemic throughout FMC European dialysis clinics. This tool can have significant implications for public health practice in that it represents a robust strategy to assess the level of community transmission of COVID-19 and to guide the selection and implementation of mitigation measures. The same framework can be applied in other networked settings, such as healthcare facilities or schools to improve early detection and forecasting of SARS-CoV-2 transmission. Finally, the implementation of our surveillance system can guide preparedness efforts for future pandemics.

Author Contributions: Conceptualization: F.B. and L.N.; data curation: M.G. and F.M.-M.; formal analysis: P.C., M.G. and F.M.-M.; supervision: S.S.; validation: F.B., L.N. and S.S.; writing—original draft: P.C. and C.L.; writing—review and editing: F.B., P.C., C.L. and L.N. All authors have read and agreed to the published version of the manuscript.

Funding: This research was funded by Fresenius Medical Care Deutschland GmbH.

Institutional Review Board Statement: The study was conducted according to the guidelines of the Declaration of Helsinki. IRB approval was not necessary because all input data for modeling were aggregated statistics concerning COVID-19 infection distribution and practice patterns across dialysis centers (i.e., cumulative number of infections in countries, number of prescribed laboratory tests in dialysis centers, number of new cases in dialysis centers). No patients' personal information has been used for the present study.

Informed Consent Statement: No patients' personal information has been used for the present study since all input data for modeling were aggregated statistics concerning COVID-19 infection distribution and practice patterns across dialysis centers (i.e., cumulative number of infections in countries, number of prescribed laboratory tests in dialysis centers, number of new cases in dialysis centers).

Data Availability Statement: Open source datasets adopted for the study have been referenced throughout the manuscript. Restrictions apply to the availability of these data. Data was obtained from Fresenius Medical Care and may be available for specific, well-motivated requests, from the corresponding author with the permission of Fresenius Medical Care.

Conflicts of Interest: C.L. received consultancy fees from Fresenius Medical Care Deutschland GmbH. All remaining authors are full time employees of Fresenius Medical Care Deutschland GmbH.

Appendix A

Table A1. Variables included in the model.

Category	Variable	Reference Time
Epidemic Status in the Country/Region (prefix: RG)		
	cumulative cases	previous 7 days and last 7 days
	number of hospitalized	previous 7 days and last 7 days
	number of ICU patients	previous 7 days and last 7 days
	cumulative fatalities	previous 7 days and last 7 days
	cumulative recovered	previous 7 days and last 7 days
	trend of cumulative cases	last 7 days/previous 7 days
Category	**Variable**	**Reference Time**
	trend of hospitalized patients	last 7 days/previous 7 days
	trend of ICU patients	last 7 days/previous 7 days
	trend of cumulative recovered in the last week	last 7 days/previous 7 days
	trend of cumulative fatalities	last 7 days/previous 7 days
epidemic status in the clinic (prefix: CL)		
	number of suspected COVID-19 cases	previous 14 days, previous 7 days, and last 7 days
	change in suspected cases	last 7 days–previous 7 days
	change in suspected cases	last 14 days–previous 14 days

Table A1. *Cont.*

Category	Variable	Reference Time
distance-weighted information of the adjacent clinics (prefix: CL)		
	number of COVID-19 suspected cases in the closest clinics	previous 14d, previous 7 days, and last 7 days
	change in COVID-19 suspected cases in the closest clinics	last 7 days–previous 7 days
	change in COVID-19 suspected cases in the closest clinics	last 14 days–previous 14 days
other parameters related to the clinic (prefix: CL)		
	change in the number of treated patients	last 28 days–last 14 days
	change in the number of treatments	last 28 days–last 14 days
	change in the weekly dialysis frequency per clinic	last 28 days–last 14 days
	change in the weekly dialysis frequency per patient	last 28 days–last 14 days
	change in the number of treatments with pre/post-BT	last 28 days–last 14 days
	change in the number of treatments with pre/post-BT > 37 °C	last 28 days–last 14 days
	change in the percentage of treatments with pre/post-BT > 37 °C	last 28 days–last 14 days
	change in the mean value of pre/post-dialysis BT	last 28 days–last 14 days
	change in the number of treatments with pre-dyalisis diastolic BP	last 28 days–last 14 days
	change in the mean value of pre-dialysis diastolic BP	last 28 days–last 14 days
	change in the number of treatments with dialysis time	last 28 days–last 14 days
	change in the mean value of dialysis time	last 28 days–last 14 days
	change in the number of treatments with IDWG	last 28 days–last 14 days
	change in the mean value of IDWG	last 28 days–last 14 days
	change in the number of treatments with O2 sat	last 28 days–last 14 days
	change in the mean value of O2 sat	last 28 days–last 14 days
	change in the number of patients with lab tests	last 28 days–last 14 days
	change in the number of lab tests	last 28 days–last 14 days
	change in the number of lab tests with Albumin	last 28 days–last 14 days
	change in the mean value of Albumin	last 28 days–last 14 days
	change in the number of lab tests with lymphocytes	last 28 days–last 14 days
	change in the mean value of lymphocytes	last 28 days–last 14 days
	change in the number of lab tests with monocytes	last 28 days–last 14 days
	change in the mean value of monocytes	last 28 days–last 14 days
	change in the number of lab tests with neutrophils	last 28 days–last 14 days
	change in the mean value of neutrophils	last 28 days–last 14 days
	change in the number of lab tests with platelets	last 28 days–last 14 days
	change in the mean value of platelets	last 28 days–last 14 days
	change in the number of lab tests with PDW	last 28 days–last 14 days

Table A1. *Cont.*

Category	Variable	Reference Time
	change in the mean value of PDW	last 28 days–last 14 days
	change in the number of lab tests with leukocytes	last 28 days–last 14 days
	change in the mean value of leukocytes	last 28 days–last 14 days
	change in the number of lab tests with D-dimer	last 28 days–last 14 days
	change in the mean value of D-dimer	last 28 days–last 14 days
	change in the number of lab tests with CRP	last 28 days–last 14 days
	change in the mean value of CRP	last 28 days–last 14 days
	change in the number of lab tests with IL-6	last 28 days–last 14 days
	change in the mean value of IL-6	last 28 days–last 14 days
	change in the number of lab tests with ANP	last 28 days–last 14 days
	change in the mean value of ANP	last 28 days–last 14 days
	change in the number of lab tests with BNP	last 28 days–last 14 days
	change in the mean value of BNP	last 28 days–last 14 days
	change in the number of lab tests with Ferritin	last 28 days–last 14 days
	change in the mean value of Ferritin	last 28 days–last 14 days
	Number of patients with at least one hospitalization	last 14 days
	Number of hospitalizations	last 14 days

References

1. Li, J.; Huang, D.Q.; Zou, B.; Yang, H.; Hui, W.Z.; Rui, F.; Yee, N.T.S.; Liu, C.; Nerurkar, S.N.; Kai, J.C.Y.; et al. Epidemiology of COVID-19: A systematic review and meta-analysis of clinical characteristics, risk factors, and outcomes. *J. Med. Virol.* **2021**, *93*, 1449–1458. [CrossRef]
2. Muller, C.P. Do asymptomatic carriers of SARS-COV-2 transmit the virus? *Lancet Reg. Health* **2021**, *4*, 100082. [CrossRef]
3. He, X.; Lau, E.H.Y.; Wu, P.; Deng, X.; Wang, J.; Hao, X.; Lau, Y.C.; Wong, J.Y.; Guan, Y.; Tan, X.; et al. Temporal dynamics in viral shedding and transmissibility of COVID-19. *Nat. Med.* **2020**, *26*, 672–675. [CrossRef] [PubMed]
4. Byambasuren, O.; Cardona, M.; Bell, K.; Clark, J.; McLaws, M.-L.; Glasziou, P. Estimating the extent of asymptomatic COVID-19 and its potential for community transmission: Systematic review and meta-analysis. *JAMMI Off. J. Assoc. Med. Microbiol. Infect. Dis. Can.* **2020**, *5*, 223–234. [CrossRef]
5. Galvani, A.P.; May, R.M. Epidemiology: Dimensions of superspreading. *Nature* **2005**, *438*, 293–295. [CrossRef] [PubMed]
6. Lemieux, J.; Siddle, K.J.; Shaw, B.M.; Loreth, C.; Schaffner, S.; Gladden-Young, A.; Adams, G.; Fink, T.; Tomkins-Tinch, C.H.; Krasilnikova, L.A.; et al. Phylogenetic analysis of SARS-CoV-2 in the Boston area highlights the role of recurrent importation and superspreading events. *medRxiv* **2020**, PMC7457619. [CrossRef]
7. Lewis, D. Superspreading drives the COVID pandemic-and could help to tame it. *Nature* **2021**, *590*, 544–546. [CrossRef]
8. Chu, D.K.; Akl, E.A.; Duda, S.; Solo, K.; Yaacoub, S.; Schünemann, H.J.; El-harakeh, A.; Bognanni, A.; Lotfi, T.; Loeb, M.; et al. Physical distancing, face masks, and eye protection to prevent person-to-person transmission of SARS-CoV-2 and COVID-19: A systematic review and meta-analysis. *Lancet* **2020**, *395*, 1973–1987. [CrossRef]
9. Regmi, K.; Lwin, C.M. Impact of non-pharmaceutical interventions for reducing transmission of COVID-19: A systematic review and meta-analysis protocol. *BMJ Open* **2020**, *10*, e041383. [CrossRef]
10. Apata, I.W.; Cobb, J.; Navarrete, J.; Burkart, J.; Plantinga, L.; Lea, J.P. COVID-19 infection control measures and outcomes in urban dialysis centers in predominantly African American communities. *BMC Nephrol.* **2021**, *22*, 81. [CrossRef]
11. Weiner, D.E.; Watnick, S.G. Hemodialysis and COVID-19: An Achilles' Heel in the Pandemic Health Care Response in the United States. *Kidney Med.* **2020**, *2*, 227–230. [CrossRef]
12. Meijers, B.; Messa, P.; Ronco, C. Safeguarding the Maintenance Hemodialysis Patient Population during the Coronavirus Disease 19 Pandemic. *Blood Purif.* **2020**, *49*, 259–264. [CrossRef]
13. Li, S.Y.; Tang, Y.S.; Chan, Y.J.; Tarng, D.C. Impact of the COVID-19 pandemic on the management of patients with end-stage renal disease. *J. Chin. Med. Assoc.* **2020**, *83*, 628–633. [CrossRef]
14. Lamarche, C.; Iliuta, I.A.; Kitzler, T. Infectious Disease Risk in Dialysis Patients: A Transdisciplinary Approach. *Can. J. Kidney Health Dis.* **2019**, *6*, 2054358119839080. [CrossRef] [PubMed]

15. Clarke, C.L.; Prendecki, M.; Dhutia, A.; Gan, J.; Edwards, C.; Prout, V.; Lightstone, L.; Parker, E.; Marchesin, F.; Griffith, M.; et al. Longevity of SARS-CoV-2 immune responses in hemodialysis patients and protection against reinfection. *Kidney Int.* **2021**, *99*, 1470–1477. [CrossRef]
16. Lisowska, K.A.; Pindel, M.; Pietruczuk, K.; Kuźmiuk-Glembin, I.; Storoniak, H.; Dębska-Ślizień, A.; Witkowski, J.M. The influence of a single hemodialysis procedure on human T lymphocytes. *Sci. Rep.* **2019**, *9*, 5041. [CrossRef] [PubMed]
17. Betjes, M.G.H. Immune cell dysfunction and inflammation in end-stage renal disease. *Nat. Rev. Nephrol.* **2013**, *9*, 255–265. [CrossRef] [PubMed]
18. Williamson, E.J.; Walker, A.J.; Bhaskaran, K.; Bacon, S.; Bates, C.; Morton, C.E.; Curtis, H.J.; Mehrkar, A.; Evans, D.; Inglesby, P.; et al. Factors associated with COVID-19-related death using OpenSAFELY. *Nature* **2020**, *584*, 430–436. [CrossRef] [PubMed]
19. Thakur, B.; Dubey, P.; Benitez, J.; Torres, J.P.; Reddy, S.; Shokar, N.; Aung, K.; Mukherjee, D.; Dwivedi, A.K. A systematic review and meta-analysis of geographic differences in comorbidities and associated severity and mortality among individuals with COVID-19. *Sci. Rep.* **2021**, *11*, 8562. [CrossRef]
20. Wu, Z.; McGoogan, J.M. Characteristics of and Important Lessons From the Coronavirus Disease 2019 (COVID-19) Outbreak in China: Summary of a Report of 72 314 Cases From the Chinese Center for Disease Control and Prevention. *JAMA* **2020**, *323*, 1239–1242. [CrossRef] [PubMed]
21. Jager, K.J.; Kramer, A.; Chesnaye, N.C.; Couchoud, C.; Sánchez-Álvarez, J.E.; Garneata, L.; Collart, F.; Hemmelder, M.H.; Ambühl, P.; Kerschbaum, J.; et al. Results from the ERA-EDTA Registry indicate a high mortality due to COVID-19 in dialysis patients and kidney transplant recipients across Europe. *Kidney Int.* **2020**, *98*, 1540–1548. [CrossRef] [PubMed]
22. Steil, H.; Amato, C.; Carioni, C.; Kirchgessner, J.; Marcelli, D.; Mitteregger, A.; Moscardo, V.; Orlandini, G.; Gatti, E. EuCliD®—A Medical Registry. *Methods Inf. Med.* **2004**, *43*, 83–88. [PubMed]
23. Merello Godino, J.I.; Rentero, R.; Orlandini, G.; Marcelli, D.; Ronco, C. Results from EuCliD®(European Clinical Dialysis Database): Impact of shifting treatment modality. *Int. J. Artif. Organs* **2002**, *25*, 1049–1060. [CrossRef]
24. European Commission Joint Research Centre—ISPRA-Space, Security and Migration Directorate (JRC). Available online: https://covid-statistics.jrc.ec.europa.eu/ (accessed on 12 July 2020).
25. Chen, T.; Guestrin, C. XGBoost: A Scalable Tree Boosting System. In Proceedings of the 22nd ACM SIGKDD International Conference on Knowledge Discovery and Data Mining, San Francisco, CA, USA, 13–17 August 2016.
26. Available online: https://github.com/dmlc/xgboost (accessed on 21 December 2019).
27. Van Rossum, G. *Python Tutorial*; CreateSpace Independent Publishing Platform; (online publisher); 1995.
28. Ling, C.X.; Huang, J.; Zhang, H. AUC: A better measure than accuracy in comparing learning algorithms. In *Advances in Artificial Intelligence. Canadian AI 2003*; Lecture Notes in Computer Science (Lecture Notes in Artificial Intelligence); Springer: Berlin/Heidelberg, Germany, 2003; Volume 2671, pp. 329–341.
29. Lundberg, S.M.; Lee, S.-I. Unified Approach to Interpreting Model Predictions. In Proceedings of the 31st Conference on Neural Information Processing Systems (NIPS 2017), Long Beach, CA, USA, 4–9 December 2017; 2017.
30. Abbas, M.; Robalo Nunes, T.; Martischang, R.; Zingg, W.; Iten, A.; Pittet, D.; Harbarth, S. Nosocomial transmission and outbreaks of coronavirus disease 2019: The need to protect both patients and healthcare workers. *Antimicrob. Resist. Infect. Control* **2021**, *10*, 7. [CrossRef]
31. Leeds, C. COVID 19: Health care workers, risks, protection and transmission. *Lancet Reg. Health* **2021**, *1*, 100022. [CrossRef]
32. La Milia, V.; Bacchini, G.; Bigi, M.C.; Casartelli, D.; Cavalli, A.; Corti, M.; Crepaldi, M.; Limardo, M.; Longhi, S.; Manzoni, C.; et al. COVID-19 Outbreak in a Large Hemodialysis Center in Lombardy, Italy. *Kidney Int. Rep.* **2020**, *5*, 1095–1099. [CrossRef]
33. Kliger, A.S.; Silberzweig, J. Mitigating risk of COVID-19 in dialysis facilities. *Clin. J. Am. Soc. Nephrol.* **2020**, *15*, 707–709. [CrossRef] [PubMed]
34. Basile, C.; Combe, C.; Pizzarelli, F.; Covic, A.; Davenport, A.; Kanbay, M.; Kirmizis, D.; Schneditz, D.; Van Der Sande, F.; Mitra, S. Recommendations for the prevention, mitigation and containment of the emerging SARS-CoV-2 (COVID-19) pandemic in haemodialysis centres. *Nephrol. Dial. Transplant.* **2020**, *35*, 737–741. [CrossRef]
35. Kliger, A.S.; Cozzolino, M.; Jha, V.; Harbert, G.; Ikizler, T.A. Managing the COVID-19 pandemic: International comparisons in dialysis patients. *Kidney Int.* **2020**, *98*, 12–16. [CrossRef]
36. Marcelli, D. EuCliD (European Clinical Database): A database comparing different realities. *J. Nephrol.* **2001**, *14*, S94–S100.
37. Richards, N.; Ayala, J.A.; Cesare, S.; Chazot, C.; Di Benedetto, A.; Gassia, J.P.; Merello, J.I.; Rentero, R.; Scatizzi, L.; Marcelli, D. Assessment of quality guidelines implementation using a continuous quality improvement programme. *Blood Purif.* **2007**, *25*, 221–228. [CrossRef]
38. Marcelli, D.; Moscardó, V.; Steil, H.; Day, M.; Kirchgessner, J.; Mitteregger, A.; Orlandini, G.; Gatti, E. Data management and quality assurance for dialysis network. *Contrib. Nephrol.* **2002**, *137*, 293–299. [CrossRef]
39. Delamater, P.L.; Street, E.J.; Leslie, T.F.; Yang, Y.T.; Jacobsen, K.H. Complexity of the basic reproduction number (R0). *Emerg. Infect. Dis.* **2019**, *25*, 1–4. [CrossRef]
40. Corbett, R.W.; Blakey, S.; Nitsch, D.; Loucaidou, M.; McLean, A.; Duncan, N.; Ashby, D.R.; Appelbe, M.; Brown, E.; Cairns, T.; et al. Epidemiology of COVID-19 in an urban dialysis center. *J. Am. Soc. Nephrol.* **2020**, *31*, 1815–1823. [CrossRef]
41. Meyers, L.A.; Pourbohloul, B.; Newman, M.E.J.; Skowronski, D.M.; Brunham, R.C. Network theory and SARS: Predicting outbreak diversity. *J. Theor. Biol.* **2005**, *232*, 71–81. [CrossRef]

42. Frieden, T.R.; Lee, C.T. Identifying and interrupting superspreading events-implications for control of severe acute respiratory syndrome coronavirus 2. *Emerg. Infect. Dis.* **2020**, *26*, 1061–1066. [CrossRef] [PubMed]
43. Herrera, J.L.; Srinivasan, R.; Brownstein, J.S.; Galvani, A.P.; Meyers, L.A. Disease Surveillance on Complex Social Networks. *PLoS Comput. Biol.* **2016**, *12*, e1004928. [CrossRef] [PubMed]
44. Zwald, M.L.; Lin, W.; Sondermeyer Cooksey, G.L.; Weiss, C.; Suarez, A.; Fischer, M.; Bonin, B.J.; Jain, S.; Langley, G.E.; Park, B.J.; et al. Rapid Sentinel Surveillance for COVID-19—Santa Clara County, California, March 2020. *Morb. Mortal. Wkly. Rep.* **2020**, *69*, 419–421. [CrossRef]
45. Colman, E.; Holme, P.; Sayama, H.; Gershenson, C. Efficient sentinel surveillance strategies for preventing epidemics on networks. *PLoS Comput. Biol.* **2019**, *15*, e1007517. [CrossRef]
46. Monaghan, C.; Larkin, J.; Chaudhuri, S.; Han, H.; Jiao, Y.; Bermudez, K.; Weinhandl, E.; Dahne-Steuber, I.; Belmonte, K.; Neri, L.; et al. Artificial Intelligence for COVID-19 Risk Classification in Kidney Disease: Can Technology Unmask an Unseen Disease? *medRxiv* **2020**. [CrossRef]

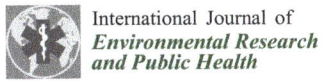

Review

Sharing Is Caring—Data Sharing Initiatives in Healthcare

Tim Hulsen

Department of Professional Health Solutions & Services, Philips Research, 5656AE Eindhoven, The Netherlands; tim.hulsen@philips.com

Received: 28 February 2020; Accepted: 24 April 2020; Published: 27 April 2020

Abstract: In recent years, more and more health data are being generated. These data come not only from professional health systems, but also from wearable devices. All these 'big data' put together can be utilized to optimize treatments for each unique patient ('precision medicine'). For this to be possible, it is necessary that hospitals, academia and industry work together to bridge the 'valley of death' of translational medicine. However, hospitals and academia often are reluctant to share their data with other parties, even though the patient is actually the owner of his/her own health data. Academic hospitals usually invest a lot of time in setting up clinical trials and collecting data, and want to be the first ones to publish papers on this data. There are some publicly available datasets, but these are usually only shared after study (and publication) completion, which means a severe delay of months or even years before others can analyse the data. One solution is to incentivize the hospitals to share their data with (other) academic institutes and the industry. Here, we show an analysis of the current literature around data sharing, and we discuss five aspects of data sharing in the medical domain: publisher requirements, data ownership, growing support for data sharing, data sharing initiatives and how the use of federated data might be a solution. We also discuss some potential future developments around data sharing, such as medical crowdsourcing and data generalists.

Keywords: data sharing; data management; data science; big data; healthcare

1. Introduction

The past years have seen a steep rise in the amount of health data being generated. These data come not only from professional health systems (MRI scanners, pathology slides, DNA tests, etc.) but also from wearable devices. All these data combined form 'big data' that can be utilized to optimize treatments for each unique patient ('precision medicine') [1]. To achieve this precision medicine, it is necessary that hospitals, academia and industry work together to bridge the 'valley of death' of translational medicine [2]. However, hospitals and academia often have problems with sharing their data, even though the patient is actually the owner of his/her own health data, and data sharing is associated with increased citation rate [3,4]. Academic hospitals usually want to be the first ones to publish papers on the data, because they spent a lot of time in setting up clinical trials and collecting the data. Society benefits the most if the patient's data are shared as soon as possible so that other researchers can work with it [5], but this idea has not settled in yet. Some datasets are publicly available (e.g., in prostate cancer [6]), but these are usually only shared after studies are finished and/or publications have been written based on the data, which means a severe delay of months or even years before others can use the data for analysis. One solution is to incentivize the hospitals [7,8] to share their data with (other) academic institutes and the industry. Besides this academic reluctance, data is also being shared less because of stricter privacy laws such as the EU General Data Protection Regulation (GDPR) [9] and the California Consumer Privacy Act (CCPA) [10]. At the moment, only around 10% of the world's population has it personal information covered by the GDPR or similar laws, but Gartner Research predicts that this will be around 50% by 2022 [11]. There is an increasingly urgent need to balance the opportunity big data provides for improving healthcare, against the right of individuals to control their own data [1]. Scientists should maximize their efforts to improve healthcare, but they should also only use data with appropriate informed consent. This open science vs. privacy balance will remain an increasing challenge for the coming years.

The topic of data sharing has received more attention in recent years. In 1980, only 46 articles (0.0186% of the total) published in PubMed contained the keyword "data sharing", while in 2019 there were 5960 articles (0.4253% of the total) containing this keyword (Figure 1). It is also interesting to see the sudden rise of interest in the subject since 2016, the year of the approval of the GDPR, and another peak in 2018, the year of its enforcement.

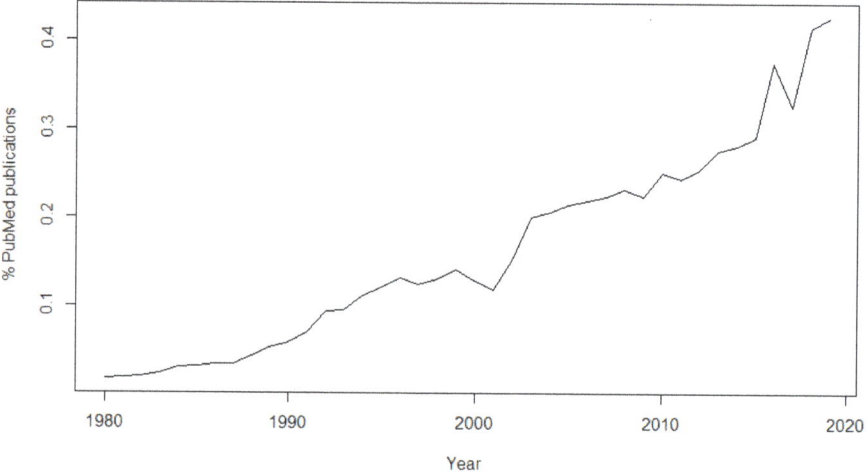

Figure 1. Graph of the number of abstracts of PubMed publications containing the keyword "data sharing" as a percentage of the total, per year since 1980.

If we use PubMed to find terms related to "data sharing", there are some interesting observations (Figure 2). Mostly used are obviously terms such as "patients", "health", "study" and "information", but closely behind these are "use" (or "used"/"using"), "treatment", "care" "analysis" and "rights". "Use" might point to the fact that data collection and sharing is closely connected to the usage of the data, i.e., in the consent form it should be mentioned in detail what the health data will be used for. "Treatment", "care" and "analysis" point to one of the main uses of the data: analysis in order to improve treatment and care, for example in clinical decision support (CDS) systems. "Rights" is probably related to the patients' privacy rights when it comes to data sharing, an issue that is discussed in detail in this manuscript.

There have been some studies on the conditions and challenges for sharing data. For example, for the BigData@Heart platform of the Innovative Medicines Initiative (IMI), a descriptive case study into the condition for data sharing was carried out [12]. Principle investigators of the participating databases were requested to send any kind of documentation that possibly specified the conditions for data sharing, which were then qualitatively reviewed for conditions related to data sharing and data access. This review revealed overlap on the conditions: (1) only to share health data for scientific research, (2) in anonymized/coded form, (3) after approval from a designated review committee, and while (4) observing all appropriate measures for data security and in compliance with the applicable laws and regulations. These challenges give thought to the design of an ethical governance framework for data sharing platforms. The conclusion of the case study was that current data sharing initiatives should concentrate on: (1) the scope of the research questions that may be addressed, (2) how to deal with varying levels of de-identification, (3) determining when and how review committees should come into play, (4) align what policies and regulations mean by "data sharing" and (5) how to deal with datasets that have no system in place for data sharing.

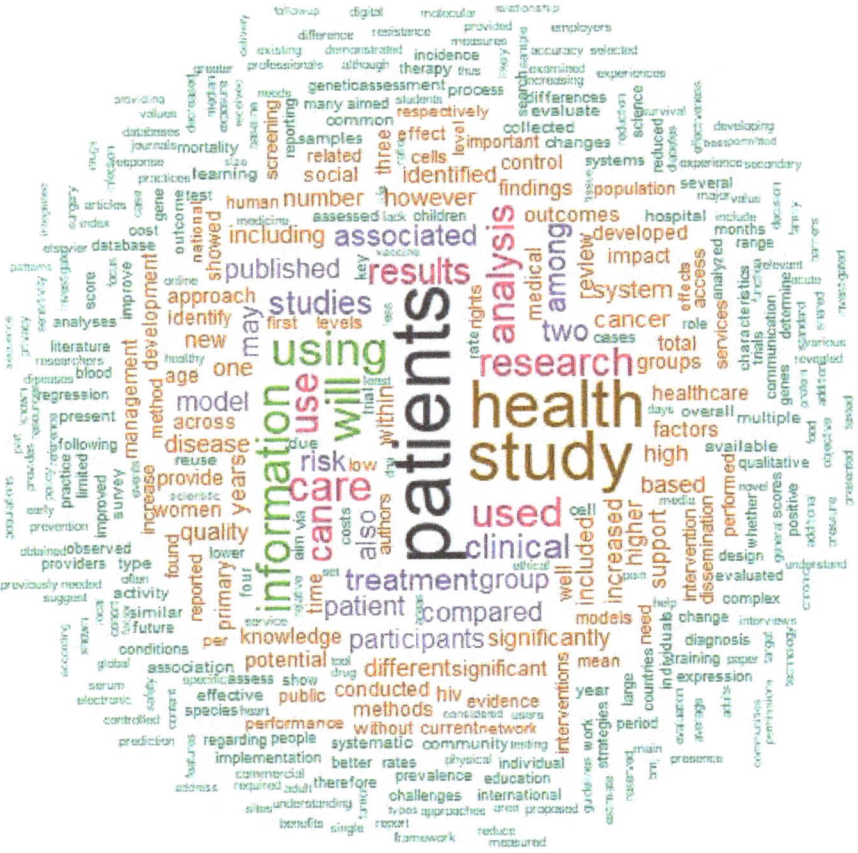

Figure 2. Wordcloud of all abstracts of PubMed publications containing the keyword "data sharing", generated by the R package PubMedWordcloud [13].

Sharing data should not just be a one-way street from the clinician to the researcher; ideally the clinician, the researcher and the patient (or patient organization) would work together on setting up the study, so that there is an agreement on data usage upfront, and expectations are managed. Sharing data will also increase confidence and trust in the conclusions drawn from clinical trials [14]. It will help to enable the independent confirmation of results (reproducibility), an essential part of the scientific process. It will foster the development and testing of new hypotheses. Sharing clinical trial data should also make progress more efficient by making the most of what may be learned from each trial and by avoiding unwarranted repetition. It will help to satisfy the moral obligation of researchers towards study participants, and it will benefit patients, investigators, sponsors, and society. In this review, we discuss several aspects of data sharing in the medical domain. The Section 2 is about publisher requirements, which shows what guidelines have been created by publishers and editors to promote the sharing of data. Since academics rely on publication of their data, these are important measures and a logical first topic to be discussed. The Section 3 shows that there is an ongoing discussion about data ownership, which influences the way that regulations are being implemented. The Section 4 shows the growing support for data sharing, making the link to open science and the reproducibility of results. The Section 5 shows data sharing initiatives that have been undertaken recently. The Sections 6 and 7 discusses how the use of federated data might be a solution of the privacy and reproducibility issues mentioned in the Sections 2–4.

2. Publisher Requirements

Most publishers strongly recommend sharing research data. For this section, the publisher requirements of five major publishers are discussed, as well as the most widely used sets of guidelines from publishers and editors.

Nature states that data sharing makes new types of research possible [15], for example through the pooling of patient cohorts, and hints to future developments: sharing data is not only a way to improve the reproducibility and robustness of the science that is taking place today, but can drive new science for tomorrow. By browsing through existing datasets, new hypotheses can be formed, which can then be tested in new studies. Because nobody can predict how valuable a dataset will be in the future, data should be made available to future scientists whenever possible. The Science journals support the efforts of databases that aggregate published data for the use of the scientific community [16]. Therefore, before publication, large data sets must be deposited in an approved database and an accession number or a specific access address must be included in the published paper. The Science journals also encourage compliance with Minimum Information for Biological and Biomedical Investigations (MIBBI) guidelines [17]. British Medical Journal (BMJ) journals have three different data sharing policies ("tiers"), dependent of the journal [18]. They encourage researchers to make available as much of the underlying data from an article as possible (without compromising the privacy of the patients). The BMJ journals also consider reproducibility: all data that are needed to reproduce the results presented in the associated article should be made available. When submitting a manuscript to a publisher such as BioMed Central (BMC), the researcher even "agrees to make the raw data and materials described in your manuscript freely available to any scientist wishing to use them for non-commercial purposes, as long as this does not breach participant confidentiality" [19]. Public Library of Science (PLOS) journals require authors "to make all data necessary to replicate their study's findings publicly available without restriction at the time of publication. When specific legal or ethical restrictions prohibit public sharing of a data set, authors must indicate how others may obtain access to the data" [20]. Other publishers have similar guidelines in place, promoting data sharing on a global level.

In 2015, the Transparency and Openness Promotion (TOP) guidelines [21] were published. The guidelines were developed to translate scientific norms and values into concrete actions and change the current incentive structures to drive researchers' behavior toward more openness. The TOP guidelines have eight standards: (1) citation standards; (2) data transparency; (3) analytics methods (code) transparency; (4) research materials transparency; (5) design and analysis transparency; (6) preregistration of studies; (7) preregistration of analysis plans; and (8) replication. For each standard, there are three levels with increasing stringency. Currently, over 1000 scientific journals have implemented the TOP guidelines [22].

The International Committee of Medical Journal Editors (ICMJE) also recommends the sharing of data [14]. In 2016, they proposed to require authors to share with others the deidentified individual-patient data (IPD) underlying the results presented in the article no later than 6 months after publication. The data underlying the results are defined as "the IPD required to reproduce the article's findings, including necessary metadata". Since 2019, the ICMJE requires investigators to register a data-sharing plan when registering a trial as well. This plan must include where the researchers will house the data and, if not in a public repository, the mechanism by which they will provide others access to the data, whether data will be freely available to anyone upon request or only after application to and approval by a learned intermediary, whether a data use agreement will be required, etc. Declaring the plan for sharing data prior to their collection will further enhance transparency in the conduct and reporting of clinical trials by exposing when data availability following trial completion differs from prior commitments. However, ICMJE also stresses that the rights of investigators and trial sponsors must be protected. To achieve this, the following four rules apply: (1) editors will not consider the deposition of data in a registry to constitute prior publication; (2) authors of secondary analyses using these shared data must attest that their use was in accordance with the terms (if any) agreed to upon their receipt; (3) authors of secondary analyses must reference the source of the data using a unique identifier of a clinical trial's data set to provide appropriate credit to those who generated it and allow searching for the studies it has supported; (4) authors of secondary analyses must explain completely how theirs differ from previous analyses. In addition, those who generate and then share clinical trial data sets deserve substantial credit for their efforts. Those using data collected by others should seek collaboration with those who collected the data.

By providing the guidelines and rules set out above, the publishers and editors contribute to the acceptance of data sharing by researchers. Not only does it help solve their problem of a lack of reproducibility of the scientific results published in their journals, increasing confidence and trust in these results; it will also help the scientists in the generation of new hypotheses, and avoiding unnecessary repetition. In the end, publishers, as well as scientists, patients and societies will benefit from complying with these rules.

3. Data Ownership

When discussing the sharing of data, it is important to realize that there is not much consensus on who is actually the owner of that data. This section briefly discusses this issue of data ownership in the light of recent privacy laws. These laws have a very large impact on the topic of data sharing.

Institutions tend to believe that they own the patient data, since they collected it. However, these institutions are in fact just "data custodians"; the data is the property of the patient and the access and use of that data outside of the clinical institute usually requires patient consent [1]. This limits the exploitation of the "big data" that are available in the clinical records, because the data should be destroyed (or sufficiently anonymized) after the end of the study. Big data techniques such as machine learning and deep learning use thousands to millions of data points, which may have required considerable processing. It would be a waste to lose such valuable data at the end of the project. Therefore, it is advised to ask the patient for consent to store and use their data for future scientific research. Although it is not possible to use the data from a large number of retrospective datasets in this manner, this will make sure that at least the prospectively collected data can be used in future studies. The dilemma of the use of patient data versus privacy rights has gotten much attention because of the implementation of the GDPR in 2018 (as well as the CCPA in 2020), initiating an international debate on the sharing of big data in the healthcare domain [23]. Earlier laws such as the Health Insurance Portability and Accountability Act (HIPAA) Privacy Rule [24] of the USA and the Personal Information Protection and Electronic Documents Act (PIPEDA) [25] of Canada already gave more rights to patients regarding their data, but the GDPR and CCPA have taken it to another level. However, GDPR and similar laws do not say much about data ownership. The GDPR's main entities are the data controller and the data processor [9]. "Data controller" means the natural or legal person, public authority, agency or other body which, alone or jointly with others, determines the purposes and means of the processing of personal data. "Data processor" means a natural or legal person, public authority, agency or other body which processes personal data on behalf of the controller. In countries outside of the European Union, where GDPR does not apply, there is also not much agreement on data ownership, making it even more justifiable to always ask for the consent of the patient.

4. Growing Support for Data Sharing

The idea that data should be shared as much as possible to enable scientific progress is gaining momentum, mostly because of the power of big data analyses, machine learning, deep learning, etc. In this section, some developments are discussed which show this growing support for data sharing.

Some of them were already known to the author, whereas others were a result from the literature analysis mentioned in the introduction.

Science in Transition [26] claims that "science has become a self-referential system where quality is measured mostly in bibliometric parameters and where societal relevance is undervalued", emphasizing that researchers tend to care mostly about publications instead of using the data to solve real-life problems. It also gives attention to the reproducibility problem in science: more than 70% of researchers have tried and failed to reproduce another scientist's experiments, and more than half have even failed to reproduce their own experiments [27]. This problem is not only caused by a lack of data sharing, but also because researchers do not share methodologies used to combine and analyse datasets. In many projects, data from several sources (possibly collected using different protocols and standards) need to be combined before the data analysis can take place. If these methodologies, as well as the analysis scripts, are not shared, results cannot be reproduced even if the data is available. This reproducibility issue could be resolved by 'Open Science', which is defined as the practising of science in a sustainable manner which gives others the opportunity to work with, contribute to and make use of the scientific process. This allows users from outside science to influence the research world with questions and ideas and help gather research data [28]. The Open Science movement stimulates not only open access to data, but also open access publishing, open source scientific software and open educational resources [29].

The Mayo Clinic Platform [30] is a new cloud-based clinical data analytics platform, storing de-identified patient data, which providers, payers and pharmaceutical companies outside of Mayo can link up to via application programming interfaces (APIs), as well as establishing standard templates for compliance and legal agreements. The first partner of the Mayo Clinic Platform is Nference, a software startup that Mayo is an investor in. Nference develops analytics, machine learning and natural language processing tools that "augment" the work of data scientists, in order to help research organizations and pharmaceutical companies conduct "research at scale". Mayo Clinic hopes to work with pharma to commercialize new therapies. Mayo itself wouldn't commercialize those therapies, though the system could receive royalties from insights generated on the platform. These royalties would be re-invested into Mayo's clinical practice, research and education work.

Healthcare Business and Technology wrote about how data sharing could change the entire healthcare industry [31]. It discusses the partnership announced by Apple in 2018 with 13 major healthcare systems, including Johns Hopkins and the University of Pennsylvania, that will allow Apple to download patients' electronic health data onto its devices (with consent of the patients). This type of data sharing could transform the U.S. healthcare industry by empowering patients in new ways and improving care. It could even reduce organizational costs by streamlining care processes, because hospital staff would need to spend less time on making data available to patients. And artificial intelligence (AI) could use the patient data to answer patients' questions and direct them to the healthcare services they need.

The 'Ten Commandments of Translational Research Informatics' [32] are some guidelines related to data management and data integration in translational research projects. Some of the commandments relate to the sharing of data: clear arrangements about data access need to be made (commandment 4), agree about de-identification and anonymization (commandment 5), the FAIR guiding principles [33] should be adhered to (commandment 8), and researchers should think about what will happen to the data after the project (commandment 10): e.g., research can be shared in a public repository.

5. Data Sharing Initiatives

There are many initiatives around the world supporting the sharing of medical data, leading the way to open science while still respecting the privacy rights of the patients. This paragraph gives some recent examples of these initiatives, resulting from the literature analysis from the introduction.

GIFT-Cloud [34] is a platform for data sharing and collaboration in medical imaging research. The goal of GIFT-Cloud is to provide a flexible, clinician- and researcher-friendly system for anonymising and sharing data across multiple institutions. It was built to support the Guided Instrumentation for Fetal Therapy and Surgery (GIFT-Surg) project, an international research collaboration that is developing novel imaging methods for fetal surgery, but it also has general applicability to other areas of imaging research. It simplifies the transfer of imaging data from clinical to research institutions, facilitating the development and validation of medical research software and the sharing of results back to the clinical partners. GIFT-Cloud supports collaboration between multiple healthcare and research institutions while satisfying the demands of patient confidentiality, data security and data ownership. It achieves this by building upon existing, well-established cross-platform technologies. GIFT-Cloud stores data from each institution in a separate data group and access to these groups can be individually configured for each account, corresponding with what is arranged in the data sharing agreements.

Another development in data sharing is the Personalized Consent Flow [35]: a new consent model that allows people to control their personally collected health data and determine to what extent they want to share these for research purposes. Three main features characterize the consent flow: (1) Users are asked general questions about sharing data. When they wish to share data for scientific research, they may opt for "narrow" consent (treating each study separately) or "broad" consent (for multiple studies). Furthermore, users can decide which data will be shared for specific studies and with whom. (2) Users can choose to share existing data that they have collected passively, to share prospectively, collect data, or both. For prospective studies, researchers can invite specific users to collect selected data during a specific time period. Users can also be notified about future studies by signing up for the research program. (3) Expiration dates are connected to each consent choice, which ensures that a user reconsiders his decision. A default expiration date of one year will be assigned, but users may also select personal expiration dates, such as an expiration date connected to the duration of the study. Users can choose to quit sharing data at any time, as required by GDPR regulations. During all steps, users are informed about implications of consent options.

In the United States, the Sync for Science (S4S) [36] collaboration between Electronic Health Record (EHR) vendors, the National Institutes of Health (NIH), the Office of the National Coordinator for Health IT (ONC), and Harvard Medical School's Department of Biomedical Informatics was started in 2016. S4S allows individuals to access their health data and share these data with researchers to support studies that generate insights into human health and disease [37]. Different EHRs collect and store health data differently, so S4S has focused on promoting both authorization and healthcare data standards to make it possible for EHR systems to release, upon patient approval, high quality data that researchers can readily consume. The All of Us Research Program [38] was the first study to adopt S4S technology in a pilot program. The program began national enrollment in 2018 and is expected to last at least 10 years. An initiative like Sync for Science gives the power to the patient: the patient can decide what information to share with researchers, and under what conditions. Much like many countries now have organ donation registration systems in place, this 'data donation registration' might be something that will be implemented around the world in the near future.

In the EU, the 1+ Million Genomes Initiative [39] is a good example of how many datasets could be combined into one large database, enabling the study of, e.g., rare diseases. The declaration aims to bring together fragmented infrastructure and expertise supporting a shared and tangible goal: one million genomes accessible in the EU by 2022. The 22 participating European countries envision that the digital transformation of genomic medicine (and healthcare in general) will help health systems to meet the challenges they face and become more sustainable, thereby improving the provision of high-quality health services and the effectiveness of treatments. They believe that this requires a concerted effort to overcome data silos, lack of interoperability and fragmentation of initiatives across the EU. Another recent example of such a large-scale collaborative data sharing effort is the Pan-Cancer Analysis of Whole Genomes (PCAWG) [40], which was facilitated by international data sharing using compute clouds. PCAWG contains 2658 whole-cancer genomes and their matching normal tissues across 38 tumour types. More than 1300 scientists and clinicians from 37 countries were involved in the project.

Data sharing goes beyond the academic world. Many public-private partnerships have been set up, in order to make sure that discoveries are not only published, but also applied in a product such as a medical device, a medicine or a computer program. Funding programmes, such as the Horizon 2020 Research and Innovation Programme of the European Union, very much stimulate data sharing with companies. In May 2016, it was announced that Deepmind, a company owned by Google and most famous for its innovative use of AI, was given access to the healthcare data of up to 1.6 million patients from three hospitals run by a major London NHS trust [41]. And in January 2018, Apple announced that they created a pact with 13 prominent health systems, including prestigious centers like Johns Hopkins and the University of Pennsylvania, allowing Apple to download the electronic health data of patients onto its devices, with consent [42]. Of course, when sharing data with commercial parties, privacy needs to be taken into account. For example, if GDPR applies, the patient needs to 'opt-in' for sharing their data for commercial use. Besides industry using data generated by academia, the opposite is also possible; these collaborations are called "data collaboratives" [43]. Data collaboratives are a new form of partnership in which privately held data are made accessible for analysis and use by external parties working in the public interest. By having researchers from both industry and academia work on the data, new insights and innovations can be created, and the potential of privately-owned data can be unlocked.

6. Federated Data

Data federation is a recent development in medical science, which is a possible solution for the data sharing vs. patient privacy dilemma. In this section, three examples of federated data systems for sharing medical data are discussed, resulting from the literature analysis from the introduction.

When applying machine learning methods on healthcare data, large samples sizes are required. Often these sizes can only be achieved by combining data from several studies. But this kind of pooling of information is difficult because of patient privacy and data protection needs. Privacy preserving distributed learning technology has the potential to overcome these limitations. The general idea behind distributed learning is that sites share a statistical model and its parameters, instead of sharing sensitive data. Each site runs computations on a local data store that generate these aggregated statistics. In this setting, organizations can collaborate by exchanging aggregated data/statistics while keeping the underlying data safely on site and undisclosed. VANTAGE6 [44] provides a way to use distributed learning technology, using open source software. It is one of the federated data systems that has recently become available in order to share data while preserving the patients' privacy rights.

The Personal Health Train (PHT) [45,46] is another example of a federated data system; it aims to connect distributed health data and create value by increasing the use of existing health data for citizens, healthcare, and scientific research. The key concept in the Personal Health Train is to bring algorithms ('trains') to the data where they happen to be ('stations'), rather than bringing all data together in a central database. The Personal Health Train is designed to give controlled access to heterogeneous data sources, while ensuring privacy protection and maximum engagement of individual subjects. As a prerequisite, health data are made FAIR (Findable, Accessible, Interoperable and Reusable) [33]. Stations containing FAIR data may be controlled by individuals, (general) physicians, biobanks, hospitals and public or private data repositories. The Personal Health Train was applied recently to a project with 20,000+ lung cancer patients [47] and will also be used in the Coronary ARtery disease: Risk estimations and Interventions for prevention and EaRly detection (CARRIER) project [48]. Likely more projects will follow.

Another example of a federated data system is DataSHIELD [49]. It provides a novel technological solution that can circumvent some of the most basic challenges in facilitating the access of researchers and other healthcare professionals to individual-level data. It facilitates research in settings where sharing the data itself is not possible (due to government restrictions, intellectual property issues, or data size). Commands are sent from a central analysis computer (AC) to several data computers (DCs) storing the data to be co-analysed. The data sets are analysed simultaneously but in parallel. The separate parallelized analyses are linked by non-disclosive summary statistics and commands transmitted back and forth between the DCs and the AC. DataSHIELD has been used by the Healthy Obese Project and the Environmental Core Project of the Biobank Standardisation and Harmonisation for Research Excellence in the European Union (BioSHaRE-EU [50]) for the federated analysis of 10 datasets across eight European countries.

7. Conclusions

This review discusses the current state of data sharing in healthcare. It shows that data sharing is widely supported by governments, funding programs and publishers, but that there are also issues. Clinicians or researchers might be reluctant to share data, because of publication pressure and fear for competition. This might be solved by the "open science" initiatives mentioned in this paper, which need to be supported by governments as well as the scientific communities itself in order to make it a success. Next to this, there are also patient-related issues such as stricter privacy laws. A possible (technical) solution here is the use of federated data systems such as the Personal Health Train, which enable algorithms to reach out the data without having the need to bring all data together. The challenges around privacy might also be solved by non-technical means such as using standardized consent forms to enable future use of data for research and/or commercial purposes. For the (near) future, there are some more developments that might be influential on the acceptance of open science and the sharing of data. One of these developments is medical crowdsourcing [51], which offers hope to patients who suffer from complex health conditions or rare diseases that are difficult to diagnose. Medical crowdsourcing platforms empower patients to use the "wisdom of the crowd" by providing access to a large pool of diverse medical information. One example medical crowdsourcing platform is CrowdMed [52]. This platform was appreciated by some patients with undiagnosed illnesses, because they received helpful guidance from crowdsourcing their diagnoses during their difficult diagnostic journeys [53]. Greater participation in crowdsourcing increases the likelihood of encountering a correct solution, and this might help to encourage patients to share their data. However, more participation can also lead to more noise, making the identification of the most likely solution from a broader pool of recommendations difficult. The challenge for medical crowdsourcing platforms is to increase participation of both patients and solution providers, while simultaneously increasing the efficacy and accuracy of solutions. Moreover, caution should be taken when giving people without a medical background the power to diagnose others. Another future development is the increase in "data generalists"; experts that focus entirely on data sharing and communication [54]. A data generalist takes on all responsibility for the sharing of data and needs critical thinking skills to integrate, evaluate and communicate the benefits and drawbacks of providing open data. They also have a role in data analysis. The emergence of this role should encourage better sharing of data. In a time where much attention is going to the data scientist, it could be the data generalist that really has the job of the future.

Funding: This research received no external funding.

Conflicts of Interest: Tim Hulsen is employed by Philips Research.

References

1. Hulsen, T.; Jamuar, S.S.; Moody, A.; Karnes, J.H.; Orsolya, V.; Hedensted, S.; Spreafico, R.; Hafler, D.A.; McKinney, E. From Big Data to Precision Medicine. *Front. Med.* **2019**, *6*, 34. [CrossRef] [PubMed]
2. Butler, D. Translational research: Crossing the valley of death. *Nature* **2008**, *453*, 840–842. [CrossRef] [PubMed]
3. Piwowar, H.A.; Day, R.S.; Fridsma, D.B. Sharing detailed research data is associated with increased citation rate. *PLoS ONE* **2007**, *2*, e308. [CrossRef] [PubMed]
4. Piwowar, H.A.; Vision, T.J. Data reuse and the open data citation advantage. *PeerJ* **2013**, *1*, e175. [CrossRef]

5. Packer, M. Data sharing in medical research. *BMJ* **2018**, *360*, k510. [CrossRef]
6. Hulsen, T. An overview of publicly available patient-centered prostate cancer datasets. *Transl. Androl. Urol.* **2019**, *8* (Suppl. 1), S64. [CrossRef]
7. Olfson, M.; Wall, M.M.; Blanco, C. Incentivizing Data Sharing and Collaboration in Medical Research-The S-Index. *JAMA Psychiatry* **2017**, *74*, 5–6. [CrossRef]
8. Rowhani-Farid, A.; Allen, M.; Barnett, A.G. What incentives increase data sharing in health and medical research? A systematic review. *Res. Integr. Peer Rev.* **2017**, *2*, 4. [CrossRef]
9. The European Parliament and the Council of the European Union. Regulation (EU) 2016/679 of the European Parliament and of the Council of 27 April 2016 on the protection of natural persons with regard to the processing of personal data and on the free movement of such data, and repealing Directive 95/46/EC (General Data Protection Regulation). *Off. J. Eur. Union* **2016**, *59*, 1–88.
10. State of California, The California Consumer Privacy Act of 2018. 2018. Available online: https://leginfo.legislature.ca.gov/faces/billTextClient.xhtml?bill_id=201720180AB375 (accessed on 25 April 2020).
11. Henein, N.; Willemsen, B. The State of Privacy and Personal Data Protection, 2019–2020. Gartner Research (2019). Available online: https://www.gartner.com/en/documents/3906874/the-state-of-privacy-and-personal-data-protection-2019-2 (accessed on 25 April 2020).
12. Kalkman, S.; Mostert, M.; Udo-Beauvisage, N.; van Delden, J.J.; van Thiel, G.J. Responsible data sharing in a big data-driven translational research platform: Lessons learned. *BMC Med. Inf. Decis. Mak.* **2019**, *19*, 283. [CrossRef]
13. Fan, F.Y. *PubMedWordcloud: 'Pubmed' Word Clouds*, R package Version 0.3.6; 2019. Available online: https://CRAN.R-project.org/package=PubMedWordcloud (accessed on 25 April 2020).
14. Taichman, D.B.; Backus, J.; Baethge, C.; Bauchner, H.; de Leeuw, P.W.; Drazen, J.M.; Fletcher, J.; Frizelle, F.A.; Groves, T.; Haileamlak, A.; et al. Sharing Clinical Trial Data—A Proposal from the International Committee of Medical Journal Editors. *N. Engl. J. Med.* **2016**, *374*, 384–386. [CrossRef] [PubMed]
15. Kowalczyk, S.; Shankar, K. Data sharing and the future of science. *Nat. Commun.* **2018**, *9*, 2817.
16. Science Journals: Editorial Policies. 2020. Available online: https://www.sciencemag.org/authors/science-journals-editorial-policies (accessed on 25 April 2020).
17. Taylor, C.F.; Field, D.; Sansone, S.A.; Aerts, J.; Apweiler, R.; Ashburner, M.; Ball, C.A.; Binz, P.A.; Bogue, M.; Booth, T.; et al. Promoting coherent minimum reporting guidelines for biological and biomedical investigations: The MIBBI project. *Nat. Biotechnol.* **2008**, *26*, 889–896. [CrossRef]
18. BMJ Author Hub-Data Sharing. 2019. Available online: https://authors.bmj.com/policies/data-sharing/ (accessed on 25 April 2020).
19. BioMed Central. Structuring Your Data, Materials, and Software. 2019. Available online: https://www.biomedcentral.com/getpublished/writing-resources/structuring-your-data-materials-and-software (accessed on 25 April 2020).
20. Public Library of Science. Data Availability. 2019. Available online: https://journals.plos.org/plosone/s/data-availability (accessed on 25 April 2020).
21. Nosek, B.A.; Alter, G.; Banks, G.C.; Borsboom, D.; Bowman, S.D.; Breckler, S.J.; Buck, S.; Chambers, C.D.; Chin, G.; Christensen, G.; et al. Promoting an open research culture. *Science* **2015**, *348*, 1422–1425. [CrossRef] [PubMed]
22. The Center for Open Science (COS). The TOP Guidelines. 2020. Available online: https://cos.io/top/ (accessed on 25 April 2020).
23. Knoppers, B.M.; Thorogood, A.M. Ethics and big data in health. *Curr. Opin. Syst. Biol.* **2017**, *4*, 53–57. [CrossRef]
24. U.S. Congress. Health Insurance Portability and Accountability Act-Privacy Rule. 1996. Available online: https://www.hhs.gov/hipaa/for-professionals/privacy/index.html (accessed on 25 April 2020).
25. Parliament of Canada. Personal Information Protection and Electronic Documents Act. 2000. Available online: https://www.canlii.org/en/ca/laws/stat/sc-2000-c-5/latest/sc-2000-c-5.html (accessed on 25 April 2020).
26. Dijstelbloem, H.; Huisman, F.; Miedema, F.; Mijnhardt, W. Why Science Does Not Work as It Should And What To Do about It. 2013. Available online: http://www.scienceintransition.nl/app/uploads/2013/10/Science-in-Transition-Position-Paper-final.pdf (accessed on 25 April 2020).
27. Baker, M. 1500 scientists lift the lid on reproducibility. *Nature* **2016**, *533*, 452–454. [CrossRef] [PubMed]

28. Nationaal Programma Open Science. Open Science. Available online: https://www.openscience.nl/en/open-science (accessed on 25 April 2020).
29. De la Fuente, G.B. What is Open Science? Introduction. 2020. Available online: https://www.fosteropenscience.eu/node/1420 (accessed on 25 April 2020).
30. Cohen, J.K. Mayo Clinic's New Data-Sharing Initiative Launches First Project. 2020. Available online: https://www.modernhealthcare.com/information-technology/mayo-clinics-new-data-sharing-initiative-launches-first-project (accessed on 25 April 2020).
31. Ketchum, K. How Data Sharing Could Change the Entire Healthcare Industry. 2018. Available online: http://www.healthcarebusinesstech.com/data-sharing/ (accessed on 25 April 2020).
32. Hulsen, T. The ten commandments of translational research informatics. *Data Sci.* **2019**, *2*, 341–352. [CrossRef]
33. Wilkinson, M.D.; Dumontier, M.; Aalbersberg, I.J.; Appleton, G.; Axton, M.; Baak, A.; Blomberg, N.; Boiten, J.W.; Santos, L.B.d.; Bourne, P.E.; et al. The FAIR Guiding Principles for scientific data management and stewardship. *Sci. Data* **2016**, *3*, 160018. [CrossRef]
34. Doel, T.; Shakir, D.I.; Pratt, R.; Aertsen, M.; Moggridge, J.; Bellon, E.; David, A.L.; Deprest, J.; Vercauteren, T.; Ourselin, S. GIFT-Cloud: A data sharing and collaboration platform for medical imaging research. *Comput. Methods Programs Biomed.* **2017**, *139*, 181–190. [CrossRef]
35. Rake, E.A.; van Gelder, M.; Grim, D.C.; Heeren, B.; Engelen, L.; van de Belt, T.H. Personalized Consent Flow in Contemporary Data Sharing for Medical Research: A Viewpoint. *Biomed. Res. Int.* **2017**, *2017*, 7147212. [CrossRef]
36. Sync for Science-Helping Patients Sharing EHR Data with Researchers. 2017. Available online: http://syncfor.science/ (accessed on 25 April 2020).
37. Mandel, J. Sync for Science: Empowering Individuals to Participate in Health Research. 2018. Available online: https://blog.verily.com/2018/03/sync-for-science-empowering-individuals.html (accessed on 25 April 2020).
38. The All of Us Research Program Investigators. The "All of Us" Research Program. *New Engl. J. Med.* **2019**, *381*, 668–676. [CrossRef] [PubMed]
39. European Commission. Declaration of Cooperation-Towards access to at Least 1 Million Sequenced Genomes in the European Union by 2022. 2018. Available online: https://ec.europa.eu/newsroom/dae/document.cfm?doc_id=50964 (accessed on 25 April 2020).
40. The ICGC/TCGA Pan-Cancer Analysis of Whole Genomes Consortium, Pan-cancer analysis of whole genomes. *Nature* **2020**, *578*, 82–93. [CrossRef] [PubMed]
41. Quinn, B. Google Given access to Healthcare Data of up to 1.6 Million Patients. 2016. Available online: https://www.theguardian.com/technology/2016/may/04/google-deepmind-access-healthcare-data-patients (accessed on 25 April 2020).
42. Blumenthal, D.; Chopra, A. Apple's Pact with 13 Health Care Systems Might Actually Disrupt the Industry. 2018. Available online: https://hbr.org/2018/03/apples-pact-with-13-health-care-systems-might-actually-disrupt-the-industry (accessed on 25 April 2020).
43. GovLab. Wanted: Data Stewards-(Re-)Defining the Roles and Responsibilities of Data Stewards for an Age of Data Collaboration. 2020. Available online: http://thegovlab.org/wanted-data-stewards-re-defining-the-roles-and-responsibilities-of-data-stewards-for-an-age-of-data-collaboration/ (accessed on 25 April 2020).
44. VANTAGE6. Available online: http://vantage6.ai (accessed on 25 April 2020).
45. Dutch Techcentre for Life Sciences (DTL). Personal Health Train. 2019. Available online: https://www.dtls.nl/fair-data/personal-health-train/ (accessed on 25 April 2020).
46. van Soest, J.; Sun, C.; Mussmann, O.; Puts, M.; van den Berg, B.; Malic, A.; van Oppen, C.; Towend, D.; Dekker, A.; Dumontier, M. Using the Personal Health Train for Automated and Privacy-Preserving Analytics on Vertically Partitioned Data. *Stud. Health Technol. Inf.* **2018**, *247*, 581–585.
47. Deist, T.M.; Dankers, F.J.W.M.; Ojha, P.; Marshall, M.S.; Janssen, T.; Faivre-Finn, C.; Masciocchi, C.; Valentini, V.; Wang, J.; Chen, J.; et al. Distributed learning on 20,000+ lung cancer patients. *Pers. Health Train. Radiother. Oncol.* **2020**, *144*, 189–200. [CrossRef] [PubMed]
48. Commit2Data. CARRIER-Coronary ARtery Disease: Risk Estimations and Interventions for Prevention and EaRly Detection. 2019. Available online: https://commit2data.nl/en/commit2data-program/gezondheid/big-data-health-early-detection-and-prevention-of-cardiovasculair-diseases/carrier-coronary-artery-disease-risk-estimations-and-interventions-for-prevention-and-early-detection (accessed on 25 April 2020).

49. Gaye, A.; Marcon, Y.; Isaeva, J.; LaFlamme, P.; Turner, A.; Jones, E.M.; Minion, J.; Boyd, A.W.; Newby, C.J.; Nuotio, M.-L.; et al. DataSHIELD: Taking the analysis to the data, not the data to the analysis. *Int. J. Epidemiol.* **2014**, *43*, 1929–1944. [CrossRef] [PubMed]
50. Kaye, J.; Moraia, L.B.; Curren, L.; Bell, J.; Mitchell, C.; Soini, S.; Hoppe, N.; Oien, M.; Rial-Sebbag, E. Consent for Biobanking: The Legal Frameworks of Countries in the BioSHaRE-EU Project. *Biopreserv. Biobank.* **2016**, *14*, 195–200. [CrossRef] [PubMed]
51. Dissanayake, I.; Nerur, S.; Singh, R.; Lee, Y. Medical Crowdsourcing: Harnessing the "Wisdom of the Crowd" to Solve Medical Mysteries. *J. Assoc. Inf. Syst.* **2019**, *20*, 4.
52. CrowdMed. CrowdMed. 2020. Available online: https://www.crowdmed.com/ (accessed on 25 April 2020).
53. Meyer, A.N.D.; Longhurst, C.A.; Singh, H. Crowdsourcing Diagnosis for Patients With Undiagnosed Illnesses: An Evaluation of CrowdMed. *J. Med. Internet. Res.* **2016**, *18*, e12. [CrossRef]
54. Lupton, E. Looking to the Future of Data Sharing. 2019. Available online: https://researchdata.springernature.com/users/208739-emily-lupton/posts/43809-looking-to-the-future-of-data-sharing (accessed on 25 April 2020).

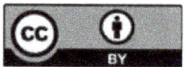

© 2020 by the author. Licensee MDPI, Basel, Switzerland. This article is an open access article distributed under the terms and conditions of the Creative Commons Attribution (CC BY) license (http://creativecommons.org/licenses/by/4.0/).

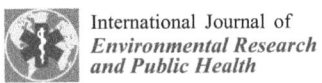

Article

Digital Training for Non-Specialist Health Workers to Deliver a Brief Psychological Treatment for Depression in Primary Care in India: Findings from a Randomized Pilot Study

Shital S. Muke [1], Deepak Tugnawat [1], Udita Joshi [1], Aditya Anand [1], Azaz Khan [1], Ritu Shrivastava [1], Abhishek Singh [1], Juliana L. Restivo [2], Anant Bhan [1], Vikram Patel [2,3] and John A. Naslund [2,*]

[1] Sangath, 120 Deepak Society, Chuna Bhatti, Kolar Road, Bhopal 462016, India; shital.muke@sangath.in (S.S.M.); deepak.tugnawat@sangath.in (D.T.); udita.joshi@sangath.in (U.J.); aditya.a@sangath.in (A.A.); azaz.khan@sangath.in (A.K.); ritu.shrivastava@sangath.in (R.S.); abhishek.singh@sangath.in (A.S.); anant.bhan@sangath.in (A.B.)
[2] Department of Global Health and Social Medicine, Harvard Medical School, Boston, MA 02115, USA; Juliana_Restivo@hms.harvard.edu (J.L.R.); vikram_patel@hms.harvard.edu (V.P.)
[3] Department of Global Health and Population, Harvard TH Chan School of Public Health, Boston, MA 02115, USA
* Correspondence: john_naslund@hms.harvard.edu

Received: 30 June 2020; Accepted: 28 August 2020; Published: 1 September 2020

Abstract: *Introduction*: Task sharing holds promise for scaling up depression care in countries such as India, yet requires training large numbers of non-specialist health workers. This pilot trial evaluated the feasibility and acceptability of a digital program for training non-specialist health workers to deliver a brief psychological treatment for depression. *Methods*: Participants were non-specialist health workers recruited from primary care facilities in Sehore, a rural district in Madhya Pradesh, India. A three-arm randomized controlled trial design was used, comparing digital training alone (DGT) to digital training with remote support (DGT+), and conventional face-to-face training. The primary outcome was the feasibility and acceptability of digital training programs. Preliminary effectiveness was explored as changes in competency outcomes, assessed using a self-reported measure covering the specific knowledge and skills required to deliver the brief psychological treatment for depression. Outcomes were collected at pre-training and post-training. *Results*: Of 42 non-specialist health workers randomized to the training programs, 36 including 10 (72%) in face-to-face, 12 (86%) in DGT, and 14 (100%) in DGT+ arms started the training. Among these participants, 27 (64%) completed the training, with 8 (57%) in face-to-face, 8 (57%) in DGT, and 11 (79%) in DGT+. The addition of remote telephone support appeared to improve completion rates for DGT+ participants. The competency outcome improved across all groups, with no significant between-group differences. However, face-to-face and DGT+ participants showed greater improvement compared to DGT alone. There were numerous technical challenges with the digital training program such as poor connectivity, smartphone app not loading, and difficulty navigating the course content—issues that were further emphasized in follow-up focus group discussions with participants. Feedback and recommendations collected from participants informed further modifications and refinements to the training programs in preparation for a forthcoming large-scale effectiveness trial. *Conclusions*: This study adds to mounting efforts aimed at leveraging digital technology to increase the availability of evidence-based mental health services in primary care settings in low-resource settings.

Keywords: depression; psychological treatment; task sharing; primary care; pilot study; non-specialist health worker; training; digital technology; mental health

1. Introduction

According to the global burden of disease study, nearly 200 million people were living with mental disorders in India by 2017, which represents 14.3% of the total population of the country [1]. This includes over 45 million people living with depressive disorder, the leading mental health contributor to the global disease burden, comprising approximately 3.3% of the total population of the country [1]. The National Mental Health Survey of India 2015–16 found that the prevalence of depression was about 2.7% and the lifetime prevalence was 5.3% in the study population [2]. Several studies have reported a significant gap between those living with depression and those who have access to adequate care [3,4]. The National Mental Health Survey estimated that the care gap for current depression was 79.1% [2], while in some regions of the country this gap exceeds 90% [5].

The World Health Organization's (WHO) Mental Health Gap Action Programme (mhGAP) recommends brief psychological interventions as first-line treatments for depression [6]. However, access to brief psychological treatments remains a significant challenge, particularly in lower-income countries like India. This is partly due to the limited number of available specialist providers to deliver these treatments or supervise care, as well as to train other therapists [7,8]. Task sharing involves building the capacity of non-specialist health workers, which include a broad range of frontline health workers who do not have specialized training in mental health care, to deliver brief evidence-based psychological treatments for common mental disorders [9]. This approach appears to be a key strategy to address the care gap for depression, as reflected by mounting evidence that non-specialist health workers can effectively deliver brief psychological treatments for depression across a range of lower resource settings [10–12].

In India, the formation of the National Mental Health Policy of India in 2014 [13] and enforcement of the Mental Health Care Act 2017 [14], as well as revised guidelines of the National Mental Health Program (NMHP) [15], are major drivers at the policy and health system level for expanding and integrating mental health services in primary health care [16]. These recent legislative developments have highlighted the importance of task sharing as being critical to achieving universal coverage of basic mental health services. A major barrier to the successful implementation and scale up of task sharing is the need to adequately train sufficient non-specialist health workers to deliver brief psychological treatments and to ensure that this workforce achieves the necessary clinical competencies to sustain delivery of high-quality care [17–19].

In India, conventional face-to-face residential training requiring extended stays at government training facilities is the typical approach for training non-specialist health workers, such as ASHAs (Accredited Social Health Activists) through the National Health Mission [20–23]. However, there are financial and logistical challenges, such as the need for expert trainers to lead the training, as well as the requirement of significant travel across long distances for participants to attend the training [7,24]. Therefore, this method of training health workers is limited by poor scalability. The increasing availability and use of digital technologies, such as smartphones, among non-specialist health workers offer new opportunities to support training and skill-building without requiring in-person instruction [25,26]. For instance, mobile internet penetration continues to increase rapidly in many low-resource countries, with close to 450 million people in 2020 in India having internet access from their phones [27]. While many frontline health workers do not have access to or own smartphones, this is changing in several parts of India as government health systems are now providing smartphones to health workers to support them in their work [28,29].

To date, there have been promising initial efforts demonstrating the feasibility of using digital technology as a tool for enhancing in-person training programs for non-specialist health workers in a low-resource setting in rural Pakistan [30]. Additionally, prior studies have demonstrated promising findings using digital technology to support task-sharing mental health services in low-resource settings through the use of digital tools for diagnosis, guiding clinical decision making, and facilitating supervision [25]. Specifically in India, recent studies have reported on a successful digital decision-support platform for supporting community health workers and primary care providers in the screening, diagnosis, and management of common mental disorders [31]; the use of an Android app with tailored video content for training community volunteers about mental health, connecting individuals with available services, and raising awareness [32]; and the initial feasibility and acceptability of a digital game accessible from a smartphone app involving a problem-solving intervention for adolescent mental health [33]. These studies highlight the viability and promise of digital interventions for mental health in low-resource settings such as India; however, there remains an immediate need to generate evidence on the feasibility, acceptability, and potential effectiveness of using a fully remote digital training program delivered on a smartphone application to non-specialist health workers in a rural area of a low-resource setting.

In earlier formative research, we demonstrated the interest in using digital technology for accessing a training program to deliver a brief psychological treatment for depression among non-specialist health workers in Madhya Pradesh, India [34]. We found that a digital platform was feasible for use among non-specialist health workers, and through a series of focus group discussions, we gained valuable stakeholder insights about what features could make a digital training program interesting and appealing for this target group. Specifically, participants provided suggestions for simplifying the language in the program contents and materials, and using familiar terms tailored to the local context; they also recommended adding more images or graphics and interactive features to create a more engaging training program [34]. Drawing from these findings, our team developed a digital program for training non-specialist health workers to deliver the Healthy Activity Program (HAP), a brief evidence-based psychological treatment for depression in primary care [35].

Our next step, and primary objective of this pilot study, was to determine the feasibility and acceptability of this digital training program compared to conventional face-to-face training. In this pilot study, our goal was to collect data on the use of the digital training, such as navigating the smartphone app and accessing the training content, as well as participant feedback to inform refinements to the digital training as well as our study procedures in preparation for a larger fully powered effectiveness trial. Specifically, we conducted this three-arm randomized pilot trial to explore the acceptability and feasibility of two digital training programs (digital training alone and digital training with remote support), and to explore changes in competency outcomes compared to conventional face-to-face training for non-specialist health workers, to deliver the evidence-based HAP treatment for depression in Sehore, a rural district in Madhya Pradesh, India.

We included a third arm in this pilot study to test the use of remote support for enhancing engagement and completion of the digital training program. Our rationale for using remote support stems from the existing online education literature highlighting that additional support can promote participant engagement and completion in online learning programs [36,37]. While this study was primarily focused on determining the feasibility and acceptability of the digital training program, we also collected a measure of competency to assess preliminary effectiveness, which was defined by the acquisition of the knowledge and skills required to deliver HAP.

2. Material and Methods

This exploratory three-arm randomized pilot study followed the extension of CONSORT guidelines to pilot studies [38]. In this study, non-specialist health workers were recruited from three community health centers (i.e., Doraha, Bilkishganj, and Shyampur) in the Sehore district of Madhya Pradesh, India. This study site was selected because Sangath, the research organization leading this project, has a close partnership and an established Memorandum of Understanding with the state government. Additionally, the goal was to create a model of depression care that could be successfully delivered by non-specialist health workers in Sehore district and then scaled up to other districts in the state, and also to other regions of India. Madhya Pradesh is a large, centrally located state with over 72 million people, of which nearly 73% reside in rural areas [39]. Relative to many other Indian states, Madhya Pradesh ranks lower with respect to human development and availability of resources [40,41]. According to the 2016 National Mental Health Survey of India, the care gap for mental disorders in Madhya Pradesh exceeds 90% [5]. Ethics review boards at Sangath, India (VP_2017_028), and Harvard Medical School, USA (IRB17-0092), approved all study procedures.

2.1. Sample

The target sample for this pilot trial was 45 non-specialist health workers. This sample size was considered sufficient for achieving our primary goal of assessing acceptability and feasibility of the training programs [42] and was also selected to ensure we had the minimum number of participants for in-person instruction in the face-to-face training (n = 15). The sample included Accredited Social Health Activists (ASHAs), ASHA Facilitators and Multi-Purpose Health Workers (MPWs) employed in the National Health Mission (Madhya Pradesh state) in India. ASHAs are all women, and a cadre of community health workers in India, introduced by the National Health Mission (NHM) in 2005 with the goal to serve as health activists in the community, create awareness on health and its social determinants, as well as to mobilize the community especially marginalized populations to increase utilization and accountability of the existing health services [43]. Each ASHA covers a population of 1000 and receives performance-based and service-based incentives as compensation for facilitating immunization, referral, and escort services for institutional deliveries [44]. ASHA Facilitators work as a support mechanism to ASHAs to provide mentoring and support and to monitor performance. One ASHA Facilitator typically works with 10 to 20 ASHAs [43]. MPWs are male health workers who are appointed primarily for the control of communicable diseases and are a key functionary at Sub-Health Centers, which are the most peripheral health facilities covering a population of 5000 to deliver preventative health services to the community [43].

Eligible non-specialist health workers who met the inclusion criteria of having age ≥18 years (the minimum age required for employment by the National Health Mission [22,45]); being a certified non-specialist health worker (i.e., ASHA, ASHA Facilitator, or MPW); having a minimum education level of 8th standard (i.e., to ensure they can read and write to access the digital program, written training materials, and complete study assessments); willing to provide written informed consent; and, willing to complete the full training program and stay in the study area during the pilot trial period. Non-specialist health workers were excluded if they had participated in prior formative research activities conducted by our research team (due to prior exposure to the training content), which we confirmed by referring to the list of non-specialist health workers provided by a National Health Mission official in the district (see below), or if they had significant speech, sight, or hearing impairment, or were unable to read or write. Smartphone ownership was not required to participate, as participants were provided with a smartphone to access the digital training programs.

2.2. Recruitment Procedure

A district National Health Mission official provided the list of non-specialist health workers from the three community health centers. Community health centers represent secondary level health services facilities designed to provide referrals as well as specialist care to rural populations [46,47]. We screened the list containing 377 health workers based on the criteria of age (18 years and above), education (8th standard and above), and non-participation in earlier formative research activities. We found a total of 302 potentially eligible health workers. From this list, our data manager randomly selected 92 potentially eligible health workers using the Research Electronic Data Capture (REDCap) software [48]. Research assistants then contacted these potentially eligible health workers by phone to confirm their interest and availability to participate in this pilot study.

Potentially eligible non-specialist health workers were invited to attend a group information session at a nearby community health center to learn more about the study. The research team organized the group information session to describe the purpose of the study and to inform participants that this study involves collaboration with the National Health Mission. The information session also served as a way to explain what the training involves, the study procedures, and the pre- and post-training assessments. This was also an opportunity for participants to ask questions about the study, and to emphasize that their decision to participate was completely voluntary. After the group information session, non-specialist health workers who expressed interest in participating confirmed their eligibility criteria (age and education), and were provided with an information sheet and completed individual written-informed consent. During the individual consent process, health workers were informed that their decision to participate or withdraw from the study at any time would not have any adverse consequences on their current standing as a health worker or their employment status, and that any data collected during the study would be kept confidential and that no identifiable results would be shared with the health system or others outside the research team.

2.3. Randomization

Participants were randomly allocated to one of three training programs based on stratification variables of age, education, and type of non-specialist health worker (i.e., ASHA, ASHA Facilitator, MPW). The study data manager conducted the randomization using the randomizer package available in R software. The age range of recruited ASHAs (24–42 years), ASHA Facilitators (31–46 years), and MPWs (39–52 years) varied widely, hence it was decided to keep different cut-off points for stratification based on the average age for each category of health worker. Two strata for age variables for ASHAs were age ≤35 and age >35; for ASHA Facilitators were age ≤37 and age >37; and for MPWs were age ≤47 and age >47. Similarly, stratification for education for ASHAs was 8th standard and >8th standard; for ASHA Facilitators was 8–12th standard and >12th standard; and for MPWs was 8–12th standard and >12th standard. In total, there were 12 strata to maintain a balance of participant characteristics across study arms. This also served as an opportunity to pilot test our randomization procedures in preparation for the forthcoming larger trial.

2.4. Training Programs

The training programs in this study were designed to provide instruction to non-specialist health workers to gain the clinical skills and competencies necessary to deliver the Healthy Activity Program (HAP) for treatment of depression [49]. The HAP is an evidence-based brief psychological treatment for depression designed and tested in Goa, India, that has demonstrated effectiveness and cost-effectiveness in primary care settings in India [35], as well as sustained clinical benefits [50]. The success of the HAP for treating depression has also been demonstrated in other lower-resource contexts, including among people receiving treatment for multidrug-resistant tuberculosis [51] and people with severe depression in primary care settings in Nepal [52], and as part of recent efforts to scale up mental health services in Madhya Pradesh [53]. The HAP consists of two manuals covering general counseling skills and treatment specific skills. These manuals are open source and available online (http://www.sangath.in/). These manuals were adapted to the local context of Madhya Pradesh and converted into digital and F2F training programs (i.e., covering the same content using different teaching strategies). In this pilot study, we compared three different training programs: conventional face-to-face (F2F) training; digital training (DGT); and digital training with remote support (DGT+).

2.4.1. Conventional Face-to-Face Training (F2F)

The conventional F2F training consists of a six-day classroom training facilitated by two experienced counselors with certification as Master Trainers, meaning that they have significant experience delivering the HAP to patients with depression in clinical settings, have completed instruction in being an effective trainer, and have provided training to other health workers in the delivery of the HAP. This conventional in-person training is considered the 'gold-standard' in training non-specialist health workers based on the prior methods employed in the evaluation and delivery of the HAP treatment [35]. The six-day training is hosted in a community setting and follows the content in the HAP manuals. This form of in-person training is consistent with the type of training currently available to non-specialist health workers in the district.

2.4.2. Digital Training (DGT)

DGT consists of a digitized version of the HAP manuals hosted on the Moodle Learning Management System and accessible through a smartphone app [54]. The training program content was divided across 16 modules following the same structure as the F2F instruction. The modules consisted of expert lecture videos, role-play videos showing clinical scenarios, PowerPoint presentations, reading materials, interactive quizzes embedded within the modules, and assessment questions at the end of each module. Duration of digital training content was matched to the duration of the F2F training, and consisted of approximately 48 h, covering the time required to view the content, read the accompanying materials, and complete the interactive quizzes and assessment questions. Participants were provided with a smartphone to access the training program and were invited to attend a short orientation session to learn how to use the phone, access the instructional content through the smartphone app, and navigate the Learning Management System interface. Participants were provided with a 30-day window to complete the digital training. Throughout the training, participants could contact our research team for technical assistance regarding any concerns or challenges with using the smartphone or accessing the training program content.

2.4.3. Digital Training with Remote Support (DGT+)

The DGT+ training program includes access to the same smartphone app, digital training content, and technical support described above for the DGT program. DGT+ included the addition of remote support from the research team. This involved weekly phone calls from a research assistant to participants. The purpose of the support phone calls was to check in with participants about their progress with the training, and whether they had experienced any challenges or had questions about the digital platform or program content. The research assistant also provided participants with encouragement and praise during the calls as a way to motivate participants and support engagement in the training.

2.5. Outcome Assessment

We collected outcomes on acceptability and feasibility of the training programs and preliminary effectiveness of the training on competency outcomes. After informed consent, a unique participant ID number was assigned to each participant. This number was used on all subsequent data collection forms, with no participant name or identifiable information used on any of the data collection forms. Prior to the outcome assessment, participants were informed of the purpose of using participant ID numbers for their identification throughout the study duration, rather than using their names. Study outcomes were collected before and after the training using paper-based forms distributed in-person at the community health center. The average duration of completing the outcome assessment was approximately 2 h. We used paper-based forms instead of digital data collection to avoid giving an unfair advantage to participants in the digital training programs, as the F2F training participants may not have had equivalent exposure to use of digital technology. Members of our research team who were blind to arm allocation, and who were not involved in the development of the training programs, collected the outcome assessments.

2.5.1. Acceptability and Feasibility Indicators

We collected process indicators to determine participant engagement and use of each of the training programs. This included: daily attendance at the F2F training; metrics collected from the Learning Management System for the digital training programs (for both the DGT and DGT+ programs), including the number of days to complete the training program and the number of modules completed; the number of phone calls made by the participants for seeking technical assistance (for both the

DGT and DGT+ programs) from the research team; and the number of phone calls initiated by the research team to participants for follow up with their queries and types of challenges or questions that commonly were mentioned (for the DGT+ only).

After completing the training (end line), we also collected a satisfaction and acceptability questionnaire adapted from an existing measure of motivation and engagement in face-to-face and online education programs called the MUSIC® model of motivation inventory [55–58]. The 26-item questionnaire asks about the level of satisfaction with the training, acceptability of the content and method of instruction, and feasibility of completing the training. The items are rated on a six-point Likert scale, and relate to feasibility, acceptability, adoption, and appropriateness of the training programs. The questionnaire was translated into Hindi and modified for the F2F and digital (DGT and DGT+) training programs. The items are rated on a six-point Likert scale, with 1 being the lowest and 6 the highest score. The questionnaire covers the domains of acceptability, appropriateness, adoption, and feasibility. The average score of each domain was calculated by adding the score of all the items in the domain divided by the number of questions in the domain.

We also conducted one focus group discussion for all the participants in each arm to obtain feedback about the training and to ask questions pertaining to acceptability and appropriateness of the content, methods of instruction, and engagement in the training, as well as the feasibility of accessing and navigating the digital training platform on the smartphone app, and providing recommendations for what could be improved in the training program. The focus group discussions lasted about 45–60 min, were facilitated by a qualitative researcher and were audio-recorded for analysis. Another researcher from our team observed the focus groups to collect field notes to identify key recommendations from participants for modifying the training programs.

2.5.2. Preliminary Effectiveness Outcome

Competency outcomes were collected before (baseline) and after (end line) the training to determine the preliminary effectiveness of the different training programs. Competency was assessed using a questionnaire consisting of short clinical vignettes followed by multiple-choice questions covering the core skills and competencies needed to deliver the HAP. The measure was based on prior research showing that self-assessment can reliably assess therapist competency following training [24,59,60]. Three equivalent versions of the questionnaire were used to allow repeat testing. The measure focuses on testing knowledge of the HAP treatment as well as applied knowledge of how to deliver the treatment, an essential aspect of provider competence. This questionnaire is scored from 0 to 100, with higher scores reflecting higher levels of knowledge and competency. The questionnaire was translated into Hindi for this study, and modifications were made to fit the local context, such as simplifying complex or technical language and using local terms. Experienced counselors reviewed the Hindi translation to ensure that it was appropriate for administering to non-specialist health workers in the local context in Madhya Pradesh. To avoid "teaching to the test" [61], none of the individuals involved in the development of the HAP training materials had access to the competency assessment questionnaire.

2.6. Data Analysis

Descriptive statistics were computed for socio-demographic characteristics between the three training programs. Process indicators and the satisfaction questionnaires were summarized in tables. Field notes were collected during the focus group discussions to capture key feedback for supporting refinements to the programs. As this was a pilot study with the primary goal of determining feasibility and acceptability of the training programs and to inform improvements to the instructional content and delivery of the training programs, we did not conduct an in-depth thematic analysis of the qualitative data. Rather, we followed guidance from the person-based approach to intervention development [33,62], which enabled the combination of quantitative and qualitative data to inform modifications to the training programs. Specifically, we used a framework analysis approach [63] to guide our identification of common topics within the qualitative data, following a coding framework with the four core domains outlined from the satisfaction and acceptability questionnaire (i.e., appropriateness, acceptability, adoption, and feasibility) [55]. One researcher from our team who was not involved in the development of the training programs coded the transcripts following this *a priori* framework and categorized key observations from participants according to each of the broad domains. Two additional researchers from our team who supported the development of the training programs reviewed the classification of participants' observations and the key recommendations for improving the program. This second round of review provided an opportunity to expand on any observations that were not clear, and to draw from the field notes to supplement the description of the recommendations. A fourth researcher who was external to this process then reviewed the tables summarizing the qualitative feedback to ensure that actionable steps could be identified for improving the usability and acceptability of the training programs in preparation for a subsequent large scale randomized controlled effectiveness study.

As part of an exploratory analysis of change in the competency assessment outcome, we used a paired *t*-test to determine if there was a statistically significant mean difference between the competency scores obtained before and after the training. We also explored pre- and post-training differences in the competency assessment scores within the three training programs using a non-parametric Wilcoxon signed-rank test [64]. This method was selected to account for the small sample size. Due to the heteroscedasticity, since the *p*-value for the Bartletts's test for homogeneity of variance was less than 0.05, we used Welch's one-way ANOVA test to determine if the change in competency assessment scores obtained before and after the training program was different for the three arms, followed with a Games–Howell post-hoc test. All analyses were completed using STATA (StataCorp LLC, College Station, TX, USA), and $p < 0.05$ was considered statistically significant.

3. Results

Out of 92 potentially eligible non-specialist health workers, we contacted a total of 73 until reaching our recruitment target of 45. These 45 non-specialist health workers were invited to attend the group information session to learn more about the study. As outlined in Figure 1, 42 consented and enrolled in the study and were randomly allocated to the three study arms. This included 23 ASHAs, 10 ASHA Facilitators, and 9 MPWs. Participant characteristics are summarized in Table 1. Of the 42 enrolled participants, 36 started the training programs to which they were randomized ($n = 10$ in F2F; $n = 12$ in DGT; $n = 14$ in DGT+) and 36 (86%) participants completed post-training assessments ($n = 11$ in F2F; $n = 12$ in DGT; $n = 13$ in DGT+). We found that there were no differences in participant baseline characteristics (such as type of health worker, mean age, education, and gender) between those who completed the training compared with those who did not complete the training. No harms were recorded for any participants throughout the duration of this pilot study.

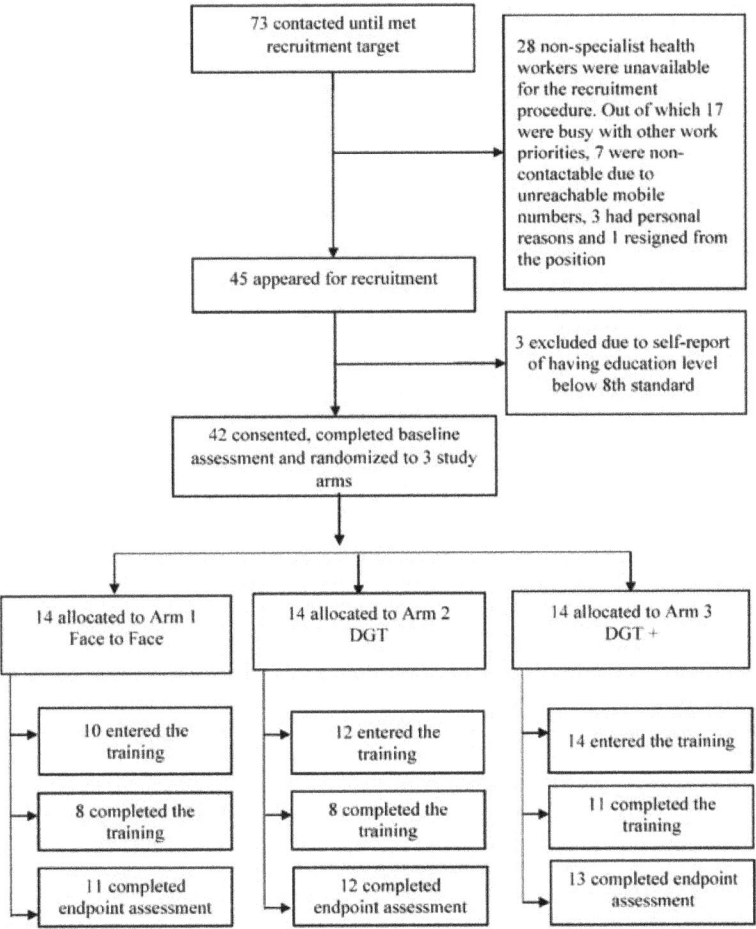

Figure 1. Participant flow diagram. DGT: Digital Training.

Table 1. Baseline socio-demographic characteristics of study participants.

Socio-Demographic Characteristics	F2F n n = 14	DGT n n = 14	DGT+ n n = 14	p-Value
Gender				1
Female	11 (79%)	11 (79%)	11 (79%)	
Male	3 (21%)	3 (21%)	3 (21%)	
Designation				1
ASHA	8 (57%)	7 (50%)	8 (57%)	
ASHA Facilitator	3 (21%)	4 (29%)	3 (21%)	
MPW	3 (21%)	3 (21%)	3 (21%)	
Education				0.51
8th to 10th	8 (57%)	9 (64%)	6 (43%)	
Above 10th	6 (43%)	5 (36%)	8 (57%)	
Experience in years mean (95% CI) *	9.73 (6.71, 12.76)	8.96 (5.37, 12.55)	8.38 (5.32, 11.44)	0.8153
Age in years mean (95% CI) *	36.07 (31.34, 40.80)	37.71 (32.43, 42.99)	36 (31.31, 40.68)	0.8341
Type of mobile phone owned #				0.931
Ordinary mobile phone	7 (50%)	6 (43%)	6 (43%)	
Smartphone	7 (50%)	7 (50%)	8 (57%)	
Family Size (number of persons in household) mean (95% CI)	5.3 (4.19, 6.42)	4.85 (3.07,6.63)	5.35 (3.62, 7.09)	0.868
Previous Experience in Mental Health Training **	(n = 11)	(n = 12)	(n = 14)	0.591
Yes	5 (46%)	8 (67%)	8 (57%)	
No	6 (54%)	4 (33%)	6 (43%)	
How many years before took part in the training mean (95% CI) *	3 (0.67, 5.32)	3 (2.22, 3.77)	3.13 (1.6, 4.66)	0.9814

one missing value in DGT arm. * Means ± CIs are presented for continuous variables, counts for categorical variables. ** The non-specialist health workers had previously learned about mental health issues associated with domestic violence during their routine trainings. However, they have not received any formal training on delivering brief psychological treatments for mental health problems such as depression. We collected the data for this question after the baseline assessment; hence, the number of respondents is lower. F2F: Face-to-Face; DGT: Digital Training; ASHA: Accredited Social Health Activists; MPW: Multi-Purpose Workers.

3.1. Acceptability and Feasibility Indicators

Process indicators are listed in Table 2. Six participants never started the training program, out of which 5 were the MPWs and 1 was an ASHA. The reasons for not starting the training were largely due to other work commitments, and other personal or family commitments. Further, several participants ($n = 9$) started the training but could not complete it. This was similarly due to other family or work commitments, and inclement weather as the training happened during the monsoon season (making it difficult to travel to the training facility for F2F participants). Thus, 27 (64%) participants completed the full training program, with 8 (57%) in F2F, 8 (57%) in DGT, and 11 (79%) in DGT+. We observed differences in program completion between the different types of non-specialist health workers, where 16 (70%) ASHAs, 8 (80%) ASHA Facilitators, and 3 (33%) MPWs completed the training.

Table 2. Summary of process indicators across the three different training programs.

Number of Participants	F2F (n = 14)	DGT (n = 14)	DGT+ (n = 14)
Started the training	10 (71%)	12 (86%)	14 (100%)
Completed the full training (all modules)	8 (57%)	8 (57%)	11 (79%)
Did not complete all of the modules in the training	2 (14%)	4 (29%)	3 (21%)
Number of phone calls made by participants for seeking technical assistance	NA	149	57
Number of phone calls made by the research team to participants for follow up on their queries	NA	106	87

F2F: Face-to-Face; DGT: Digital Training.

There were a total of 399 support calls related to technical assistance for the digital training programs. Among the DGT participants, there were 255 calls. This involved calls made by the participants and calls made by the research team to respond to the participants. In total, 58% of the calls (149 out of 255) were from participants to the research team. While 42% of the calls (106 out of 255) were from the research team in response to participants' queries. For DGT+ participants, the major difference was that our research team initiated the calls (as opposed to participants initiating calls). Among DGT+ participants, there were 144 calls. In total, our research team initiated 60% of the calls (87 out of 144) to participants, while 40% of the calls (57 out of 144) were from participants to our research team. The number of calls per participant ranged from 4 to 37. The calls primarily related to technical challenges, as summarized in Table 3, such as poor connectivity, the mobile app not loading or being deleted from the phone, and challenges with navigating the course content.

Table 3. Common technical challenges mentioned by participants during phone calls with the research team in the digital training programs.

Registered Queries by Phone	Specific Technical Challenges Encountered
Internet related	• Internet is not working • There is no phone connectivity network in the area • Internet speed is slow • Internet data is over, should I recharge it • Course is not opening even connecting on Wi-Fi
Smartphone handling related	• How to operate smartphone features • Don't know how to use a smartphone • App has been deleted/removed from phone
Moodle Learning Management System app related	• Got logged out from course • The app is requiring me to enter the password • The app is showing an error on the screen • Videos are not opening in the app • Quizzes are not showing up in the app • Videos are running very slow, show continuous booting
Course navigation related	• How to attempt quizzes and in which order to attempt them • How to erase the wrong answer if entered mistakenly in the assessment quiz • How to see in the app how much of the course is completed • How to know what grades I have scored • Completed all three given attempts but would like to attempt more to increase my scores, how to do it
Smartphone hardware/software related	• Phone screen has been broken • Phone is lost

Table 4 summarizes participants' responses to the satisfaction and acceptability questionnaire for each training program. Mean score across the domains was generally 5 or greater (out of a possible score of 6), indicating that participants rated the training programs favorably for feasibility, acceptability, and adoption. Across study arms, appropriateness was ranked lowest, suggesting that additional efforts are necessary to promote engagement with the program content. Findings from the focus group discussions ($n = 28$ participants) were grouped within the same four domains from the satisfaction and acceptability questionnaire, as highlighted in Table 5. Recommendations for improving the F2F training including increasing the duration of the training and clarifying some of the training manual content. For the digital training programs, the main recommendations were related to ensuring that the entire course could be accessed offline due to poor internet connectivity in the region, as well as providing a more comprehensive orientation session at the beginning of the program to provide an overview of the smartphone app and navigating the digital program interface, as well as extending the availability of telephone support from the research team.

Table 4. Participant ratings of satisfaction and acceptability with the training programs *.

Domains of Satisfaction and Acceptability (F2F and DGT)	F2F (n = 11) Mean (SD)	Study Arms DGT (n = 12) Mean (SD)	DGT+ (n = 13) Mean (SD)
Acceptability			
The instructor was available to answer my questions about the coursework (F2F)./I could find answers to questions I had about the coursework (DGT).	5.6 (0.44)	5.2 (1.10)	5.5 (0.52)
The instructor was willing to assist me if I needed help in the course (F2F)./Answers to questions about the coursework were easy to understand (DGT).	5.6 (0.51)	5.1 (1.16)	5.5 (0.51)
The instructor cared about how well I did in this course (F2F)./The instructor in the recorded lecture cared about helping me to learn (DGT).	5.4 (0.51)	5.3 (1.40)	5.2 (1.14)
The instructor was respectful of me (F2F)./The instructor in the recorded lecture used a respectful tone (DGT).	5.4 (1.26)	5.3 (1.21)	5.5 (0.66)
The instructor was friendly (F2F)./The instructor in the recorded lecture used a friendly tone (DGT).	5.7 (0.48)	5.3 (1.21)	5.5 (0.66)
I believe that the instructor cared about my feelings (F2F)./The recorded lecture used familiar language and expressions (DGT).	5.7 (0.48)	4.8 (1.40)	5.2 (1.16)
	5.6 (0.51)	5.4 (1.24)	5.8 (0.6)
Appropriateness			
The coursework held my attention (F2F/DGT).	4.9 (0.57)	5.0 (0.74)	5.1 (0.64)
The instructional methods used in this course held my attention (F2F/DGT).	5.4 (0.51)	5.3 (0.65)	5.3 (1.10)
I enjoyed the instructional methods used in this course (F2F/DGT).	4.9 (1.59)	5.0 (1.27)	4.9 (1.38)
The instructional methods engaged me in the course (F2F/DGT).	5.3 (0.48)	5.3 (0.98)	5.5 (0.77)
I enjoyed completing the coursework (F2F/DGT).	2.7 (1.88)	3.3 (1.82)	4.0 (1.77)
The coursework was interesting to me (F2F/DGT).	5.7 (0.48)	5.3 (1.13)	5.5 (0.66)
	5.5 (0.52)	5.6 (0.66)	5.5 (0.51)
Adoption			
In general, the coursework was useful to me (F2F/DGT).	5.5 (0.38)	5.5 (0.79)	5.6 (0.43)
The coursework was beneficial to me (F2F/DGT).	5.2 (0.42)	5.5 (0.52)	5.5 (0.51)
I found the coursework to be relevant to my future (F2F/DGT).	5.3 (0.48)	5.7 (0.65)	5.7 (0.48)
I will be able to use the knowledge I gained in this course (F2F/DGT).	5.7 (0.48)	5.4 (0.79)	5.6 (0.50)
The knowledge I gained in this course is important for my future (F2F/DGT).	5.6 (0.51)	5.4 (1.24)	5.6 (0.50)
	5.6 (0.51)	5.6 (1.16)	5.6 (0.50)
Feasibility			
I had the opportunity to decide for myself how to meet the course goals (F2F/DGT).	5.2 (0.40)	5.4 (0.81)	5.5 (0.42)
I was confident that I could succeed in the coursework (F2F/DGT).	4.9 (1.10)	5.7 (0.49)	5.8 (0.43)
I had the freedom to complete the coursework my own way (F2F/DGT).	5.1 (1.19)	5.3 (1.21)	5.6 (0.50)
I felt that I could be successful in meeting the academic challenges in this course (F2F/DGT).	5.4 (0.51)	5.3 (0.65)	5.8 (0.43)
I had options on how to achieve the goals of the course (F2F/DGT).	5.3 (0.48)	5.2 (1.19)	5.2 (1.21)
I was capable of getting a high grade in this course (F2F/DGT).	4.4 (1.26)	5.4 (0.79)	5.2 (1.09)
I had control over how I learned the course content (F2F/DGT).	5.5 (0.52)	5.0 (1.53)	5.5 (0.66)
Throughout the course, I felt that I could be successful on the coursework (F2F/DGT).	5.0 (1.15)	5.2 (1.33)	5.5 (0.66)
I had flexibility in what I was allowed to do in this course (F2F/DGT).	5.3 (0.48)	5.4 (1.16)	5.6 (0.51)
	5.5 (0.52)	5.8 (0.38)	5.6 (0.51)

* The satisfaction and acceptability questionnaire was adapted from an existing measure of motivation and engagement in education programs called the MUSIC® model of motivation inventory [55–58]. The measure consists of 26 items and was tailored to the Face-to-Face (F2F) or digital (DGT) training and translated into Hindi for use in this study. The items are rated on a six-point Likert scale, with 1 being the lowest and 6 the highest score. The questionnaire covers the domains of acceptability, appropriateness, adoption, and feasibility. The average score of each domain was calculated by adding the score of all the items in the domain divided by the number of questions in the domain. F2F: Face-to-Face; DGT: Digital Training.

Table 5. Summary of key findings from the focus group discussions with participants in the three training programs.

Focus Group Discussion Themes	F2F (n = 8)	DGT (n = 9) and DGT+ (n = 11)
Acceptability		
Facilitators	<ul><li>Became aware about depression; before the training, did not know much about it</li><li>Felt happy and good about having the chance of being part of training on mental health and depression</li><li>Pleased with the way trainers conducted the training</li></ul>	<ul><li>Enjoyed the subject of the training and found it useful to help people with stress and tension</li><li>Able to relate to the training subject as they had experienced symptoms of depression in their own lives or among people around them</li><li>Pleased to learn about depression and mental illness as it was a new subject for them</li><li>Learned how to do the training on smartphones</li><li>Digital training app was easy to understand and navigate</li><li>Digital training app was attractive, interactive, and well-designed</li></ul>
Challenges and/or suggestions to address the challenges		<ul><li>Some participants sought help from family members (i.e., husband, children, neighbor, etc.) to address challenges faced while using the smartphone and understanding the app</li></ul>
Appropriateness		
Facilitators	<ul><li>Trainers taught the course and were able to address participants' questions</li><li>The role plays and group activities were helpful to learn the topic and helped to decrease hesitation while performing role plays</li><li>Participants used training materials to supplement role plays and group activities</li><li>Liked to learn about the HAP model, PHQ-9, and counseling skills (e.g., how to provide mental support and talk to the person with stress, how to sit during a session, how to ask questions, etc.)</li></ul>	<ul><li>Understandable language</li><li>Learning through video lectures was helpful for learning the content and more quickly</li><li>Interesting to learn about symptoms of depression and how to identify them, suicide risks, PHQ-9, and counseling processes and counseling skills (e.g., how to build rapport and how to talk with patients)</li><li>Provision of a list of all modules was useful</li><li>Multiple chances for attempting questions was helpful to answer the questions correctly and learn more about particular topics</li><li>Did not use the help tab given on the digital training app when facing problems, instead phoned to seek support from the research team</li><li>The support provided by the research team was helpful in addressing questions and challenges</li><li>Active support from the research team worked as a motivating factor</li><li>Interactive questions were interesting and kept participants engaged with the course</li><li>Some participants found the training manual helpful, others did not feel the need to use it</li></ul>
Challenges and/or suggestions to address challenges	<ul><li>Some participants did not use training manual during training</li><li>The training manual should contain details of all sessions of HAP modules explaining practical guidelines to carry out HAP activities and sessions instead of theoretical HAP details</li><li>Training was too packed and heavy, felt like a lot of content taught in six days</li><li>Training days can be increased but that will not be feasible, hence the alternative is to organize refresher training after every 3 or 6 months</li></ul>	<ul><li>Learning PHQ-9 and interpretation of the PHQ-9 score and activity chart was challenging to understand for some participants during the first time viewing the course content; but participants were able to understand the content after reviewing the content again</li><li>Did not check the notifications and messages sent on the digital training app</li><li>Found it difficult to comprehend messages on the phone that were in the English language</li><li>At the time of orientation to the training program, the purpose and use of the help option on the digital training app should be explained</li><li>Calling hours from 10 am to 5 pm to seek support should be extended as health workers remain busy with their work schedules during these hours</li><li>Some of the participants suggested to add subtitles to the videos</li></ul>

Table 5. *Cont.*

Focus Group Discussion Themes	F2F (*n* = 8)	DGT (*n* = 9) and DGT+ (*n* = 11)
Adoption		
Facilitators	• HAP training will be useful to identify the people with stress or tension (i.e., local term for depression) in the community and help them through counseling • Training will be useful for health workers to also address their own mental health issues	• This training can be helpful in providing counseling to people and especially to pregnant women with stress and tension
Challenges and/or suggestions to address challenges		• Wanted the course on their mobile device after completing the training so that they can relearn the training if they forget anything
Feasibility		
Facilitators		• Convenient and flexible to learn the training in the time allotted • Can learn and re-learn the content if needed
Challenges and/or suggestions to address challenges	• Some words in the training were difficult to understand	• Poor internet connectivity created disturbance in learning, and irritation and sometimes frustration lowered motivation to learn • Make the entire course offline to address the issue of poor internet connectivity • Poor mobile network in some of the villages • Use a different mobile service provider to address connectivity issues • Difficulty in understanding how to submit the answers online • Include digital orientation training as part of the course to address the technical challenges • Deleted the digital training app by mistake • Due to the challenge of poor internet connectivity, unable to access all content from the modules as all videos did not play

F2F: Face-to-Face; DGT: Digital Training; HAP: Healthy Activity Program; PHQ-9: 9-item Patient Health Questionnaire.

3.2. Preliminary Effectiveness Outcome

Using a paired *t*-test to explore whether there was a statistically significant mean difference between the competency scores obtained pre- and post-training for all participants (all three training programs combined), we found that participants (N = 36) overall scored better on the post-training assessment (Mean = 35.43; SD = 11.39) compared to the pre-training (baseline) assessment (Mean = 25.82; SD = 7.42), with a maximum attainable score of 100. This represents a significant increase of 9.61 points (95% CI: 5.17 to 14.04), $t(35) = 4.401$, $p < 0.0005$, suggesting that competency scores increased after completing the training program regardless of training format (F2F or digital). For the F2F training, the Wilcoxon signed-rank test showed a significant change in participants' competency scores ($Z = 2.934$, $p = 0.0033$). For the DGT training participants, the change was not significant ($Z = 0.863$, $p = 0.3882$), whereas, for the DGT+ training participants, the change was statistically significant ($Z = 2.271$, $p = 0.0231$), as illustrated in Figure 2. For F2F, the mean competency score improved by 13.8 (SD = 6.6) points, while for the DGT and DGT+ arms it was 2.5 (SD = 7.8) points and 12.7 (SD = 18.2) points, respectively.

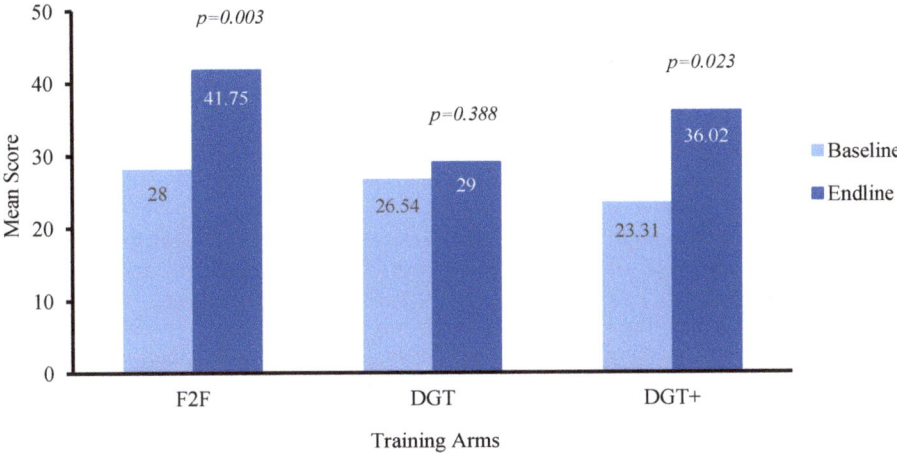

Figure 2. Change in competency assessment scores within each training program. Note: this Figure includes scores from the $n = 11$ in F2F, $n = 12$ in DGT, and $n = 13$ DGT+ participants who completed the post-training (endline) competency measure; though, some of these participants did not complete the training programs. F2F: Face-to-Face; DGT: Digital Training.

Next, we explored changes in scores on the competency measure between training groups. We conducted a Welch's ANOVA test, which showed that there was a statistically significant difference in change in the competency score obtained before and after the training between the three groups, $F(2,21) = 7.0358$, $p = 0.00455$. Following up with a Games–Howell post-hoc test, we found that there was a statistically significant difference in the scores on the competency assessment obtained pre- and post-training between the F2F and DGT arm with $p < 0.01$, but not between the F2F and DGT+ arms.

4. Discussion

This pilot study evaluated the feasibility and acceptability of conventional F2F training compared with digital training programs to build the capacity of non-specialist health workers for delivering HAP, a brief evidence-based psychological treatment for depression. The primary goals of this study were to test the study procedures and, importantly, to inform modifications and refinements to the training programs in preparation for a large-scale fully powered effectiveness trial. While we previously demonstrated the interest in using digital technology for accessing training programs among non-specialist health workers, the current study substantially expanded on our prior work by testing these programs in the field, allowing the opportunity to gain insights about the use of the training programs in real world settings.

This study highlighted the need for several significant modifications to the digital training program. These included: the need to modify the timing and structure of the F2F training to accommodate participants' long commutes from distant villages, as well as to account for their family responsibilities such as childcare; the need to ensure that the digital program content could be accessed entirely offline given the low internet connectivity in rural areas in the Sehore district; the need for a more comprehensive orientation session for using the smartphone app to access the training program and navigating the Learning Management System, including use of more pictures and screenshots of 'how to' examples to account for low digital literacy among participants (this was also reflected by the large number of technical assistance calls received during this pilot study); and modifications to the provision of technical support, to allow early identification of participants who may be struggling to complete the digital training and enable a more timely response to technical challenges that could arise. The challenge of poor internet connectivity was similarly reported in a prior trial from Pakistan, where efforts to address this concern also involved ensuring access to the training content in an offline format [30]. This prior study reported that the online training approach required a stable internet connection that may not be available in many remote, rural, resource-poor settings; hence, to increase the feasibility of the online training program, the researchers used an offline tablet-based application to deliver the training to frontline health workers [30]. Following the focus group discussions, we made substantial modifications to the remote support component of the DGT+ arm, given that participants expressed high interest in having a member of our research team contact them to provide encouragement and motivation on a regular basis.

Our study aligns with an emphasis in the digital mental health research literature that it is necessary to consider the perspectives of users in order to support adoption, engagement, and sustained use of digital interventions [65–67]. Despite the large number of technical challenges that participants mentioned throughout this pilot study, we were reassured by participants' continued interest in learning about the mental health treatment related content. This was consistent between participants in the digital training programs and F2F training, suggesting recognition among non-specialist health workers of the importance of depression care in their communities. This is an essential first step towards successfully scaling up mental health services in primary care settings in the Sehore district, as well as across the state and nation.

Another important finding in this study was about which cadre of non-specialist health workers would be most suitable for completing the training program based on their availability. We learned that the MPWs had too many other competing demands, and were frequently called away by their superiors for attending to urgent duties, which is reflected in their low completion rates across the three training programs. However, for non-specialist health workers who are frequently required to travel for other work related activities, use of a digital training program may offer the opportunity for these individuals to gain the necessary skills to deliver mental health services while accommodating their already busy workload. In addition, digital training holds the potential to train all types of health workers on depression care, as the program can be accessed on a smartphone, which could potentially expand access to mental health services at the community level, thereby advancing efforts to achieve the Mental Health Care Policy goal of providing universal mental health care services for all [13].

While this was a pilot study primarily focused on assessing the feasibility and acceptability of the different training programs, we found that scores on the competency assessment improved for the F2F and DGT+ participants. This is a promising finding, suggesting that digital training with added support may be equally effective compared to the regular classroom or in-person training in terms of gaining knowledge and skills. Also, digital training is potentially more convenient, feasible, and scalable for building the capacity of non-specialist health workers when compared to conventional in-person training, which is supported by similar studies and recent reviews from other low-income and middle-income countries [30,68,69]. Additionally, the findings also indicate that the training content is appropriate for gaining the knowledge and skills related to HAP delivery, as reflected by improved scores on the competency measure. However, the DGT participants did not show significant improvements, suggesting that the use of digital technology alone may not be sufficient for contributing to knowledge acquisition. Importantly, the addition of support initiated by our research team appeared to greatly improve program completion for DGT+ participants (79%) compared to DGT participants (57%). This is consistent with prior studies of online education programs that have demonstrated that the use of digital training is most effective when supplemented with access to remote or in-person support [30,36]. For example, the recent study of the Technology-Assisted Cascaded Training and Supervision system for Lady Health Workers, conducted in rural areas in Pakistan, found that use of digital technology in combination with in-person support and training contributed to comparable improvements in competence as conventional face-to-face training [30]. Additionally, a study in Zambia using technology to train community health workers highlighted a similar finding that in-person support is required to address technical challenges related to poor network coverage, mobile hardware, and software [70]. If these challenges are not addressed, it can negatively impact the delivery process and training outcomes [70]. Further, a recent review of mobile technologies for education and the training of community health workers in low-income and middle-income countries indicated the value of digital training methods for augmenting periodic in-person training activities, while highlighting that digital training programs could be embedded within existing health care services to allow opportunities for continuing education among community health workers [69].

Several limitations with this study warrant consideration. Firstly, this was a pilot study looking at acceptability and feasibility of the training program, and therefore the sample size was small and not adequately powered to detect differences in competency outcomes between groups. Additionally, participants' satisfaction and acceptability ratings were generally very positive, suggesting a potential desirability bias. On the other hand, appropriateness was ranked lower, suggesting the need for improvements to the training programs to promote engagement and sustained interest, which was further reflected during the focus group discussions. The self-report measure used to assess competency outcomes was translated into Hindi and adapted to the local context, though the psychometric properties of this measure have not yet been established for use in rural India. It will be important that further efforts seek to validate this self-report competency measure to support its widespread use in diverse contexts in India. While more scalable and efficient to administer, the use of a self-report measure for competency presents other disadvantages compared to conventional competency assessment methods such as role plays or direct observation because it may not capture the application of skills during direct interactions between the health worker and patient. Furthermore, we made conscious efforts to limit potential bias during the quantitative and qualitative data collection. For instance, the quantitative surveys about satisfaction and acceptability with the training programs may have been subject to social desirability bias, where participants may have reported highly positive responses. To minimize this potential risk, members of our research team overseeing data collection were not involved in the intervention development, and they also reassured participants that there are no right or wrong answers to the questions about program satisfaction because honest feedback is most important for finding ways to improve the training program and content for the future. To minimize a similar risk of social desirability bias in the qualitative data collection, we ensured that the facilitators of the focus group discussions and note taking were also not members of our team involved in the training program development, as they may have influenced participants' responses. Members of our research team who were not involved in the development of the training program conducted the focus group discussions and collected field notes. Given that our study was primarily aimed at informing a subsequent large-scale trial, we did not conduct an in-depth thematic analysis of our qualitative findings. Therefore, in future research developing digital applications, we can build on our approach presented here to strengthen the qualitative methods for analysis and interpretation of participants' feedback and recommendations about program design.

We made an effort to recruit only participants who had not previously participated in our formative research as a method to minimize prior exposure. However, there is still a possible risk of contamination [71], which we did not assess, though we believe that this risk was low. Furthermore, the non-specialist health workers were recruited from real world settings; therefore, it is not possible to fully minimize contamination in such settings, as health workers may look up information about the training materials on the Internet or may talk to each other about the program content in routine encounters in the workplace. Participants were recruited from three community health centers in a single district in Madhya Pradesh, indicating that these findings may not generalize to other settings in India in terms of context and culture, or other settings globally. However, many of the findings reported here relate to the use of digital training in a low-resource setting and overcoming challenges such as low digital literacy and poor bandwidth likely apply to many other settings. Our finding that some cadres of health workers, such as the MPWs, were not able to complete the training due to their prior engagement with work commitments highlights potential challenges for scaling up this type of training program due to competing priorities. Therefore, our findings may only generalize to health workers who have the time available and who are interested and willing to learn about treatment for depression.

To achieve the goal of universal access to mental health services, it will be necessary to consider what cadres of health workers are available and ideally positioned to successfully complete the training program and provide care for depression and other mental disorders as part of their routine service delivery. Furthermore, we restricted our sample to non-specialist health workers with minimum 8th standard education to ensure that they were literate and able to follow the written training materials, to access and navigate the training program on the smartphone app, and to answer the questions on the competency assessment measure. This type of training would likely not be suitable for health workers who may be illiterate, or who may not be able to operate a smartphone. Even though we found that roughly half of the sample had ever used a smartphone, all participants randomized to either of the digital training programs were able to learn to use the smartphone and access the training program content. This further attests to the interest among non-specialist health workers to use digital technology to support their work, which has been consistently reported in prior studies [68,69].

5. Conclusions

The findings and observations from this pilot study offer insights that can inform modifications and improvements to the face-to-face and digital training programs for non-specialist health workers in preparation for a larger fully powered effectiveness trial. A potentially important finding from this pilot study was the apparent motivation for enrollment and starting the training on depression care among non-specialist health workers ($n = 36$ out of $n = 42$) and the motivation to complete this training ($n = 27$ out of $n = 36$), and specifically among ASHAs and ASHA Facilitators. Based on our findings, there seems to be a demand for training in depression care that will be further explored in the forthcoming trial. With digital technologies becoming an increasingly important tool in health systems in many low-resource settings in India, as reflected by efforts to finance the adoption of smartphones among frontline health workers to support care delivery [29], future research can expand on the findings reported here to determine how technology can support the scale up of mental health care. Importantly, it will be necessary to determine how to effectively leverage digital technology to enable supervision and quality assurance for the sustained delivery of high quality psychological treatment for depression, as this will be critical to support task-sharing mental health services in low-resource settings towards addressing the care gap [72].

Author Contributions: Prepared the study outline and manuscript proposal, S.S.M. and J.A.N.; wrote the first draft of the manuscript, S.S.M., D.T., and J.A.N.; data collection, S.S.M. and U.J.; data analysis, S.S.M., A.A., R.S. and A.K.; interpretation of the study findings, S.S.M., A.A., A.K., R.S. and J.A.N.; development and field-testing of the digital training program, A.K., R.S., and D.T.; oversaw the project and supervision, A.B., D.T., V.P. and J.A.N.; reviewed drafts of the manuscript and provided critical and intellectual inputs, A.K., U.J., J.L.R., A.S., A.B. and V.P. All authors have read and agreed to the published version of the manuscript.

Funding: This work was supported by the National Institute of Mental Health (NIMH), USA (grant no. U19MH113211). The funder had no role in study design, data collection and analysis, decision to publish, or preparation of the manuscript.

Acknowledgments: We would like to acknowledge Dinesh Chandke, Kamlesh Sharma, and Narendra Verma, for their contribution to participant recruitment and coordination of endpoint assessments. In addition, we acknowledge Deepali Vishwakarma and Pooja Dhurve, for providing technical support and ensuring effective delivery of the training programs to participants. We would also like to acknowledge the contributions of Medha Upadhye, Miriam Sequeira, and Urvita Bhatia for supporting the development of the training program content. We wish to acknowledge our advisors, collaborators, researchers, and clinicians who have supported our efforts with the ESSENCE project, including Zafra Cooper, Sona Dimidjian, Christopher Fairburn, Steven Hollon, Chunling Lu, Lauren Mitchell, Abhijit Nadkarni, Rohit Ramaswamy, Daisy Singla, and Donna Spiegelman. Additionally, we acknowledge our study participants; the non-specialist health workers for their participation, time, and contribution to this study; and our collaborators from National Health Mission, Madhya Pradesh State and National Health Systems Resource Center, Delhi, India for their support.

Conflicts of Interest: The authors declare no competing interests.

References

1. Sagar, R.; Dandona, R.; Gururaj, G.; Dhaliwal, R.; Singh, A.; Ferrari, A.; Dua, T.; Ganguli, A.; Varghese, M.; Chakma, J.K. The burden of mental disorders across the states of India: The Global Burden of Disease Study 1990–2017. *Lancet Psychiatry* **2020**, *7*, 148–161. [CrossRef]
2. Arvind, B.A.; Gururaj, G.; Loganathan, S.; Amudhan, S.; Varghese, M.; Benegal, V.; Rao, G.N.; Kokane, A.M.; Chavan, B.; Dalal, P. Prevalence and socioeconomic impact of depressive disorders in India: Multisite population-based cross-sectional study. *BMJ Open* **2019**, *9*, e027250. [CrossRef] [PubMed]
3. Pathare, S.; Brazinova, A.; Levav, I. Care gap: A comprehensive measure to quantify unmet needs in mental health. *Epidemiol. Psychiatr. Sci.* **2018**, *27*, 463–467. [CrossRef]
4. Patel, V.; Xiao, S.; Chen, H.; Hanna, F.; Jotheeswaran, A.; Luo, D.; Parikh, R.; Sharma, E.; Usmani, S.; Yu, Y. The magnitude of and health system responses to the mental health treatment gap in adults in India and China. *Lancet* **2016**, *388*, 3074–3084. [CrossRef]
5. Kokane, A.; Pakhare, A.; Gururaj, G.; Varghese, M.; Benegal, V.; Rao, G.N.; Arvind, B.; Shukla, M.; Mitra, A.; Yadav, K. Mental Health Issues in Madhya Pradesh: Insights from National Mental Health Survey of India 2016. In *Healthcare*; Multidisciplinary Digital Publishing Institute: Basel, Switzerland, 2019.
6. World Health Organization. *mhGAP Intervention Guide Mental Health Gap Action Programme Version 2.0 for Mental, Neurological and Substance use Disorders in Non-Specialized Health Settings*; World Health Organization: Geneva, Switzerland, 2016; pp. 1–173.
7. Fairburn, C.G.; Patel, V. The global dissemination of psychological treatments: A road map for research and practice. *Am. J. Psychiatry* **2014**, *171*, 495–498. [CrossRef] [PubMed]
8. Kazdin, A.E. Addressing the treatment gap: A key challenge for extending evidence-based psychosocial interventions. *Behav. Res. Ther.* **2017**, *88*, 7–18. [CrossRef]
9. Raviola, G.; Naslund, J.A.; Smith, S.L.; Patel, V. Innovative Models in Mental Health Delivery Systems: Task Sharing Care with Non-specialist Providers to Close the Mental Health Treatment Gap. *Curr. Psychiatry Rep.* **2019**, *21*, 44. [CrossRef]
10. Singla, D.R.; A Kohrt, B.; Murray, L.K.; Anand, A.; Chorpita, B.F.; Patel, V. Psychological Treatments for the World: Lessons from Low- and Middle-Income Countries. *Annu. Rev. Clin. Psychol.* **2017**, *13*, 149–181. [CrossRef]
11. Hoeft, T.J.; Fortney, J.C.; Patel, V.; Unützer, J. Task-Sharing Approaches to Improve Mental Health Care in Rural and Other Low-Resource Settings: A Systematic Review. *J. Rural. Heal.* **2016**, *34*, 48–62. [CrossRef]
12. Barbui, C.; Purgato, M.; Abdulmalik, J.; Acarturk, C.; Eaton, J.; Gastaldon, C.; Gureje, O.; Hanlon, C.; Jordans, M.; Lund, C.; et al. Efficacy of psychosocial interventions for mental health outcomes in low-income and middle-income countries: An umbrella review. *Lancet Psychiatry* **2020**, *7*, 162–172. [CrossRef]
13. Ministry of Health & Family Welfare. *New Pathways New Hope National Mental Health Policy of India*; Ministry of Health & Family Welfare, Government of India: New Delhi, India, 2014.
14. Ministry of Law and Justice. *The Mental Health Care Act 2017*; Ministry of Law and Justice, Government of India: New Delhi, India, 2017.
15. Directorate General of Health Services. *National Mental Health Programme*; Ministry of Health & Family Welfare, Government of India: New Delhi, India, 2017.
16. Ahuja, S.; Shidhaye, R.; Khan, A.; Roberts, T.; Jordans, M.; Thornicroft, G.; Petersen, I. Understanding mental health system governance in India: Perspectives of key stakeholders. *Preprints* **2020**. [CrossRef]
17. Barnett, M.L.; Lau, A.S.; Miranda, J. Lay health worker involvement in evidence-based treatment delivery: A conceptual model to address disparities in care. *Annu. Rev. Clin. Psychol.* **2018**, *14*, 185–208. [CrossRef] [PubMed]
18. Barnett, M.L.; Gonzalez, A.; Miranda, J.; Chavira, D.A.; Lau, A.S. Mobilizing Community Health Workers to Address Mental Health Disparities for Underserved Populations: A Systematic Review. *Adm. Policy Ment. Health* **2018**, *45*, 195–211. [CrossRef] [PubMed]
19. Padmanathan, P.; De Silva, M.J. The acceptability and feasibility of task-sharing for mental healthcare in low and middle income countries: A systematic review. *Soc. Sci. Med.* **2013**, *97*, 82–86. [CrossRef]
20. National Health Mission. *Update on ASHA Programme*; Ministry of Health and Family Welfare, Government of India: New Delhi, India, 2017.

21. Ministry of Health and Family Welfare, Government of India. *National Rural Health Mission*; Ministry of Health and Family Welfare, Government of India: New Delhi, India, 2011.
22. Ved, R.; Scott, K.; Gupta, G.; Ummer, O.; Singh, S.; Srivastava, A.; George, A. How are gender inequalities facing India's one million ASHAs being addressed? Policy origins and adaptations for the world's largest all-female community health worker programme. *Hum. Resour. Health* **2019**, *17*, 3. [CrossRef]
23. National Rural Health Mission. *ASHA: Which way forward? Evaluation of ASHA Programme*; National Rural Health Mission, National Health Systems Resource Center, National Institute of Health and Family Welfare, Government of India: New Delhi, India, 2011.
24. Fairburn, C.G.; Cooper, Z. Therapist competence, therapy quality, and therapist training. *Behav. Res. Ther.* **2011**, *49*, 373–378. [CrossRef]
25. Naslund, J.A.; Shidhaye, R.; Patel, V. Digital Technology for Building Capacity of Nonspecialist Health Workers for Task Sharing and Scaling Up Mental Health Care Globally. *Harv. Rev. Psychiatry* **2019**, *27*, 181–192. [CrossRef]
26. Naslund, J.A.; Aschbrenner, K.A.; Araya, R.; Marsch, L.A.; Unützer, J.; Patel, V.; Bartels, S.J. Digital technology for treating and preventing mental disorders in low-income and middle-income countries: A narrative review of the literature. *Lancet Psychiatry* **2017**, *4*, 486–500. [CrossRef]
27. Keelery, S. Mobile Phone Internet Users in India 2015–2023. Available online: https://www.statista.com/statistics/558610/number-of-mobile-internet-user-in-india/ (accessed on 7 August 2020).
28. Modi, D.; Dholakia, N.; Gopalan, R.; Venkatraman, S.; Dave, K.; Shah, S.; Desai, G.; Qazi, S.A.; Sinha, A.; Pandey, R.M. mHealth intervention "ImTeCHO" to improve delivery of maternal, neonatal, and child care services—A cluster-randomized trial in tribal areas of Gujarat, India. *PloS Med.* **2019**, *16*, e1002939. [CrossRef]
29. Saha, S.; Kotwani, P.; Pandya, A.; Patel, C.; Shah, K.; Saxena, D.; Puwar, T.; Desai, S.; Patel, D.M.; Sethuraman, A. Addressing comprehensive primary healthcare in Gujarat through mHealth intervention: Early implementation experience with TeCHO+ programme. *J. Fam. Med. Prim. Care* **2020**, *9*, 340. [CrossRef]
30. Rahman, A.; Akhtar, P.; Hamdani, S.U.; Atif, N.; Nazir, H.; Uddin, I.; Nisar, A.; Huma, Z.; Maselko, J.; Sikander, S. Using technology to scale-up training and supervision of community health workers in the psychosocial management of perinatal depression: A non-inferiority, randomized controlled trial. *Glob. Ment. Health* **2019**, *6*, e8. [CrossRef] [PubMed]
31. Maulik, P.K.; Kallakuri, S.; Devarapalli, S.; Vadlamani, V.K.; Jha, V.; Patel, A. Increasing use of mental health services in remote areas using mobile technology: A pre–post evaluation of the SMART Mental Health project in rural India. *J. Glob. Health* **2017**, *7*, 010408. [CrossRef] [PubMed]
32. Shields-Zeeman, L.; Pathare, S.; Walters, B.H.; Kapadia-Kundu, N.; Joag, K. Promoting wellbeing and improving access to mental health care through community champions in rural India: The Atmiyata intervention approach. *Int. J. Ment. Health Syst.* **2017**, *11*, 6. [CrossRef] [PubMed]
33. Gonsalves, P.P.; Hodgson, E.S.; Kumar, A.; Aurora, T.; Chandak, Y.; Sharma, R.; Michelson, D.; Patel, V. Design and development of the 'POD Adventures' smartphone game: A blended problem-solving intervention for adolescent mental health in India. *Front. Public Health* **2019**, *7*, 238. [CrossRef] [PubMed]
34. Muke, S.; Shrivastava, R.; Mitchell, L.; Khan, A.; Murhar, V.; Tugnawat, D.; Shidhaye, R.; Patel, V.; Naslund, J.A. Acceptability and feasibility of digital technology for training community health workers to deliver evidence-based psychosocial treatment for depression in rural India. *Asian J. Psychiatry* **2019**, *45*, 99–106. [CrossRef]
35. Patel, V.; Weobong, B.; Weiss, H.A.; Anand, A.; Bhat, B.; Katti, B.; Dimidjian, S.; Araya, R.; Hollon, S.D.; King, M. The Healthy Activity Program (HAP), a lay counsellor-delivered brief psychological treatment for severe depression, in primary care in India: A randomised controlled trial. *Lancet* **2017**, *389*, 176–185. [CrossRef]
36. Homitz, D.J.; Berge, Z.L. Using e-mentoring to sustain distance training and education. *Learn. Organ.* **2008**, *15*, 326–335. [CrossRef]
37. Friedman, L.W.; Friedman, H. Using social media technologies to enhance online learning. *J. Educ. Online* **2013**, *10*, 1–22. [CrossRef]
38. Eldridge, S.M.; Chan, C.L.; Campbell, M.J.; Bond, C.M.; Hopewell, S.; Thabane, L.; Lancaster, G.A. CONSORT 2010 statement: Extension to randomised pilot and feasibility trials. *BMJ* **2016**, *355*, i5239. [CrossRef]

39. Directorate of Census Operations Madhya Pradesh. *Census of India 2011: Provisional Population Totals Madhya Pradesh*; Ministry of Home Affairs, Government of India: New Delhi, India, 2011.
40. Suryanarayana, M.; Agrawal, A.; Seeta Prabhu, K. *Inequality-Adjusted Human Development Index for India's States*; United Nations Development Programme (UNDP): New Delhi, India, 2011.
41. Menon, P.; Deolalikar, A.; Bhaskar, A. *India State Hunger Index: Comparisons of Hunger Across States*; International Food Policy Research Institute: Washington, DC, USA, 2009.
42. Billingham, S.A.; Whitehead, A.L.; Julious, S.A. An audit of sample sizes for pilot and feasibility trials being undertaken in the United Kingdom registered in the United Kingdom Clinical Research Network database. *BMC Med. Res. Methodol.* **2013**, *13*, 104. [CrossRef]
43. National Health Mission. *Nation Health Mission (M.P.)*; National Health Mission: New Delhi, India, 2018.
44. Saprii, L.; Richards, E.; Kokho, P.; Theobald, S. Community health workers in rural India: Analysing the opportunities and challenges Accredited Social Health Activists (ASHAs) face in realising their multiple roles. *Hum. Resour. Health* **2015**, *13*, 1–13. [CrossRef] [PubMed]
45. Scott, K.; George, A.S.; Ved, R.R. Taking stock of 10 years of published research on the ASHA programme: Examining India's national community health worker programme from a health systems perspective. *Health Res. Policy Syst.* **2019**, *17*, 29. [CrossRef] [PubMed]
46. Satpathy, S. Indian public health standards (IPHS) for community health centres. *Indian J. Public Health* **2005**, *49*, 123–126. [PubMed]
47. Directorate General of Health Services. *Indian Public Health Standard (IPHS) For Community Health Centres (Revised 2010)*; Directorate General of Health Services, Ministry of Health & Family Welfare, Government of India: New Delhi, India, 2010.
48. Harris, P.A.; Taylor, R.; Minor, B.L.; Elliott, V.; Fernandez, M.; O'Neal, L.; McLeod, L.; Delacqua, G.; Delacqua, F.; Kirby, J. The REDCap consortium: Building an international community of software platform partners. *J. Biomed. Inform.* **2019**, *95*, 103208. [CrossRef] [PubMed]
49. Chowdhary, N.; Anand, A.; Dimidjian, S.; Shinde, S.; Weobong, B.; Balaji, M.; Hollon, S.D.; Rahman, A.; Wilson, G.T.; Verdeli, H. The Healthy Activity Program lay counsellor delivered treatment for severe depression in India: Systematic development and randomised evaluation. *Br. J. Psychiatry* **2016**, *208*, 381–388. [CrossRef] [PubMed]
50. Weobong, B.; Weiss, H.A.; McDaid, D.; Singla, D.R.; Hollon, S.D.; Nadkarni, A.; Park, A.-L.; Bhat, B.; Katti, B.; Anand, A. Sustained effectiveness and cost-effectiveness of the Healthy Activity Programme, a brief psychological treatment for depression delivered by lay counsellors in primary care: 12-month follow-up of a randomised controlled trial. *PLoS Med.* **2017**, *14*, e1002385. [CrossRef] [PubMed]
51. Walker, I.F.; Khanal, S.; Hicks, J.P.; Lamichhane, B.; Thapa, A.; Elsey, H.; Baral, S.C.; Newell, J.N. Implementation of a psychosocial support package for people receiving treatment for multidrug-resistant tuberculosis in Nepal: A feasibility and acceptability study. *PLoS ONE* **2018**, *13*, e0201163. [CrossRef]
52. Jordans, M.J.; Luitel, N.P.; Garman, E.; Kohrt, B.A.; Rathod, S.D.; Shrestha, P.; Komproe, I.H.; Lund, C.; Patel, V. Effectiveness of psychological treatments for depression and alcohol use disorder delivered by community-based counsellors: Two pragmatic randomised controlled trials within primary healthcare in Nepal. *Br. J. Psychiatry* **2019**, *215*, 485–493. [CrossRef]
53. Shidhaye, R.; Baron, E.; Murhar, V.; Rathod, S.; Khan, A.; Singh, A.; Shrivastava, S.; Muke, S.; Shrivastava, R.; Lund, C. Community, facility and individual level impact of integrating mental health screening and treatment into the primary healthcare system in Sehore district, Madhya Pradesh, India. *BMJ Glob. Health* **2019**, *4*, e001344. [CrossRef]
54. Khan, A.; Shrivastava, R.; Tugnawat, D.; Singh, A.; Dimidjian, S.; Patel, V.; Bhan, A.; Naslund, J.A. Design and Development of a Digital Program for Training Non-specialist Health Workers to Deliver an Evidence-Based Psychological Treatment for Depression in Primary Care in India. *J. Technol. Behav. Sci.* **2020**. [CrossRef]
55. Jones, B.D. User Guide for Assessing the Components of the MUSIC® Model of Motivation. Available online: https://www.themusicmodel.com/ (accessed on 15 November 2018).
56. Jones, B.D. Motivating students to engage in learning: The MUSIC model of academic motivation. *International. J. Teach. Learn. High. Educ.* **2009**, *21*, 272–285.
57. Jones, B.D. An examination of motivation model components in face-to-face and online instruction. *Electron. J. Res. Educ. Psychol.* **2010**, *8*, 915–944. [CrossRef]

58. Jones, B.D. *Motivating Students by Design: Practical Strategies for Professors*, 2nd ed.; CreateSpace: Charleston, SC, USA, 2018.
59. Cooper, Z.; Doll, H.; Bailey-Straebler, S.; Bohn, K.; de Vries, D.; Murphy, R.; O'Connor, M.E.; Fairburn, C.G. Assessing therapist competence: Development of a performance-based measure and its comparison with a web-based measure. *JMIR Ment. Health* **2017**, *4*, e51. [CrossRef] [PubMed]
60. Restivo, J.L.; Mitchell, L.; Joshi, U.; Anand, A.; Gugiu, P.C.; Hollon, S.D.; Singla, D.R.; Patel, V.; Naslund, J.A.; Cooper, Z. Assessing health worker competence to deliver a brief psychological treatment for depression: Development and validation of a scalable measure. *J. Behav. Cogn. Ther.* **2020**, in press.
61. Popham, W.J. Teaching to the Test? *Educ. Leadersh.* **2001**, *58*, 16–21.
62. Yardley, L.; Morrison, L.; Bradbury, K.; Muller, I. The person-based approach to intervention development: Application to digital health-related behavior change interventions. *J. Med. Internet Res.* **2015**, *17*, e30. [CrossRef]
63. Gale, N.K.; Heath, G.; Cameron, E.; Rashid, S.; Redwood, S. Using the framework method for the analysis of qualitative data in multi-disciplinary health research. *BMC Med. Res. Methodol.* **2013**, *13*, 117. [CrossRef]
64. Rey, D.; Neuhäuser, M. Wilcoxon-Signed-Rank Test. In *International Encyclopedia of Statistical Science*; Gibbons, J.D., Chakraborti, S., Eds.; Springer: Berlin, Germany, 2011; pp. 1658–1659.
65. Naslund, J.A.; Gonsalves, P.P.; Gruebner, O.; Pendse, S.R.; Smith, S.L.; Sharma, A.; Raviola, G. Digital Innovations for Global Mental Health: Opportunities for Data Science, Task Sharing, and Early Intervention. *Curr. Treat. Options Psychiatry* **2019**, *6*, 337–351. [CrossRef]
66. Mohr, D.C.; Lyon, A.R.; Lattie, E.G.; Reddy, M.; Schueller, S.M. Accelerating digital mental health research from early design and creation to successful implementation and sustainment. *J. Med. Internet Res.* **2017**, *19*, e153. [CrossRef]
67. Merchant, R.; Torous, J.; Rodriguez-Villa, E.; Naslund, J.A. Digital technology for management of severe mental disorders in low-income and middle-income countries. *Curr. Opin. Psychiatry* **2020**, *33*, 501–507. [CrossRef]
68. Winters, N.; Langer, L.; Nduku, P.; Robson, J.; O'Donovan, J.; Maulik, P.; Paton, C.; Geniets, A.; Peiris, D.; Nagraj, S. Using mobile technologies to support the training of community health workers in low-income and middle-income countries: Mapping the evidence. *BMJ Glob. Health* **2019**, *4*, e001421. [CrossRef] [PubMed]
69. Winters, N.; Langer, L.; Geniets, A. Scoping review assessing the evidence used to support the adoption of mobile health (mHealth) technologies for the education and training of community health workers (CHWs) in low-income and middle-income countries. *BMJ Open* **2018**, *8*, e019827. [CrossRef] [PubMed]
70. Biemba, G.; Chiluba, B.; Yeboah-Antwi, K.; Silavwe, V.; Lunze, K.; Mwale, R.K.; Russpatrick, S.; Hamer, D.H. A mobile-based community health management information system for community health workers and their supervisors in 2 districts of Zambia. *Glob. Health Sci. Pract.* **2017**, *5*, 486–494. [CrossRef]
71. Keogh-Brown, M.; Bachmann, M.; Shepstone, L.; Hewitt, C.; Howe, A.; Ramsay, C.R.; Song, F.; Miles, J.; Torgerson, D.; Miles, S. Contamination in trials of educational interventions. *Health Technol. Assess.* **2007**, *11*, ix-107. [CrossRef] [PubMed]
72. Kemp, C.G.; Petersen, I.; Bhana, A.; Rao, D. Supervision of Task-Shared Mental Health Care in Low-Resource Settings: A Commentary on Programmatic Experience. *Glob. Health: Sci. Pract.* **2019**, *7*, 150–159. [CrossRef]

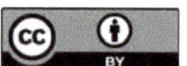

© 2020 by the authors. Licensee MDPI, Basel, Switzerland. This article is an open access article distributed under the terms and conditions of the Creative Commons Attribution (CC BY) license (http://creativecommons.org/licenses/by/4.0/).

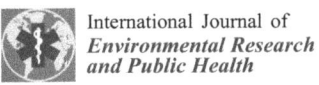

Article

Association of Metabolically Healthy Obesity and Future Depression: Using National Health Insurance System Data in Korea from 2009–2017

Yongseok Seo [1,†], Seungyeon Lee [1,†], Joung-Sook Ahn [2], Seongho Min [2], Min-Hyuk Kim [2], Jang-Young Kim [3], Dae Ryong Kang [4], Sangwon Hwang [5], Phor Vicheka [5] and Jinhee Lee [2,*]

1. Wonju College of Medicine, Yonsei University, Wonju 26426, Korea; s_ys_@naver.com (Y.S.); yeonnii96@gmail.com (S.L.)
2. Department of Psychiatry, Wonju College of Medicine, Yonsei University, Wonju 26426, Korea; jsahn@yonsei.ac.kr (J.-S.A.); mchorock@yonsei.ac.kr (S.M.); mhkim09@yonsei.ac.kr (M.-H.K.)
3. Department of Internal Medicine, Wonju College of Medicine, Yonsei University, Wonju 26426, Korea; kimjy@yonsei.ac.kr
4. Department of Precision Medicine, Wonju College of Medicine, Yonsei University, Wonju 26426, Korea; dr.kang@yonsei.ac.kr
5. Institute of AI and Big Data in Medicine, Wonju College of Medicine, Yonsei University, Wonju 26426, Korea; arsenal@yonsei.ac.kr (S.H.); phorvicheka@yahoo.com (P.V.)
* Correspondence: jinh.lee95@yonsei.ac.kr; Tel.: +82-33-741-1260
† These authors contributed equally to this work.

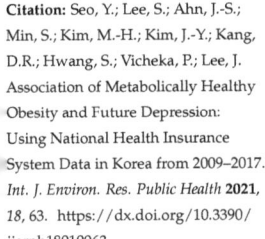

Citation: Seo, Y.; Lee, S.; Ahn, J.-S.; Min, S.; Kim, M.-H.; Kim, J.-Y.; Kang, D.R.; Hwang, S.; Vicheka, P.; Lee, J. Association of Metabolically Healthy Obesity and Future Depression: Using National Health Insurance System Data in Korea from 2009–2017. *Int. J. Environ. Res. Public Health* **2021**, *18*, 63. https://dx.doi.org/10.3390/ijerph18010063

Received: 13 October 2020
Accepted: 17 December 2020
Published: 23 December 2020

Publisher's Note: MDPI stays neutral with regard to jurisdictional claims in published maps and institutional affiliations.

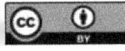

Copyright: © 2020 by the authors. Licensee MDPI, Basel, Switzerland. This article is an open access article distributed under the terms and conditions of the Creative Commons Attribution (CC BY) license (https://creativecommons.org/licenses/by/4.0/).

Abstract: (1) Background: The health implications associated with the metabolically healthy obese (MHO) phenotype, in particular related to symptoms of depression, are still not clear. the purpose of this study is to check whether depression and metabolic status are relevant by classifying them into four groups in accordance with the MHO diagnostic standard. Other impressions seen were the differences between sexes and the effects of the MHO on the occurrence of depression. (2) Methods: A sample of 3,586,492 adult individuals from the National Health Insurance Database of Korea was classified into four categories by their metabolic status and body mass index: (1) metabolically healthy non-obese (MHN); (2) metabolically healthy obese (MHO); (3) metabolically unhealthy non-obese (MUN); and (4) metabolically unhealthy obese (MUO). Participants were followed for six to eight years for new incidences of depression. The statistical significance of the general characteristics of the four groups, as well as the mean differences in metabolic syndrome risk factors, was assessed with the use of a one-way analysis of variance (ANOVA). (3) Results: The MHN ratio in women was higher than in men (men 39.3%, women 55.2%). In both men and women, depression incidence was the highest among MUO participants (odds ratio (OR) = 1.01 in men; OR = 1.09 in women). It was concluded as well that, among the risk factors of metabolic syndrome, waist circumference was the most related to depression. Among the four groups, the MUO phenotype was the most related to depression. Furthermore, in women participants, MHO is also related to a higher risk of depressive symptoms. These findings indicate that MHO is not a totally benign condition in relation to depression in women. (4) Conclusion: Therefore, reducing metabolic syndrome and obesity patients in Korea will likely reduce the incidence of depression.

Keywords: metabolically healthy obese phenotype; metabolic syndrome; obesity; depression

1. Introduction

Obesity is usually one of the metabolic syndrome conditions. It is a cluster of cardiometabolic abnormalities, including elevated high blood pressure, fasting blood glucose and dyslipidemia [1]. However, this does not mean that all obese persons are suffering from metabolic abnormalities, and there is some evidence that the impact of obesity on health can be kept away from individuals who comprise the metabolically healthy obese

(MHO) phenotype [2,3]. It is interesting to note the health implications associated with this phenotype, even though there are no consistent results across studies and the health outcomes have not been examined [4–8].

Obesity and depression are essential factors of disease burden, but the evidence that proves that these two conditions are associated with one another is still not vivid. Even though recent studies including meta-analysis of prospective cohorts have proposed that having a greater body mass index (BMI) can increase the risk of depressive symptoms, several individual studies show that there is no relationship between obesity and depressive symptoms, while another group of individual studies show that greater BMI can reduce the risk of future mental health problems and of suicide [9–12]. Metabolic syndrome has a relationship with depression, independent of obesity [13]. The analysis of the relationship between depressive symptoms and the MHO phenotype sheds light on the association of obesity and depression.

Only a few studies have investigated the relationship between depressive symptoms and the MHO phenotype [14–16]. Two of them have shown that there is not an increased risk of depressive symptoms in MHO individuals followed for two years and ten years in comparison with healthy and non-obese individuals [14,16]. However, in another study, which was a pooled analysis of eight cross-sectional studies, it was shown that there is a moderately increased risk of depressive symptoms in obese individuals with advantageous metabolic profiles in comparison with healthy and non-obese individuals [15].

The purpose of this study is to check whether depression and metabolic status are relevant by dividing them into four groups in accordance with the MHO diagnostic standard. The differences between sexes and the effects of the MHO on the occurrence of depression were observed.

2. Materials and Methods

2.1. Study Population

In this retrospective study, we used a database given by the National Health Insurance Services-Health Screening (NHIS-HEALS) Cohort in Korea. The insurance system was set by the Korean government and covers about 97.2% of the residents. Individuals aged ≥ 40 years can have a general health-screening program every 2 years. The screening has included standardized self-reporting questionnaires on routine laboratory tests of blood and urine, anthropometric and blood pressure measurements, medical history and lifestyle behaviors. The cohort profile of the NHIS-HEALS is presented elsewhere [17]. Furthermore, the NHIS gave a research-specific database from the NHIS-HEALS in accordance with the conditions set by the researchers. Our research-specific database included 2009–2011 data of participants aged 19–69 years who had at least two general health-screening programs in 2009–2011. We extracted a list of participants from the research-specific database and excluded those who were aged ≤ 40 years or ≥ 70 years in 2009 or who did not participate in a general health screening program in 2009 (n = 4,708,511). Thus, all the participants in the list have their own 2009 health screening records. Participants who had one or more missing values in the metabolic syndrome (MetS) components were excluded (n = 9448) because MetS scores were not available. To exclude participants with depression, participants who were receiving medications for depression or who had the following the 10th revision of the international classification of disease (ICD-10) codes (as a main diagnosis or a sub-diagnosis at baseline) were not included: F32.0 to F34.9 (n = 822,603). Medication status was determined by prescription records. Based on the individual's smoking information entered in the survey response, participants whose smoking information had changed or was missing were also excluded (n = 289,968). A total of 3,586,492 participants (1,936,582 men and 1,649,910 women) participated in this study (Supplementary Table S1). The institutional review board of Yonsei University, Wonju College of Medicine, Korea (IRB number: CR318350) approved a Waiver of Informed Consent for this study.

2.2. Measurements and Definitions

Healthcare institutions for screening were selected in accordance with the Framework Act on Health Examinations and the standard requirements for equipment, manpower and facilities. To lessen the measurement errors, the average values of all test data from laboratory between 2009 and 2011 were used. Values beyond the extreme outlier were considered as missing values. Height, weight and waist circumference were measured, and BMI was calculated with the formula BMI = kg/m^2, where kg is a participant's weight in kilograms and m^2 is the square of the participant's height in meters. Blood samples for serum glucose and total cholesterol (TC) level measurement were acquired following an overnight fast [18]. Low-density lipoprotein cholesterol (LDL-C) levels were calculated from TC, high-density lipoprotein cholesterol (HDL-C) and triglyceride (TG) levels or measured directly.

Obesity was defined as BMI ≥ 25 kg/m^2 and metabolically healthy as metabolic syndrome risk < 2 in the 2009–2011 health-screening program. The participant's level of alcohol consumption, frequency of physical activity, family economic status and smoking status were acquired using a set of questions. Smoking status was grouped as current smoker and not, and alcohol consumption as heavy drinker (i.e., consumption of 14 and 7 units of alcohol per week in men and women, respectively) and not. Regular exercise was interpreted as moderate to vigorous intensity physical activity for more than three days each week.

We categorized the participants into four main groups according to their metabolic status and BMI:

1. Metabolically healthy non-obese (MHN): those who have less than two metabolic syndrome risk factors and a BMI under 25 kg/m^2;
2. Metabolically healthy obese (MHO): those who have less than two metabolic syndrome risk factors and a BMI of 25 kg/m^2 or greater;
3. Metabolically unhealthy non-obese (MUN): those who have more than two metabolic syndrome risk factors and a BMI under 25 kg/m^2;
4. Metabolically unhealthy obese (MUO): those who have more than two metabolic syndrome risk factors and a BMI of 25 kg/m^2 or greater.

2.3. Study Outcome

In this study, we registered the population at risk between 2009 and 2011 and analyzed the outcomes in the follow-up period from 2014 to 2017, succeeding a 2-year washout period (2012–2013). The primary endpoint of the study was newly diagnosed depression in the follow-up period. Depression was determined by a recording of international classification of diseases (ICD)-10 codes F32.0 to F34.9 on health insurance data or the taking of an antidepressant (Supplementary Tables S2 and S3). Medication status was determined by the Anatomical Therapeutic Chemical (ATC) code provided in the National Health Insurance Survey.

2.4. Statistical Analysis

The statistical significance of the general characteristics of the four groups and the mean differences in metabolic syndrome risk factor were assessed with the use of one-way analysis of variance (ANOVA). The depression incidence among the four groups was assessed and compared with the odds ratio (OR) using multiple logistic regressions by complex sampling. We applied the multivariable-adjusted proportional hazards model: model 1 adjusted for age, while model 2 adjusted for age, alcohol consumption, exercise and smoking status. We also carried out a subgroup analysis based on the sex of the participants. We also compared the OR between seven metabolic syndrome risk factors adjusted for the participant's age with the use of multiple logistic regressions.

3. Results

3.1. Baseline Characteristics of the Study Population

There were a total of 3,586,492 participants (1,936,582 men and 1,649,910 women) enrolled in this study. Tables 1 and 2 show the baseline characteristics of both the men and women participants included in the analysis by BMI categories and metabolic status. The MHN ratio in women was higher than in men (men 39.3%, women 55.2%). According to the study, 11–12% of obese participants were described as metabolically healthy, i.e., with no more than one metabolic risk factor.

Table 1. Characteristics of the study population at the baseline (men).

	MHN	MUN	MHO	MUO
	(n = 760,561)	(n = 441,741)	(n = 213,940)	(n = 520,340)
Age (years)	50.3 ± 7.85	51.6 ± 7.78	49.4 ± 7.49	50.4 ± 7.64
Income classification				
Highest 25% (%)	13.5	16.2	11.8	15.0
Upper-middle 25% (%)	17.2	18.1	14.7	15.8
Lower-middle 25% (%)	25.9	26.4	24.2	25.4
Lowest 25% (%)	43.4	39.2	49.3	43.8
Alcohol consumption				
≥3/week (%)	20.3	28.9	19.3	26.2
2/week (%)	18.5	20.6	19.7	21.3
1/week (%)	26.2	22.4	26.8	23.4
<1/week (%)	35.1	28.2	34.3	29.1
Non-smokers (%)	24.1	19.5	25.9	21.2
Ex-smokers (%)	34.3	34.4	40.2	39.0
Current smokers (%)	41.6	46.1	33.9	39.8
Vigorous activity (%)	27.0	26.1	31.4	27.5
BMI (kg/m^2)	22.3 ± 1.78	23.0 ± 1.51	26.3 ± 1.18	27.3 ± 1.89
Waist (cm)	79.6 ± 5.06	82.5 ± 4.88	86.7 ± 3.91	91.0 ± 5.34
FBS (mg/dL)	94.1 ± 14.57	110.6 ± 28.47	94.1 ± 12.44	108.9 ± 26.01
HDL (mg/dL)	56.3 ± 18.57	51.5 ± 24.10	53.1 ± 17.94	48.8 ± 19.97
TG (mg/dL)	112.8 ± 55.50	197.9 ± 111.05	127.1 ± 61.80	210.4 ± 117.76
sBP (mmHg)	112.0 ± 10.36	129.5 ± 11.46	122.3 ± 9.72	130.3 ± 11.19
dBP (mmHg)	75.1 ± 6.99	81.8 ± 7.30	76.5 ± 6.73	82.4 ± 7.55

Mean ± standard deviation or proportions of participants are indicated. Abbreviations: BMI, body mass index; dBP, diastolic blood pressure; FBS, fasting blood sugar; HDL, high-density lipoprotein; MHN, metabolically healthy non-obese; MHO, metabolically healthy obese; MUN, metabolically unhealthy non-obese; MUO, metabolically unhealthy obese; sBP, systolic blood pressure; TG, triglyceride. Vigorous activity is defined as physical activity more than three times a week with a strength of moderate, severe or above.

Table 2. Characteristics of the study population at baseline (women).

	MHN	MUN	MHO	MUO
	(n = 910,641)	(n = 258,827)	(n = 198,719)	(n = 281,723)
Age (years)	49.5 ± 7.35	54.2 ± 7.90	51.4 ± 7.66	54.7 ± 7.94
Income classification				
Highest 25% (%)	27.9	26.7	28.8	26.7
Upper-middle 25% (%)	21.7	21.1	22.1	21.8
Lower-middle 25% (%)	20.7	22.9	22.1	24.0
Lowest 25% (%)	29.7	29.4	27.1	27.5
Alcohol consumption				
≥3/week (%)	3.1	3.1	3.3	3.1
2/week (%)	4.6	3.7	4.7	3.9
1/week (%)	15.4	11.0	14.7	11.4
<1/week (%)	76.9	82.2	77.4	81.6
Non-smokers (%)	97.0	96.6	97.5	96.8

Table 2. *Cont.*

	MHN	MUN	MHO	MUO
Ex-smokers (%)	1.1	0.9	0.9	1.0
Current smokers (%)	1.9	2.4	1.6	2.2
Vigorous activity (%)	24.4	23.8	25.1	22.9
BMI (kg/m^2)	22.0 ± 1.77	22.8 ± 1.54	26.6 ± 1.52	27.8 ± 2.35
Waist (cm)	73.0 ± 5.19	76.9 ± 5.42	81.6 ± 4.72	87.0 ± 6.08
FBS (mg/dL)	91.0 ± 10.98	104.8 ± 23.51	92.2 ± 10.78	105.3 ± 23.59
HDL (mg/dL)	62.4 ± 20.69	51.7 ± 21.93	60.6 ± 20.43	52.9 ± 20.98
TG (mg/dL)	90.4 ± 37.37	161.5 ± 81.53	101.1 ± 39.52	159.3 ± 79.25
sBP (mmHg)	116.1 ± 11.28	127.4 ± 12.84	120.3 ± 10.81	129.8 ± 12.37
dBP (mmHg)	72.2 ± 7.47	79.2 ± 8.08	74.3 ± 7.05	80.3 ± 7.86

Mean ± standard deviation or proportions of participants are indicated. Abbreviations: BMI, body mass index; dBP, diastolic blood pressure; FBS, fasting blood sugar; HDL, high-density lipoprotein; MHN, metabolically healthy non-obese; MHO, metabolically healthy obese; MUN, metabolically unhealthy non-obese; MUO, metabolically unhealthy obese; sBP, systolic blood pressure; TG, triglyceride. Vigorous activity is defined as physical activity more than three times a week with a strength of moderate, severe or above.

3.2. Relation between Metabolically Healthy Obesity and Depression

According to the pooled analysis for men participants with MHN as the reference category, a relationship with a higher risk of depressive symptoms was only shown in the MUO group (fully adjusted OR = 1.012; confidence interval (CI) = 1.002, 1.023) (Table 3).

Table 3. Odds ratio (OR) (95% CI) for the relationship between metabolic health and obesity with a risk of depression over three years of follow-up (men).

	Cases/N	Model 1 OR (95% CI)	Model 2 OR (95% CI)
Metabolically healthy non-obese (MHN)	104,143/760,561	1.000 (Ref)	1.000 (Ref)
Metabolically unhealthy non-obese (MUN)	64,297/441,741	1.012 (1.001–1.023)	1.009 (0.998–1.019)
Metabolically healthy obese (MHO)	28,149/213,940	0.999 (0.984–1.013)	1.002 (0.987–1.016)
Metabolically unhealthy obese (MUO)	72,235/520,340	1.014 (1.003–1.024)	1.012 (1.002–1.023)

Abbreviations: CI, confidence interval; Model 1: adjustment for age; Model 2: adjustment for age, alcohol consumption, exercise and smoking status.

In female participants, however, compared to MHN as the reference category, a higher risk of depressive symptoms presented in all three other groups (Table 4). The relationship with depressive symptoms was significantly higher for MUO (fully adjusted OR = 1.096; CI = 1.085, 1.107). In comparison to all non-obese participants (MHN or MUN), the depression risk for MUO (fully adjusted OR = 1.096; CI = 1.085, 1.107) was higher than for MHO (fully adjusted OR = 1.073; CI = 1.061, 1.086). Table 4 also indicates that, in comparison to all metabolically healthy participants (MHO or MHN), the depression risk for MUO (fully adjusted OR = 1.096; CI = 1.085, 1.107) was higher than for MUN (fully adjusted OR = 1.035; CI = 1.024, 1.046).

Table 4. OR (95% CI) for the relationship between metabolic health and obesity with a risk of depression over three years of follow-up (women).

	Cases/N	Model 1 OR (95% CI)	Model 2 OR (95% CI)
Metabolically healthy non-obese (MHN)	189,972/910,641	1.000 (Ref)	1.000 (Ref)
Metabolically unhealthy non-obese (MUN)	63,850/258,827	1.038 (1.027–1.049)	1.035 (1.024–1.046)
Metabolically healthy obese (MHO)	46,256/198,719	1.072 (1.060–1.085)	1.073 (1.061–1.086)
Metabolically unhealthy obese (MUO)	73,531/281,723	1.099 (1.088–1.110)	1.096 (1.085–1.107)

Abbreviations: CI, confidence interval; Model 1: adjustment for age; Model 2: adjustment for age, alcohol consumption, exercise and smoking status.

3.3. Relationship between Metabolic Syndrome Factors and Depression

Tables 5 and 6 have shown the relationship between incident depression and metabolic syndrome factors for males (Table 5) and females (Table 6). In both sexes, the conclusion was that the greater the waist circumference, the greater the frequency of depression. In male participants, fasting blood sugar is also associated with depression (fully adjusted OR = 1.001; CI = 1.001, 1.001), while, in female participants, BMI is also associated with depression (fully adjusted OR = 0.994; CI = 0.994, 0.995).

Table 5. Relationship between metabolic syndrome factors and incident depression (men).

	Model 1	Model 2
	OR (95% CI)	OR (95% CI)
BMI	0.999 (0.998–1.001)	0.978 (0.976–0.981)
Waist	1.004 (1.003–1.004)	1.011 (1.010–1.012)
FBS	1.001 (1.001–1.001)	1.001 (1.001–1.001)
HDL	1.000 (1.000–1.000)	1.000 (1.000–1.001)
TG	1.000 (1.000–1.000)	1.000 (1.000–1.000)
sBP	0.997 (0.997–0.998)	0.997 (0.996–0.998)
dBP	0.996 (0.996–0.997)	0.999 (0.998–1.000)

Abbreviations: BMI, body mass index; CI, confidence interval; dBP, diastolic blood pressure; FBS, fasting blood sugar; HDL, high-density lipoprotein; OR, odds ratio; sBP, systolic blood pressure; TG, triglyceride. Model 1: adjustment for age; Model 2: adjustment for risk factors and age of metabolic syndrome.

Table 6. Relationship between metabolic syndrome factors and incident depression (women).

	Model 1	Model 2
	OR (95% CI)	OR (95% CI)
BMI	1.013 (1.011–1.014)	0.995 (0.993–0.997)
Waist	1.008 (1.007–1.008)	1.010 (1.009–1.010)
FBS	1.001 (1.000–1.001)	1.000 (1.000–1.000)
HDL	1.000 (1.000–1.000)	1.000 (1.000–1.000)
TG	1.001 (1.001–1.001)	1.001 (1.000–1.001)
sBP	0.998 (0.998–0.998)	0.994 (0.994–0.995)
dBP	0.999 (0.999–1.000)	1.004 (1.004–1.005)

Abbreviations: BMI, body mass index; CI, confidence interval; dBP, diastolic blood pressure; FBS, fasting blood sugar; HDL, high-density lipoprotein; sBP, systolic blood pressure; TG, triglyceride. Model 1: adjustment for age; Model 2: adjustment for age and risk factors of metabolic syndrome.

4. Discussion

As far as we know, this is the first Korean population-based study to depict the relevance of both depression and metabolically healthy obesity. Even though recent studies indicate that metabolically healthy obesity (MHO) is related to an increased risk of depressive symptoms, there are still irregularities in the reports [14–16]. However, those analyses did not account for sex. In this study, we have found that the MHO group has a higher future depression risk than other subgroups in female participants, while, in male patients, there is a similar future depression risk to other subgroups.

The principal strength of this study is its nationally representative population-based study design with a huge pooled sample size. Our study is special and different from other results that can meta-analyzed based on the literature and biased by the selective publication of positive results because our current analysis was based on publicly available databases from National Health Insurance Database of Korea and not published results. It is logical to assume that the present results of these datasets generally represent Korea so they are not likely to be subject to a major publication bias.

Bi-directional associations have been outlined for the relationships between metabolic syndrome and depression, proposing that obesity, depressive symptoms and metabolic abnormalities could be associated through multiple pathways [9,19,20]. Using the NHIS-HEALS cohort, we have registered the population at risk between 2009 and 2011 and analyzed the outcomes in the follow-up period from 2014 to 2017. By excluding participants previously diagnosed with depression between 2009 and 2011, it is possible to analyze the temporal direction of the association.

In this study, complete case analysis was done by excluding participants who had one or more missing values in the MetS components (n = 9448) and whose smoking information had changed or was missing (n = 289,968). However, this study did not characterize the excluded population, which can result in bias.

The mechanisms that determine metabolically unhealthy and healthy obesity states are not popular [21,22]. One crucial factor could be where we should store the person's fat, with excess visceral fat being more harmful for metabolic health than excess subcutaneous fat [3]. Additionally, some analysis has shown that people categorized as MHO have different health characteristics to those categorized as MUO, including higher physical activity, lower smoking prevalence and higher educational levels, proposing that both behavioral and physiological factors could be involved [15]. There are also various common biological states that link metabolic factors and obesity to depression, such as impaired glycemic control, inflammation and dysregulation of the hypothalamic–pituitary–adrenocortical axis [23–28]. A different set of factors may determine the depression risk of MHO individuals from non-obese individuals, such as negative self-image, physical inactivity, functional limitations in daily life, social stigma and discrimination [29–31].

The differences in future depression between metabolically healthy obesity men and women are still not known, but there are some studies on the different effects of sex of obesity and depression. One study proposed that prenatal stress-immune programming of the different sexes effects hypothalamic-pituitary-adrenal-gonadal axes and on metabolic and cardiac functions, leading to differences between the sexes in the comorbidity of major depressive disorders and obesity/metabolic syndrome [32]. Another study has shown that obesity has a relationship with different psychosocial profiles in both men and women [33,34]. Women are associated with being overweight and having an increased risk of suicidal tendencies and clinical depression, while men are the opposite [35]. Men may favor a large muscular body rather than a skinny one and having a high body weight may not increase the risk of depression as much as being underweight. Moreover, we also noted that the greater the waist circumference, the greater the frequency of depression. However, including BMI, the incidence of depression did not affect other metabolic syndrome factors.

5. Conclusions

In conclusion, the present results from a large pooled analysis of men and women show that MUO (metabolically unhealthy obesity) has a higher risk of depressive symptoms than MHN (metabolically healthy non-obese). Furthermore, in women participants, MHO (metabolically healthy obesity) is also related to a higher risk of depressive symptoms.

These findings indicate that MHO is not a totally benign condition in relation to depression in women. Therefore, reducing metabolic syndrome and obesity patients in Korea will likely reduce the incidence of depression.

Supplementary Materials: The following are available online at https://www.mdpi.com/1660-4601/18/1/63/s1, Table S1: Study population; Table S2: List of antidepressants selected in the study; Table S3: List of ICD-10 codes selected in the study.

Author Contributions: Y.S., J.L., D.R.K., and J.-Y.K. planned and designed the study. S.L. provided statistical assistance and prepared the figures. Y.S. and S.L. drafted the manuscript. J.-S.A., S.M., S.H., P.V. and M.-H.K. revised the manuscript. All authors have read and agreed to the published version of the manuscript.

Funding: This research was funded by a grant from the Korea Health Technology R&D Project through the Korea Health Industry Development Institute (KHIDI), funded by the Ministry of Health and Welfare, Republic of Korea (grant number: HI19C1035).

Data Availability Statement: The cohort profile of the NHIS-HEALS is presented elsewhere [17].

Conflicts of Interest: The authors declare no conflict of interest.

Abbreviations

BMI	body mass index
CI	confidence interval
dBP	diastolic blood pressure
FBS	fasting blood sugar
HDL	high-density lipoprotein
HDL-C	high-density lipoprotein cholesterol
ICD	international classification of diseases
LDL-C	low-density lipoprotein cholesterol
MHO	metabolically healthy obese
MUN	metabolically unhealthy non-obese
MUO	metabolically unhealthy obese
NHIS-HEALS	National Health Insurance Services-Health Screening
OR	Odds ratio
sBP	systolic blood pressure
TC	total cholesterol
TG	triglyceride

References

1. Eckel, R.H.; Grundy, S.M.; Zimmet, P.Z. The metabolic syndrome. *Lancet* **2005**, *365*, 1415–1428. [CrossRef]
2. Stefan, N.; Haring, H.U.; Hu, F.B.; Schulze, M.B. Metabolically healthy obesity: Epidemiology, mechanisms, and clinical implications. *Lancet Diabetes Endocrinol.* **2013**, *1*, 152–162. [CrossRef]
3. Despres, J.P. What is "metabolically healthy obesity?": From epidemiology to pathophysiological insights. *J. Clin. Endocrinol. Metab.* **2012**, *97*, 2283–2285. [CrossRef] [PubMed]
4. Voulgari, C.; Tentolouris, N.; Dilaveris, P.; Tousoulis, D.; Katsilambros, N.; Stefanadis, C. Increased heart failure risk in normal-weight people with metabolic syndrome compared with metabolically healthy obese individuals. *J. Am. Coll. Cardiol.* **2012**, *58*, 1343–1350. [CrossRef] [PubMed]
5. Thomsen, M.; Nordestgaard, B.G. Myocardial infarction and ischemic heart disease in overweight and obesity with and without metabolic syndrome. *JAMA Intern. Med.* **2014**, *174*, 15–22. [CrossRef] [PubMed]
6. Hinnouho, G.M.; Czernichow, S.; Dugravot, A.; Nabi, H.; Brunner, E.J.; Kivimaki, M.; Singh-Manoux, A. Metabolically healthy obesity and the risk of cardiovascular disease and type 2 diabetes: The Whitehall II cohort study. *Eur. Heart J.* **2014**, *36*, 551–559. [CrossRef]
7. Hinnouho, G.M.; Czernichow, S.; Dugravot, A.; Batty, G.D.; Kivimaki, M.; Singh-Manoux, A. Metabolically healthy obesity and risk of mortality: Does the definition of metabolic health matter? *Diabetes Care* **2013**, *36*, 2294–2300. [CrossRef]
8. Kramer, C.K.; Zinman, B.; Retnakaran, R. Are metabolically healthy overweight and obesity benign conditions?: A systematic review and meta-analysis. *Ann. Intern. Med.* **2013**, *159*, 758–769. [CrossRef]
9. Luppino, F.S.; de Wit, L.M.; Bouvy, P.F.; Stijnen, T.; Cuijpers, P.; Penninx, B.W.; Zitman, F.G. Overweight, obesity, and depression: A systematic review and meta-analysis of longitudinal studies. *Arch. Gen. Psychiatry* **2010**, *67*, 220–229. [CrossRef]

10. Istvan, J.; Zavela, K.; Weidner, G. Bodyweight and psychological distress in NHANES I. *Int. J. Obes. Relat. Metab. Disord.* **1992**, *16*, 999–1003.
11. Crisp, A.H.; McGuiness, B. Jolly fat: Relation between obesity and psychoneurosis in general population. *BMJ* **1976**, *1*, 7–9. [CrossRef] [PubMed]
12. Magnusson, P.K.; Rasmussen, F.; Lawlor, D.A.; Tynelius, P.; Gunnell, D. Association of body mass index with suicide mortality: A prospective cohort study of more than one million men. *Am. J. Epidemiol.* **2006**, *163*, 1–8. [CrossRef] [PubMed]
13. Akbaraly, T.N.; Kivimaki, M.; Brunner, E.J.; Chandola, T.; Marmot, M.G.; Singh-Manoux, A.; Ferrie, J.E. Association between metabolic syndrome and depressive symptoms in middle-aged adults: Results from the Whitehall II study. *Diabetes Care* **2009**, *32*, 499–504. [CrossRef]
14. Hamer, M.; Batty, G.D.; Kivimaki, M. Risk of future depression in people who are obese but metabolically healthy: The English longitudinal study of ageing. *Mol. Psychiatry* **2012**, *17*, 940–945. [CrossRef] [PubMed]
15. Jokela, M.; Hamer, M.; Singh-Manoux, A.; Batty, G.D.; Kivimaki, M. Association of metabolically healthy obesity with depressive symptoms: Pooled analysis of eight studies. *Mol. Psychiatry* **2013**, *19*, 910–914. [CrossRef]
16. Hinnouho, G.-M.; Singh-Manoux, A.; Gueguen, A.; Matta, J.; Lemogne, C.; Goldberg, M.; Zins, M.; Czernichow, S. Metabolically healthy obesity and depressive symptoms: 16-year follow-up of the Gazel cohort study. *PLoS ONE* **2017**, *12*, e0174678. [CrossRef]
17. Seong, S.C.; Kim, Y.Y.; Park, S.K.; Khang, Y.H.; Kim, H.C.; Park, J.H.; Kang, H.-J.; Do, C.-H.; Song, J.-S.; Lee, E.-J.; et al. Cohort profile: The national health insurance service-national health screening cohort (NHIS-HEALS) in Korea. *BMJ Open.* **2017**, *7*, e016640. [CrossRef]
18. Kim, M.K.; Han, K.; Kim, H.-S.; Park, Y.-M.; Kwon, H.-S.; Yoon, K.-H.; Lee, S.-H. Cholesterol variability and the risk of mortality, myocardial infarction, and stroke: A nationwide population-based study. *Eur. Heart J.* **2017**, *38*, 3560–3566. [CrossRef]
19. Pan, A.; Keum, N.; Okereke, O.I.; Sun, Q.; Kivimaki, M.; Rubin, R.R.; Hu, F.B. Bidirectional association between depression and metabolic syndrome: A systematic review and meta-analysis of epidemiological studies. *Diabetes Care* **2012**, *35*, 1171–1180. [CrossRef]
20. Renn, B.N.; Feliciano, L.; Segal, D.L. The bidirectional relationship of depression and diabetes: A systematic review. *Clin. Psychol. Rev.* **2011**, *31*, 1239–1246. [CrossRef]
21. Denis, G.V.; Obin, M.S. 'Metabolically healthy obesity': Origins and implications. *Mol. Aspects Med.* **2013**, *34*, 59–70. [CrossRef] [PubMed]
22. Phillips, C.M. Metabolically healthy obesity: Definitions, determinants and clinical implications. *Rev. Endocr. Metab. Disord.* **2013**, *14*, 219–227. [CrossRef] [PubMed]
23. Raison, C.L.; Miller, A.H. The evolutionary significance of depression in Pathogen Host Defense (PATHOS-D). *Mol. Psychiatry* **2012**, *18*, 15–37. [CrossRef]
24. Capuron, L.; Su, S.; Miller, A.H.; Bremner, J.D.; Goldberg, J.; Vogt, G.J.; Maisano, C.; Jones, L.; Murrah, N.V.; Vaccarino, V. Depressive symptoms and metabolic syndrome: Is inflammation the underlying link? *Biol. Psychiatry* **2008**, *64*, 896–900. [CrossRef]
25. Kivimäki, M.; Shipley, M.J.; Batty, G.D.; Hamer, M.; Akbaraly, T.N.; Kumari, M.; Jokela, M.; Virtanen, M.; Lowe, G.D.; Ebmeier, K.P.; et al. Long-term inflammation increases risk of common mental disorder: A cohort study. *Mol. Psychiatry* **2014**, *19*, 149–150. [CrossRef]
26. Pan, A.; Ye, X.; Franco, Ó.H.; Li, H.; Yu, Z.; Zou, S.; Zhang, Z.; Jiao, S.; Lin, X. Insulin resistance and depressive symptoms in middle-aged and elderly Chinese: Findings from the nutrition and health of aging population in China study. *J. Affect. Disord.* **2008**, *109*, 75–82. [CrossRef]
27. Musselman, D.L.; Evans, D.L.; Nemeroff, C.B. The relationship of depression to cardiovascular disease: Epidemiology, biology, and treatment. *Arch. Gen. Psychiatry* **1998**, *5*, 580–592. [CrossRef]
28. Bornstein, S.R.; Schuppenies, A.; Wong, M.-L.; Licinio, J. Approaching the shared biology of obesity and depression: The stress axis as the locus of gene–environment interactions. *Mol. Psychiatry* **2006**, *11*, 892–902. [CrossRef]
29. Markowitz, S.; Friedman, M.A.; Arent, S.M. Understanding the relation between obesity and depression: Causal mechanisms and implications for treatment. *Clin. Psychol. Sci. Pract.* **2008**, *15*, 1–20. [CrossRef]
30. McElroy, S.L.; Kotwal, R.; Malhotra, S.; Nelson, E.B.; Keck, P.E.; Nemeroff, C.B. Are mood disorders and obesity related? A review for the mental health professional. *J. Clin. Psychiatry* **2004**, *65*, 634–651. [CrossRef]
31. Jokela, M.; Hintsanen, M.; Hakulinen, C.; Batty, G.D.; Nabi, H.; Singh-Manoux, A.; Kivimäki, M. Association of personality with the development and persistence of obesity: A meta-analysis based on individual-participant data. *Obes. Rev.* **2012**, *14*, 315–323. [CrossRef] [PubMed]
32. Goldstein, J.M.; Holsen, L.; Huang, G.; Hammond, B.D.; James-Todd, T.; Cherkerzian, S.; Hale, T.M.; Handa, R.J. Prenatal stress-immune programming of sex differences in comorbidity of depression and obesity/metabolic syndrome. *Dialogues Clin. Neurosci.* **2016**, *18*, 425–436.
33. Van Hout, G.C.M.; Van Oudheusden, I.; Van Heck, G.L. Psychological profile of the morbidly obese. *Obes. Surg.* **2004**, *14*, 579–588. [CrossRef] [PubMed]
34. Mahony, D. Psychological gender differences in bariatric surgery candidates. *Obes. Surg.* **2008**, *18*, 607–610. [CrossRef] [PubMed]
35. Carpenter, K.M.; Hasin, D.S.; Allison, D.B.; Faith, M.S. Relationships between obesity and DSM-IV major depressive disorder, suicide ideation, and suicide attempts: Results from a general population study. *Am. J. Public Health* **2000**, *90*, 251–257.

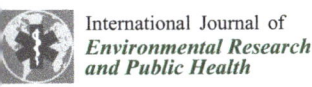

International Journal of *Environmental Research and Public Health*

Article

Assessment of Thoracic Pain Using Machine Learning: A Case Study from Baja California, Mexico

Veronica Rojas-Mendizabal [1,*], Cristián Castillo-Olea [2,*], Alexandra Gómez-Siono [1] and Clemente Zuñiga [3]

1. School of Engineering, CETYS Universidad, Mexicali 21259, Mexico; alexandra.siono@cetys.edu.mx
2. School of Medicine and Psychology, Autonomous University of Baja California, Tijuana 22800, Mexico
3. General Hospital of Tijuana, Tijuana 22000, Mexico; zclemente@hotmail.com
* Correspondence: veronica.rojas@cetys.mx (V.R.-M.); cristian.castillo2@gmail.com (C.C.-O.)

Citation: Rojas-Mendizabal, V.; Castillo-Olea, C.; Gómez-Siono, A.; Zuñiga, C. Assessment of Thoracic Pain Using Machine Learning: A Case Study from Baja California, Mexico. *Int. J. Environ. Res. Public Health* **2021**, *18*, 2155. https://doi.org/10.3390/ijerph18042155

Academic Editor: Tim Hulsen

Received: 26 December 2020
Accepted: 10 February 2021
Published: 23 February 2021

Publisher's Note: MDPI stays neutral with regard to jurisdictional claims in published maps and institutional affiliations.

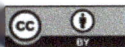

Copyright: © 2021 by the authors. Licensee MDPI, Basel, Switzerland. This article is an open access article distributed under the terms and conditions of the Creative Commons Attribution (CC BY) license (https://creativecommons.org/licenses/by/4.0/).

Abstract: Thoracic pain is a shared symptom among gastrointestinal diseases, muscle pain, emotional disorders, and the most deadly: Cardiovascular diseases. Due to the limited space in the emergency department, it is important to identify when thoracic pain is of cardiac origin, since being a symptom of CVD (Cardiovascular Disease), the attention to the patient must be immediate to prevent irreversible injuries or even death. Artificial intelligence contributes to the early detection of pathologies, such as chest pain. In this study, the machine learning techniques were used, performing an analysis of 27 variables provided by a database with information from 258 geriatric patients with 60 years old average age from Medical Norte Hospital in Tijuana, Baja California, Mexico. The objective of this analysis is to determine which variables are correlated with thoracic pain of cardiac origin and use the results as secondary parameters to evaluate the thoracic pain in the emergency rooms, and determine if its origin comes from a CVD or not. For this, two machine learning techniques were used: Tree classification and cross-validation. As a result, the Logistic Regression model, using the characteristics proposed as second factors to consider as variables, obtained an average accuracy (μ) of 96.4% with a standard deviation (σ) of 2.4924, while for F1 a mean (μ) of 91.2% and a standard deviation (σ) of 6.5640. This analysis suggests that among the main factors related to cardiac thoracic pain are: Dyslipidemia, diabetes, chronic kidney failure, hypertension, smoking habits, and troponin levels at the time of admission, which is when the pain occurs. Considering dyslipidemia and diabetes as the main variables due to similar results with machine learning techniques and statistical methods, where 61.95% of the patients who suffer an Acute Myocardial Infarction (AMI) have diabetes, and the 71.73% have dyslipidemia.

Keywords: machine learning; thoracic pain; tree classification; cross-validation

1. Introduction

Thoracic pain is one of the generally most relevant factors in people with cardiovascular problems at risk of heart attacks. However, despite its relevance in this area, chest pain may be an indicator of some other pathology not related to CVD. In 2015, the WHO (World Health Organization) recorded 17.7 million deaths related to CVD, where 42.8% were due to coronary heart disease and 36.15% to cerebrovascular accidents [1]. While the World Heart Federation in 2017 reported that in Mexico, 77% of deaths were due to NCD (Non-Communicable Diseases), where 24% of these were caused by CVD [2]. In 2018, the INEGI (National Institute of Statistical Geography) reported in Baja California 149,368 cases of death from CVD, where ischemic diseases represented 72.7%, while hypertensive diseases were 15.9%; the rest were split between pulmonary vascular disorders and acute rheumatic fever, among others [3].

Since CVDs are involved with a large percentage of the causes of death in Baja California, a decision was made to analyze a database with information from 258 patients provided by Medica Norte with variables such as Edad, Género, Fumador, HTA, Dyslipidemia, Diabetes, ERC (Cr basal), Suma FRCV, C. Isquémica previa, PPT, Rangos PPT,

Tipo dolor, TnT Ingreso, TnT Curva (4 h), ECG, Tipo Alteración, TC > 100, IC, Alta precoz, UDT, Ingreso, Ergometría, Eco stress, Cate, Angio TAC, IAM, Revascularización (See Appendix A); and thus, with the help of Orange, data analysis was carried out to find which biochemical markers or habits are mostly related to thoracic pain of cardiac origin, to more accurately locate the risk factors involved in development of a cardiac event and dismiss as an emergency those patients with chest pain who do not meet the conditions established for the development of CVD. With these results, a proposal for second parameters to take into account in emergency rooms is produced to avoid possible deaths caused by thoracic pain.

For this analysis, two variables based on troponin were considered, since it is in charge of establishing the frequency of cardiac muscle contraction, which, when affected by a heart attack, is released and can be used as a bio indicator [4]. According to a 2019 study, Troponin has a positive predictive value of 62%, while its negative predictive value is 93% for cardiac lesions [5]. Therefore, the first variable was TnT Ingreso, where troponin levels were measured in the blood of patients on arrival at the emergency room, and the second was TnT curve (4 h), which are the levels of troponin found in the blood of admitted patients four hours later.

When a patient arrives at the emergency room with chest pain, he is evaluated with an exam known as PreTest Probability (PPT), which helps choose the most accurate method of analysis to determine the type of pain in the patient. This PreTest consider variables like gender, age, and some symptoms such as typical angina, atypical angina, or non-anginal pain. Later, depending on the values of these variables, a percentage is established that can be part of one of the four ranges used, and this range will determine the probability that the pain present is due to CVD or not [6].

Among the conventional predictive methods to assess the etiology of thoracic pain are the SCORE (Systematic Coronary Risk Evaluation), ASCVD (AtheroSclerotic Cardio-Vascular Disease) Risk Estimator, and Framingham. The SCORE method is adapted from the guide for CVD prevention in 2016 carried out by a project with the same name, which is based on the calculation of risk factors for the prediction of possible CVDs at 10 years in European patients [7]. On the other hand, ASCVD Risk Estimator evaluates the risk that the patient has of atherosclerosis since this disease affects the arteries causing CVD. While the Framingham method is the most widely used and oldest, since it dates back to 1948, the risk of CVD using this method is calculated by assigning a value to variables related to the patient's condition and subsequently making a summation that will indicate the risk of developing CVD within 10 years [8].

Nowadays, machine learning technologies, deep learning, and artificial intelligence have been a meaningful tool for the healthcare industry. Thus, its classification and patterns recognition capabilities for applications enable the image processing for treatable diseases diagnosis. In addition, predictions based in mathematical models algorithms using databases to classify different diseases related with a specific system and variables correlation to find possible factors associated with high risk of mortality and chronic diseases are used as decision making tool. The way these tools work is by simulating the human brain functioning, with the greatest advantage in big data processing capabilities. This technology offers methods such as supervised learning based (Random Forest, Support Vector Machine, and Artificial Neural Network), unsupervised learning based (capable of finding patterns of unlabeled data and cluster), and hybrid methods based on trial and error (Reinforcement Learning) [9–11].

2. Materials and Methods

For the data analysis employed for this paper, we used Orange software version 3.23. This software offers a visual programming environment that allows analyzing data from statistics to machine learning by using interconnected "widgets" that indicate the flow that data must follow and functions applied to data. To analyze the database provided by Clinic Medical Norte to find the secondary variables to consider a thoracic pain with a cardiac origin, we used 17 widgets.

Five different machine learning algorithms available in the Orange data mining toolkit [12], including k-nearest neighbor (kNN), decision tree, support vector machine (SVM), random forest, and logistic regression, were employed in this study. To evaluate the classification models, we use a 10-fold cross-validation strategy, where the original samples were randomly partitioned into ten equal-sized subsamples, and we retained a single subsample as validation data for testing. For this analysis, we use the following tools of Orange:

Data

- File: Allows to upload the file to analyze. When loading the file, the value of each variable must be selected, that is, whether it is categorical, numeric, or text, and its role within the analysis, if it works as a feature, target, meta, or skip. In this case, our aims were AMI and FRCV; we registered it as categorical.
- Data table: Allows us to visualize in a table the uploaded file.

Visualize

- Scatter plot: This graphic allows us to see continuous data represented in two dimensions.
- Box plot: This graphic shows the distribution of the values of each attribute.
- Classification tree viewer: Allows us to visualize the resulting analysis of the model tree classification. It shows a classification tree that indicates the hierarchy of each value, which allows us to determine the most important.

Models

- Classification Tree.
- Logistic regression.
- Random Forest.
- kNN.
- SVM.

Evaluation:

- Tests and Scores: Analyzes the information using selected models, and shows different parameters like accuracy, Precision, F1, recall.
- Confusion Matrix: Generates a matrix presenting false positives, true positives, false negatives, and true negatives.

2.1. Description of the Database

The database (provided by the Clinic Medical Norte) contains 27 data items from 256 patients (See Appendix B). The average age of the participants included in this study is 60 years. Table 1 presents the assessment criteria used in the patients of the Clinic Medical Norte.

Table 1. Assessment criteria used for patients.

	Classic Patterns of Thoracic Pain			
Condition	Location	Radiating Pain	Duration	Type of Pain
AMI	Retroesternal	Arm, Neck	>15 min	Oppressive
Angina	Retroesternal	Arm, Neck	5–20 min	Oppressive
Aortic dissection	Retroesternal	Interescapular	Constant	Tearing
TEP	Hemithorax	-	Constant	
Pneumothorax	Hemithorax	Neck, Back	Constant	
Pericarditis	Retrosternal, shoulder, arm	Back, Neck	Constant	
Esophageal ruptura	Retrosternal	Posterior Thorax	Constant	
Esofagitis	Retrosternal	Interescapular	Minutes to hours	
Esophageal spasm	Retrosternal	Interescapular	Minutes to hours	
Musculoskeletal	Localized	-	Variable	

Note. Adapted from *Prehospital Medical Emergency Manual* (p. 334), by A. Pacheco-Rodríguez, A. Serrano-Moraza, J. Ortega-Carnicer, F. Hermoso-Gadeo, 2001 [13], Madrid, España: Aran Ediciones. Copyright 2001 by Aran Editions.

2.2. Machine Learning Models for Thoracic Pain Evaluation

Figure 1 shows the thoracic pain management guide. To create these models, we use the variables that provide post-disease information, such as medications. Furthermore, according to the clinical practice guideline, the variables used as a diagnosis were eliminated [14,15].

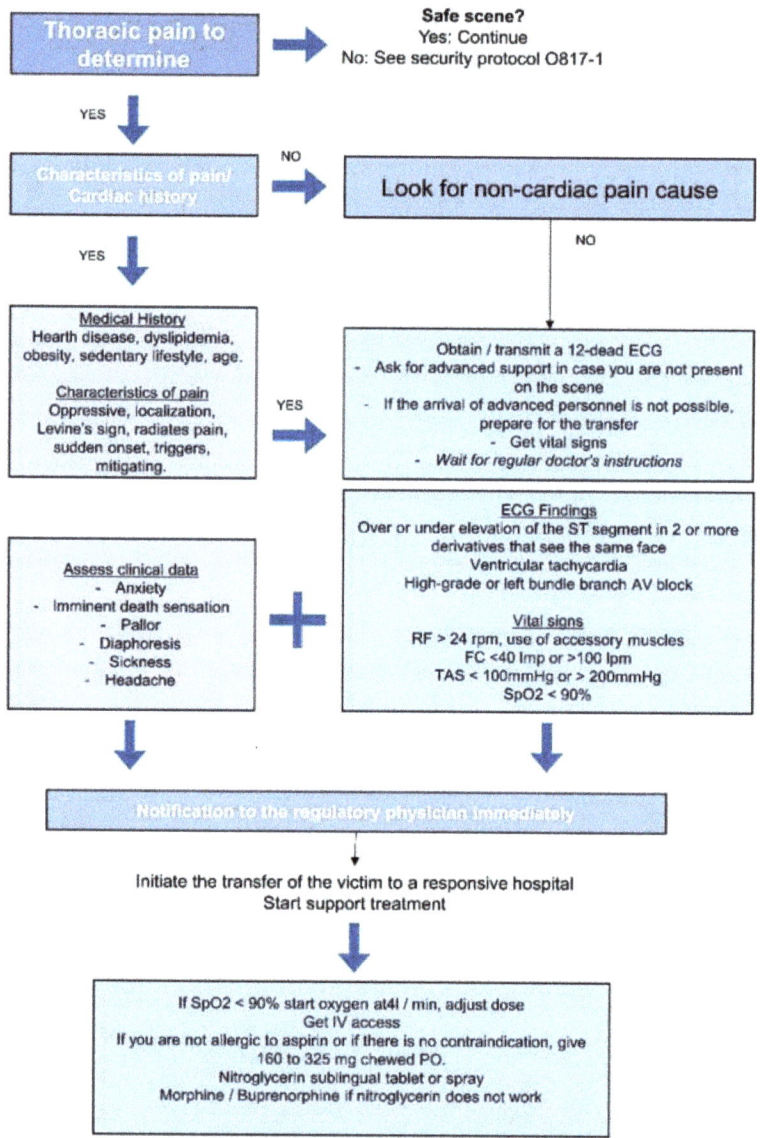

Figure 1. Thoracic pain management guide.

To identify the most influential variables in the different created models, a classification of these variables was done by assigning to each one a score, with the lower scores being indicative of greater importance. For this analysis, we considered a sample of 256 patients, and two machine learning techniques were used: Tree classification and cross-validation. For statistical analysis, the "distributions" tool from Orange was used.

3. Results

The database provided by Clinic Medical Norte is formed by 256 patients, of which 35.66% had an IAM. Of those who suffered from an IAM, 63.04% had dyslipidemia, 50% suffered from CKD, 71.74% had diabetes, 36.96% had Hypertension, 72.42% were smokers or smoke, and 54.35% were men.

3.1. Tree Classification

As mentioned before, in this model, the target was IAM where the decision tree suggested six factors to determine if the person with thoracic pain was in risk to present an IAM; these factors were found as the current considered in the emergency room when a patient with chest pain arrives. Another target examined was the variable of Risk Factors for Cardiovascular Disease (FRCV), this target was considered as a categorical variable, which showed if the patients suffered from a disease of had a negative result in clinical tests, and the result of the decision tree revealed the proposed secondary factors to evaluate if a thoracic pain has a cardiac origin or does not. In Table 2, the results from botch tree classification analysis are shown.

Table 2. Comparison between Acute Myocardial Infarction (AMI) and Risk Factors for Cardiovascular Disease (FRCV) used as a target for Tree classification.

	Tree Classification	
Level	**AMI**	**FRCV**
1	Angio TAC	Dyslipidemia
2	Ergometry	CKD
2	TnT curve 4 h	Diabetes
3	Eco-Stress	Hypertension
3	Catheterization	Smoking habits
4	PPT	Age
5	-	TnT entry
6	-	Gender

3.2. Cross-Validation

For the cross-validation analysis, 66% of the database was used to train the models, using a number of 10 folds as parameter. For this, the used classifiers were: tree classification, random forest, SVM, logistic regression and kNN. Considering the results of the FRCV decision tree, of the previous analysis, these secondary factors were used as targets, of which results are presented in Table 3.

Table 3. Metric's formulas.

Metric	Expresion
Accuracy	$Accuracy = \frac{True\ positive + True\ Negative}{True\ Positive + True\ Negative + False\ Positive + False\ Negative}$
F1	$F = 2 * \frac{Precision * Recall}{Precision + Recall}$
Precision	$Precision = \frac{True\ positive}{True\ Positive + False\ Positive}$
Recall	$Recall = \frac{True\ Positive}{True\ positive + False\ Negative}$

In Table 4, the variables determined as secondary factors to consider when a patient arrives in the emergency room with chest pain are shown. The research suggests a close relation between these diseases and habits, since one can be caused by another. Among these variables, according to the results of the machine learning analysis, dyslipidemia may be considered as the main disease responsible for possible thoracic pain with cardiac origin, followed by hypertension, smoking habits, diabetes, chronic kidney disease, and PPT ranges. In the case of the variable dyslipidemia, the best obtained result was using logistic regression with an accuracy of 0.969, F1 of 0.938, precision of 0.937, and recall of 0.940. In hypertension, we found an accuracy of 0.994, F1 of 0.966, precision of 0.966, and recall of 0.966. For smoking, we found an accuracy of 0.918, F1 of 0.799, precision of 0.796, and recall of 0.803. Lastly, for diabetes, we found an accuracy of 0.986, F1 of 0.961, precision of 0.963, and recall of 0.961. For the variable of PPT ranges, the Random Forest model showed better results, with an accuracy of 0.977, F1 of 0.880, precision of 0.881, and recall of 0.891.

Table 4. Cross-Validation results using a target FRCV decision tree results.

Variables	Classification	Accuracy	F1	Precision	Recall
Dyslipidemia	Tree classification	0.780	0.787	0.787	0.787
	SVM	0.823	0.737	0.750	0.753
	kNN	0.630	0.618	0.614	0.622
	Logistic Regression	0.969	0.938	0.937	0.940
	Random Forest	0.795	0.753	0.614	0.622
Hypertension	Tree classification	0.765	0.762	0.761	0.762
	SVM	0.846	0.757	0.757	0.758
	kNN	0.733	0.689	0.688	0.691
	Logistic Regression	0.994	0.966	0.966	0.966
	Random Forest	0.825	0.762	0.762	0.764
Smoking	Tree classification	0.691	0.580	0.578	0.586
	SVM	0.716	0.514	0.547	0.569
	kNN	0.658	0.510	0.504	0.532
	Logistic Regression	0.918	0.799	0.796	0.803
	Random Forest	0.739	0.587	0.585	0.606
Diabetes	Tree classification	0.712	0.727	0.729	0.701
	SVM	0.746	0.612	0.725	0.705
	kNN	0.546	0.602	0.590	0.625
	Logistic Regression	0.986	0.961	0.963	0.961
	Random Forest	0.733	0.704	0.706	0.724
Rangos PPT	Tree classification	0.997	0.990	0.990	0.990
	SVM	0.895	0.707	0.699	0.720
	kNN	0.992	0.855	0.954	0.960
	Logistic Regression	0.951	0.845	0.841	0.851
	Random Forest	0.977	0.880	0.881	0.891

4. Discussion

In emergency rooms, between 5% and 15% of the patients report thoracic pain, whereby 23.8% of patients with thoracic pain are related to cardiovascular pathologies [16]. Another case that was found to be alarming in the Hospital de la Línea de la Concepción in Cádiz is that 25% of the patients present an AMI (Acute Myocardial Infarction) after they left the emergency room due to a normal electrocardiogram [4], which can be construed as 1 out of 4 patients had a wrong diagnosis, which could lead to a sudden death. For this reason, it is important to find new methods to efficiently classify the origin of thoracic pain, since it can be related to cardiogenic factors either ischemic or not ischemic; and not cardiogenic factors being of gastrointestinal, pulmonar, neuromuscular, or psychological origin [17]. Due to the multiple risk factors for CVD, it is critical to find the nearest linked factor to a sudden death caused by a cardiomyopathy with thoracic pain as a symptom, considering that health conditions and lifestyle, including alimentation, have a considerable impact in CVD development. For this, machine learning techniques and tools are proposed to predict cardiopathies that could lead to sudden death [4,18]. Furthermore, studies found that when a person presents various risk factors, the probabilities to develop a CVD in a 10-year range increases significantly [19]. Hence, it is recognized as widely important to identify the risk factors present when the patient arrives at the emergency room with thoracic pain. This study suggests the use of the risk factors obtained as results in the tree classification analysis and validated by cross-validation method, in the evaluation of the thoracic pain in order to classify it as cardiac or not cardiac, considering these as secondary factors alongside those currently used in the emergency rooms. However, these results must be interpreted with caution and a series of limitations must be taken into account since the study was carried out only with elderly patients and with less than 30 variables; to achieve more precise results in future studies, the use of a database with more variables to consider and a population with different age ranges is proposed, and with this, better training in machine learning models would be achieved, which would allow for finding greater differentiation between variables.

4.1. Relationship of Secondary Factors Variables with IAM

4.1.1. Patients with Smoking Habits

Tobacco consumption increases the oxidative stress due to the free radicals generation for both passive and active consumers, and for this reason it is known as the main factor in the development of different diseases, including CVD. Among the adverse effects in health caused by tobacco consumption besides oxidative stress, studies found a relationship in the increase of the arterial pressure and cardiac frequency, increase in inflammation, developments of atherosclerosis, thrombosis, and damage in both arterial coronary systems [20,21].

Regarding chest pain, a study done with 70,208 participants, which mostly have smoking habits, discusses an experimentation using methods as pain tolerance testing and surveys, which concluded that people with smoking habits tend to have lower pain tolerance; this information is important to know regardless that the intensity has not relation with a cardiac origin pain. Moreover, it was found that the chest pain in smoking patients can be originated by, inter alia, the frequency in tobacco consumption, chronic cough and shortness of breath [22].

4.1.2. Patients with Hypertension

Hypertension is one of the most important risk factors on CVD. Worldwide, hypertension is responsible for 54% of strokes, and 47% of ischemic cardiopathy [23]. It has also been observed that after a decade of presenting hypertension, the risk of contracting any CVD has increased from 15% to 30% [24]. On the other hand, evidence of a study made in 1997 in Chile found interesting results in records of people with obesity, which suggest that obesity increases blood pressure with 6.5 mmHg, plasma cholesterol with 12 mg/dL, and 2 mg/dL of blood glucose for each 10% of accession in the patient's weight [25].

A study described in the Cuban Magazine of Health compares their findings done between 2007 and 2011 with findings made in Spain on 2011, and both results agree with the fact that Hypertension is strongly related with sudden death by a cardiac event; this, due to the development of an adaptive process initiated by blood pressure causing hypertrophy as a result of left ventricular injure. It is also stated that a combination of hypertension with smoking habits or any other risk factor as diabetes, dyslipidemia, and obesity can lead to an increase in the left ventricular hypertrophy expanding the probabilities of suffering a cardiac event [26].

4.1.3. Patients with Diabetes

Diabetes is a disease that is also tightly related with CVD and obesity, when there are no other risk factors involved it is called Diabetic Heart Disease (DHD). Amidst the possible factors of the relationships between these conditions, insulin resistance, hyperglycemia, and hyperinsulinemia were found to be responsible for the decrease in elasticity of the tissue generated by an impact in the production of collagen, which provokes myocardial damage leading to hypertrophy and fibrosis [27].

Despite the fact that in a study carried out in the Grama region, it was determined that patients with DM II who present other cardiovascular risk factors, compared to those without Diabetes, did not present chest pain as a symptom. However, the study suggests that those with DM II are exposed to cardiac failure by a factor of 2.8, since it has also been found that patients with this disease suffer from alterations in diastolic function without having any history of cardiovascular disease [28].

The chemical reactions generated by cardiac metabolism are oxidative in nature, so that as there is a lack of biological contribution to the region of cardiac tissue, ATP is stopped in cardiomyocytes, which in turn, causes a metabolic change due to the lack of oxygen and nutrients directly affecting cardiac functionality [29].

4.1.4. Patients with Chronic Kidney Disease

Chronic Kidney Disease (CRD) is another risk factor linked to CVD. Findings from a study made with dialysis patients revealed that CVD patients start their development in precocious phases of the CRD, causing problems such as left ventricular hypertrophy, atherosclerosis, and vascular calcifications [30]; therefore, early detection and treatment of this disease can reduce the chances of death from CVD, as well as decrease kidney damage, since it was revealed in a study carried out using patients with advanced ECR with and without dialysis, which those with an AMI have a very low chance of survival [31,32]. On the other hand, CKD is found in some cases related to diabetes, which is called diabetic nephropathy, which develops hypertension and kidney damage [33].

4.1.5. Patients with Dyslipidemia

Among the distributions related to patients with dyslipidemia and pain in the database from Medical Norte, 22.87% of the patients with dyslipidemia presented soft pain, while 26.74% presented moderate pain and 14.34% presented severe pain. Of the remaining individuals without dyslipidemia, only 5.81% presented severe pain. Despite these results, it is important to know, beyond pain, how dyslipidemia would affect the cardiovascular system.

Dyslipidemia is a disease where the regulation of lipids in blood is affected by the augmentation of cholesterol and triglycerides, which in turn produces the accumulation of lipids in the arterial walls causing ischemic heart disease, which can lead to death; the main reason of this disease is due to obesity, even though it can be also a genetic disease [34]. The most known disease in Mexico is obesity since, in 2012, 71.3% of the population was diagnosed with obesity, while in Baja California, 74.9% of the population presented obesity and overweight [35]. Obesity is one of the main factors for various diseases, including CVD. The relationship between dyslipidemia and obesity is very close due to the excess of fatty tissue, which produces an insulin resistance [36]; also, it is related to diseases such as Diabetes Mellitus II (DM II). According to the WHO in 2012, 44% of the people living in Baja California developed DM II due to obesity and overweight, pathology related with hypertension, dyslipidemia, CDV, osteoarthritis, and different types of cancer [37].

This documental research confirms the correlation between the proposed secondary risk factors related with possible thoracic pain with cardiac origin. In Figure 1, the diagram above shows graphically the relation between these variables, which was confirmed by both the assessment with machine learning and bibliography. The figure is divided into three main components, the blue navy hexagon in the center indicates the target, which is thoracic pain with cardiac origin, the second level with blue hexagons shows the six main conditions proposed as factors to consider in the determination of a cardiac event with thoracic pain as symptom, and the last level with light blue hexagons shows some effects that the main factors have in health. The orange lines used in Figure 2 express the relationship between the conditions.

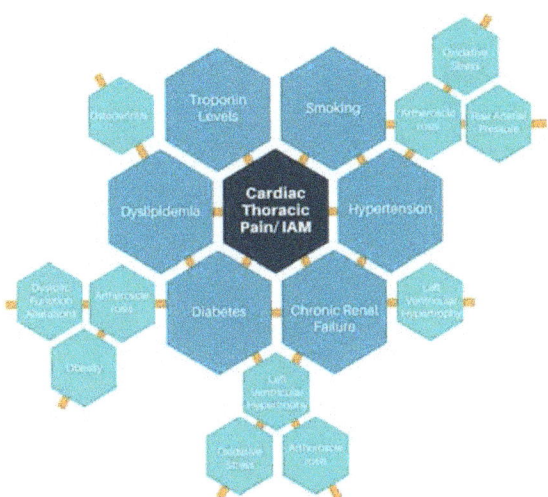

Figure 2. Relationship between secondary risk factors variables.

5. Conclusions

Among the main health problems presented in the country are deaths from obesity problems and cardiovascular diseases, which in turn are related to each other, sharing other risk factors. When considering cardiovascular problems as diseases that can cause sudden events involving a person's life, it is important to learn to recognize the patterns that these cardiac events present and to take into account the factors that have the greatest impact on their development. It is known that in emergency rooms, there are a limited number of patients to attend, and since thoracic pain is a symptom of a future cardiac event, but also a symptom of different diseases, it is important to learn to recognize when thoracic pain is of cardiac origin and non-cardiac.

Nowadays, there are different computer tools such as machine learning, deep learning, and artificial intelligence, which, through algorithms, can find patterns and classify a large number of data. This is why it was decided to carry out a machine learning analysis of a database provided by Clinic Medical Norte in Tijuana, Baja California, Mexico. The results of this analysis suggest variables that can be considered secondary conditions to classify thoracic pain as cardiac in addition to those already established in the emergency department, such as Troponin levels, smoking habits, and diseases such as dyslipidemia, chronic kidney disease, diabetes, and hypertension.

Author Contributions: Conceptualization, C.Z. and C.C.-O.; Methodology, C.C.-O., V.R.-M. and C.Z.; Software, A.G.-S. and C.C.-O.; Validation, C.C.-O., V.R.-M. and C.Z.; Formal Analysis, A.G.-S., C.C.-O. and V.R.-M.; Investigation, V.R.-M., C.C.-O.; Resources, C.Z.; Data Curation A.G.-S., C.C.-O. and V.R.-M.; Writing-Original Draft Preparation, C.C.-O., C.Z., V.R.-M. and A.G.-S.; Writing-Review & Editing, C.C.-O., C.Z., V.R.-M. and A.G.-S.; Visualization, C.Z.; Supervision, C.C.-O. and C.Z.; Project Administration, C.C.-O. and V.R.-M.; Funding Acquisition, V.R.-M. All authors have read and agreed to the published version of the manuscript.

Funding: This research was funded by the 1st Internal Call for Research Projects from CETYS University. The authors gratefully acknowledge CETYS University research coordination for the support for the realization of this project.

Institutional Review Board Statement: The study was conducted according to the guidelines of the Declaration of Helsinki and approved by the Ethics Committee of Clinic Medical Norte (protocol code 0051 and date 16/12/2019 of approval).

Informed Consent Statement: Informed consent was obtained from all subjects involved in the study.

Acknowledgments: The authors would especially like to express their gratitude to Clinic Medical Norte.

Conflicts of Interest: The authors declare no conflict of interest.

Appendix A

Table A1. Index of terms.

Term	Type	Meaning
Edad	Numeric	Age
Género	Categorical	Gender
Fumador	Categorical	Smoker
HTA	Categorical	Hypertension
Dyslipidemia	Categorical	Dislipidemia
Diabetes	Categorical	Diabetes
ERC (Cr Basal)	Categorical	Chronic Kidney Disease
Suma FRCV	Numeric	Sum of Cardiovascular Risk Factors
C. Isquémica Previa	Categorical	Previous Ischemic Heart Disease
PPT	Numeric	Pretest Probability of Ischemic Heart Disease calculated from the type of chest pain and age
Rangos PPT	Categorical	Pretest Probability Ranges
Tipo dolor	Categorical	Pain type
TnT Ingreso	Numeric	Troponin levels upon entry
TnT Curva (4 h)	Numeric	Troponin levels 4 h after entry
ECG	Categorical	Electrocardiogram
TC > 100	Categorical	Body Temperature
IC	Categorical	Ictus
Alta Precoz	Categorical	Early discharge
UDT	Categorical	Thoracic Pain Units
Ingreso	Numeric	Entry (days)
Ergometría	Categorical	Ergometry
Eco-stress	Categorical	Eco-stress
Cate	Categorical	Catheterization
Angio TAC	Categorical	Computed Tomography Angiography
AMI	Categorical	Acute Myocardial Infarction
Revascularización	Categorical	Revascularization

Appendix B

Table A2. Variables used by methods.

SCORE	ASCVD	Framingham
Age	Age	Age
Gender	Gender	Gender
Smoking habits	Race	Smoking habits
Total cholesterol (mg/dL)	Total cholesterol (mg/dL)	Total cholesterol (mg/dL)
HDL-cholesterol (mg/dL)	HDL-cholesterol (mg/dL)	HDL-cholesterol (mg/dL)
Systolic blood pressure (mmHg)	Systolic blood pressure (mmHg)	Systolic blood pressure (mmHg)
	Diastolic blood pressure (mmHg)	
	Smoking habits	
	Treated for High pressure	
	Diabetes	

Note. "Framingham risk score for estimation of 10-years of cardiovascular disease risk in patients with metabolic syndrome" by Jahangiry, L., Farhangi M.A. and Rezaei, F., 2017 (https://www.ncbi.nlm.nih.gov/pmc/articles/PMC5682637/, accessed on 17 February 2021). Copyright 2017 by Jahangiry, L., Farhangi M.A. and Rezaei, F. "ACC/AHA ASCVD Risk Calculator" by ACC/AHA, 2013 (http://www.cvriskcalculator.com/, accessed on 17 February 2021). Copyright 2013 by ACC/AHA. "SCORE Risk Charts" by European Society of Cardiology, 2020 (https://www.escardio.org/Education/Practice-Tools/CVD-prevention-toolbox/SCORE-Risk-Charts, accessed on accessed on 17 February 2021). Copyright 2020 by European Society of Cardiology.

References

1. World Health Organization (WHO). WHO Reveals Leading Causes of Death and Disability Worldwide: 2000–2019. Available online: https://www.who.int/es/news-room/fact-sheets/detail/cardiovascular-diseases-(cvds) (accessed on 15 December 2020).
2. World Heart Federation Enfermedades Cardiovasculares en México 2017. Available online: https://www.world-heart-federation.org/wp-content/uploads/2017/05/Cardiovascular_diseases_in_Mexico__Spanish_.pdf (accessed on 17 February 2021).
3. Instituto Nacional de Estadística y Geografía. *Características de las Defunciones Registradas en México durante 2018*; Instituto Nacional de Estadística y Geografía: Aguascalientes, Mexico, 2019.
4. Mair, J.; Lindahl, B.; Hammarsten, O.; Müller, C.; Giannitsis, E.; Huber, K.; Möckel, M.; Plebani, M.; Thygesen, K.; Jaffe, A.S. How is cardiac troponin released from injured myocardium? *Eur. Heart J. Acute Cardiovasc. Care* **2018**, *7*, 553–560. [CrossRef] [PubMed]

5. Cortés Valerio, A.; Cortés Bejarano, F.; Cortés Morales, E.; Duarte Núñez, D.; Quesada Campos, J. Alteraciones electrofisiológicas y/o bioquímicas del trauma cardíaco. *Med. Leg. Costa Rica* **2019**, *36*, 62–67.
6. Gallo-Villegas, J.A.; Aristizábal-Ocampo, D. La prueba de esfuerzo electrocardiográfica: Utilidad en el diagnóstico y pronóstico de la enfermedad coronaria. *Med. Lab.* **2015**, *21*, 63–84. [CrossRef]
7. Conroy, R. Estimation of ten-year risk of fatal cardiovascular disease in Europe: The SCORE project. *Eur. Heart J.* **2003**, *24*, 987–1003. [CrossRef]
8. Sarre-Álvarez, D.; Cabrera-Jardines, R.; Rodríguez-Weber, F.; Díaz-Greene, E. Enfermedad cardiovascular aterosclerótica. Revisión de las escalas de riesgo y edad cardiovascular. *Med. Interna Mex.* **2018**, *34*, 910–923.
9. Kermany, D.S.; Goldbaum, M.; Cai, W.; Valentim, C.C.S.; Liang, H.; Baxter, S.L.; McKeown, A.; Yang, G.; Wu, X.; Yan, F.; et al. Identifying Medical Diagnoses and Treatable Diseases by Image-Based Deep Learning. *Cell* **2018**, *172*, 1122–1131. [CrossRef]
10. Noorbakhsh-Sabet, N.; Zand, R.; Zhang, Y.; Abedi, V. Artificial Intelligence Transforms the Future of Health Care. *Am. J. Med.* **2019**, *132*, 795–801. [CrossRef] [PubMed]
11. Baccouche, A.; Garcia-Zapirain, B.; Castillo Olea, C.; Elmaghraby, A. Ensemble Deep Learning Models for Heart Disease Classification: A Case Study from Mexico. *Information* **2020**, *11*, 207. [CrossRef]
12. Orange Biolab Orange Biolab. Available online: https://orange.biolab.si/widget-catalog/ (accessed on 18 November 2020).
13. Pacheco Rodríguez, A. *Manual de Emergencia Médica Prehospitalaria*; Arán: Madrid, Spain, 2001; ISBN 978-84-86725-94-5.
14. Dalton, A.L.; Limmer, D.; Mistovich, J.J. *Urgencias Médicas: Evaluación, Atención y Transporte de Pacientes*; Editorial El Manual Moderno: Bogota, Colombia, 2000; ISBN 978-607-448-212-6.
15. Centro Nacional de Excelencia Tecnológica en Salud. *Guía de Práctica Clínica Diagnóstico, Estratificación y Tratamiento de Pacientes con Síndrome Coronario Agudo sin Elevación ST*; Centro Nacional de Excelencia Tecnológica en Salud: Mexico City, Mexico, 2010.
16. Hidalgo Sanjuán, M.V.; Fernández Aguirre, M.C.; Linde de Luna, F.; Rodríguez Martínez, R. Neumosur: Dolor Torácico. pp. 267–274. Available online: https://www.neumosur.net/files/EB04-21%20dolor%20toracico.pdf (accessed on 17 February 2021).
17. Ostabal-Artigas, M.I. Dolor torácico en los servicios de urgencias. *Med. Integral* **2020**, *40*, 40–49.
18. Rodríguez González, M.; Tárraga Marcos, M.L.; Madrona Marcos, F.; Sadek, I.M.; Celada Roldan, C.; Tárraga López, P.J. Efectos de la dieta mediterránea sobre los factores de riesgo cardiovascular. *J. Negat. Posit. Results* **2019**, 25–51. [CrossRef]
19. Rajesh, N.; Maneesha, T.; Hafeez, S.; Krishna, H. Prediction of Heart Disease Using Machine Learning Algorithms. *IJET* **2018**, *7*, 363. [CrossRef]
20. Pallarés-Carratalá, V.; Pascual-Fuster, V.; Godoy-Rocatí, D. Dislipidemia y riesgo vascular. Una revisión basada en nuevas evidencias. *SEMERGEN Med. Fam.* **2015**, *41*, 435–445. [CrossRef] [PubMed]
21. Alemu, R.; Fuller, E.E.; Harper, J.F.; Feldman, M. Influence of Smoking on the Location of Acute Myocardial Infarctions. *ISRN Cardiol.* **2011**, *2011*, 1–3. [CrossRef] [PubMed]
22. Ambrose, J.A.; Barua, R.S. The pathophysiology of cigarette smoking and cardiovascular disease. *J. Am. Coll. Cardiol.* **2004**, *43*, 1731–1737. [CrossRef]
23. Friedman, G.D. Cigarette Smoking and Chest Pain. *Ann. Intern. Med.* **1975**, *83*, 1. [CrossRef] [PubMed]
24. Lawes, C.M.; Hoorn, S.V.; Rodgers, A. Global burden of blood-pressure-related disease, 2001. *Lancet* **2008**, *371*, 1513–1518. [CrossRef]
25. Rodríguez, E.D.; Ramírez, R.J.T.; Jiménez, A. de la C.A. Factores de riesgo de infarto agudo del miocardio en pacientes con diagnóstico de hipertensión arterial. *Multimed* **2014**, *18*, 1–13.
26. Vilches Izquierdo, E.; Ochoa Montes, L.A.; González Lugo, M.; Ramos Marrero, L.; Tamayo Vicente, N.D.; García Ones, D.; Díaz Londres, H. Impact of essential blood hypertension and ischemic heart diseases in sudden cardiac death victims. *Rev. Cuba. Salud Pública* **2016**, *42*, 432–441.
27. Maiz Gurruchaga, A. Consecuencias patológicas de la obesidad: Hipertensión arterial, diabetes mellitus y dislipidemia. *Bol. Esc. Med.* **1997**, *26*, 18–21. [CrossRef]
28. Carabetti, J.A.M. Cardiomiopatía diabética. *Rev. Urug. Cardiol.* **2017**, *32*. [CrossRef]
29. Valdés Ramos, E.R.; Rivera Chávez, M.; Bencosme Rodríguez, N. Comportamiento del infarto agudo del miocardio en personas con diabetes mellitus de la provincia Granma. *Rev. Cuba. Endocrinol.* **2012**, *23*, 128–138.
30. Mendoza-Medellín, A.; Velázquez, G.T. Metabolismo energético del corazón normal e infartado. *Ciencia Ergo Sum* **2002**, *9*, 282–292.
31. López Gómez, J.M.; Vega Martínez, A. Alteraciones Cardiovasculares en la Enfermedad Renal Crónica | Nefrología al día. Available online: http://www.nefrologiaaldia.org/es-articulo-alteraciones-cardiovasculares-enfermedad-renal-cronica-179 (accessed on 18 November 2020).
32. Wright, S.A.; Schultz, A.E. The rising tide of artificial intelligence and business automation: Developing an ethical framework. *Bus. Horiz.* **2018**, *61*, 823–832. [CrossRef]
33. Cedeño-Mora, S.; Goicoechea, M.; Torres, E.; Verdalles, Ú.; Pérez de José, A.; Verde, E.; García de Vinuesa, S.; Luño, J. Predicción del riesgo cardiovascular en pacientes con enfermedad renal crónica. *Nefrología* **2017**, *37*, 293–300. [CrossRef] [PubMed]
34. Arrieta, F.; Iglesias, P.; Pedro-Botet, J.; Tébar, F.J.; Ortega, E.; Nubiola, A.; Pardo, J.L.; Maldonado, G.F.; Obaya, J.C.; Matute, P.; et al. Diabetes mellitus y riesgo cardiovascular: Recomendaciones del Grupo de Trabajo Diabetes y Enfermedad Cardiovascular de la Sociedad Española de Diabetes (SED, 2015). *Aten. Primaria* **2016**, *48*, 325–336. [CrossRef]

35. Centro Nacional de Programas Preventivos y Control de Enfermedades Estrategia Para la Prevención y Control del Sobrepeso. 2014. Available online: http://www.cenaprece.salud.gob.mx/programas/interior/adulto/descargas/pdf/EstrategiaSODDistritoFederal.pdf (accessed on 17 February 2021).
36. Miguel Soca, P.E. Dislipidemias. *ACIMED* **2009**, *20*, 265–273.
37. García Milian, A.J.; Creus García, E.D. La obesidad como factor de riesgo, sus determinantes y tratamiento. *Rev. Cuba. Med. Gen. Integral* **2016**, *32*, 1–13.

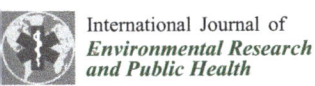

Article

Optimized Neural Network Based on Genetic Algorithm to Construct Hand-Foot-and-Mouth Disease Prediction and Early-Warning Model

Xialv Lin [1,†], Xiaofeng Wang [2,†], Yuhan Wang [1,†], Xuejie Du [2], Lizhu Jin [2], Ming Wan [2,*,‡], Hui Ge [2,*,‡] and Xu Yang [1,*,‡]

1 School of Computer Science and Technology, Beijing Institute of Technology, Beijing 100081, China; 3220201066@bit.edu.cn (X.L.); 3220180872@bit.edu.cn (Y.W.)
2 Chinese Center for Disease Control and Prevention, Beijing 102206, China; wangxf@chinacdc.cn (X.W.); duxj@chinacdc.cn (X.D.); jinlz@chinacdc.cn (L.J.)
* Correspondence: wanming@chinacdc.cn (M.W.); gehui@chinacdc.cn (H.G.); yangxu@tsinghua.edu.cn (X.Y.)
† These authors contributed equally to this work.
‡ These authors contributed equally to this work.

Abstract: Accompanied by the rapid economic and social development, there is a phenomenon of the crazy spread of many infectious diseases. It has brought the rapid growth of the number of people infected with hand-foot-and-mouth disease (HFMD), and children, especially infants and young children's health is at great risk. So it is very important to predict the number of HFMD infections and realize the regional early-warning of HFMD based on big data. However, in the current field of infectious diseases, the research on the prevalence of HFMD mainly predicts the number of future cases based on the number of historical cases in various places, and the influence of many related factors that affect the prevalence of HFMD is ignored. The current early-warning research of HFMD mainly uses direct case report, which uses statistical methods in time and space to have early-warnings of outbreaks separately. It leads to a high error rate and low confidence in the early-warning results. This paper uses machine learning methods to establish a HFMD epidemic prediction model and explore constructing a variety of early-warning models. By comparison of experimental results, we finally verify that the HFMD prediction algorithm proposed in this paper has higher accuracy. At the same time, the early-warning algorithm based on the comparison of threshold has good results.

Keywords: hand-foot-and-mouth disease; early-warning model; neural network; genetic algorithm

1. Introduction

With the intensification of global warming, climate abnormalities and natural disasters have become more and more intense, and the increasing changes in the environment have provided very favorable conditions for the spread of hand-foot-and-mouth disease (HFMD) [1,2]. Although HFMD is not a critical disease, there are still many children who have very serious complications due to this illness. If they are not treated in time, a series of complications such as myocarditis and encephalitis will occur, causing vital organ damage and even threatening their lives [3].

The prevalence of HFMD in China has continued unabated, and it has received great attention from the national health department. The prevention and treatment of HFMD should stop transmission from the root cause. However, the virus that leads to HFMD is not only many kinds, but also many types. Therefore, to carry out research on the prediction of the number of HFMD prevalence, the early-warning of epidemic trends and related factors has become the top priority of the country's HFMD epidemic control [4].

However, in previous studies on HFMD prediction and early-warning models, relevant researchers mainly conducted statistical analysis on factors related to the HFMD epidemic [5]. Including weather and demographic attributes, they explore the correlation between the different regions in the incidence of HFMD at different times of the amount of each factor and established a variety of models for prediction. However, these methods lack accurate positioning and research on the HFMD epidemic warning, and the data for establishing the prediction model is insufficient, the time and space of the data are too large, and the method used by the model is not perfect. Above shortcomings have caused many problems such as HFMD prediction and early-warning model to be inaccurate, limited to the problems of broad prediction and blind early-warning.

This paper aims to carry out accurate data analysis and standard data preprocessing based on the incidence of HFMD. At the same time, this paper also established a more accurate prediction model of the number of HFMD cases and a more reasonable early warning model. These have laid the foundation for realizing early warning of whether the regional HFMD has broken out or strengthened prevention and control.

2. Related Work

The World Health Organization (WHO) attaches great importance to the establishment of an early-warning system for infectious diseases, and develops an early-warning mechanism for infectious diseases and promoted its irreplaceable important role [6]. The principle of the early warning system is to make a judgment on whether there will be an outbreak or epidemic of infectious diseases based on the clinical information of the existing disease diagnosis patients. Their purpose is clear, just to detect abnormal health incidents promptly, quickly notify relevant health departments and staff, and take preventive and control measures in the first time. The early-warning system of such infectious diseases is the symptom monitoring system [7,8].

Since its establishment in 1946, the Centers for Disease Control and Prevention (CDC) has established a national infectious disease surveillance system for epidemic infectious diseases such as malaria and influenza. Until 1995, they began to build for all types of acute infectious disease monitoring network, in 2001 they integrated more than 100 spotty infectious disease surveillance system. Since then, the monitoring and early-warning system has been changed to "National Disease Electronic Monitoring System" [9].

The European Union (EU) has developed a group-type infectious disease monitoring and early-warning system based on the cooperation of all member states. It provides a collaborative platform for information and control and prevention for the countries in the group, and at the same time focuses on international cooperation and exchanges [10].

In January 2004, China began trial operation of the direct online reporting system for epidemics and public health emergencies, and the system was officially launched in April of the same year [11]. Afterwards, direct online reporting of various infectious diseases such as tuberculosis, dengue fever, and HFMD have been launched on the system, and public health information resources have been integrated and shared. At present, China's infectious disease early-warning model mainly uses the mobile percentile early-warning method and the spatial scanning statistical method [12,13]. However, these two methods rely too much on the direct reporting system of infectious diseases, and because the model is simple, many parameters are determined artificially. This has led to the problems of poor early-warning accuracy, repeated early-warnings, no early-warnings during epidemic periods and chaotic early-warning during non-epidemic periods, which seriously affected the early-warning work of HFMD epidemics.

At present, most researchers' research on the prevalence of HFMD relies on statistical methods such as multiple linear regression [14], cross-correlation analysis, and correlation analysis. They analyzed the correlation between related influencing factors and the incidence of HFMD, and obtained statistically significant results. This research results mostly proved the correlation between certain epidemic factors and the number of HFMD cases; at the same time, the incidence of HFMD epidemic was predicted by using the above-mentioned three infectious disease prediction methods.

Yin Ye et al. counted the daily incidence of HFMD for six years since 2011, calculated the correlation coefficient between the daily incidence of HFMD and twelve weather indicators of the day, and drew the conclusion that the daily incidence of HFMD is correlated with certain meteorological factors [15]. Jing Qinlong et al. used cross-correlation analysis methods to study relevant meteorological factors. They found that as the lag period decreases, the relationship between monthly average temperature and monthly cumulative precipitation and the number of HFMD monthly cases is the strongest [16]. Liu Yamin et al. established a variety of different prediction models using monthly incidence data from 2010 to 2015, then input the monthly incidence rate data of HFMD in 2016 as test data into the model [17]. Under the comparison of four objective evaluation indicators, they found that the seasonal autoregressive integrated moving average (SARIMA) model not only has excellent fitting generalization ability, but also has higher prediction accuracy.

As we entered the era of big data, many scholars began to design methods using big data to help build more accurate prediction or early-warning model of diseases [18,19]. So in this paper, we would present our effort at constructing a HFMD prediction and early-warning model with the help of big data.

3. Construct HFMD Prediction Algorithm Model Based on BP Neural Network

Figure 1 shows the overall process of the HFMD prevalence prediction model based on back propagation (BP) neural network constructed in this article, which will be introduced in detail below.

3.1. Data Acquisition and Analysis

This paper uses big data to build a predictive and early-warning model for HFMD through multi-dimensional data fusion. The data used mainly include two parts: incidence data and environmental data.

First of all, the incidence data comes from HFMD in Shanxi Province in 2016. There is no personal privacy data in this data, including: region (township), date of onset, age group, gender group, and population classification.

For the incidence data, we carried out exploratory data analysis to select appropriate characteristic factors affecting the HFMD epidemic in the model construction process, mainly analyzing indicators such as gender, population type, onset time, and patient age:

1. In terms of gender: As shown in Figure 2, among all HFMD patients in the province in 2016, the ratio of male to female patients was about 4:3. It can be considered that the relationship between HFMD infection and gender is very small, i.e., the chances of male and female being infected with HFMD are equal, so the ratio of men to women is not considered as a relevant factor affecting the prevalence of HFMD.
2. In terms of population types: As shown in Figure 3, there are three types of populations for all patients: kindergarten, scattered living, and other categories. The proportions of patients are 33.6%, 60.2%, and 6.2% respectively. Patients infected with HFMD are mainly concentrated in kindergartens and scattered populations, but the proportion of scattered patients is twice that of kindergarten patients, so the number of children in kindergartens cannot be a good predictor of HFMD infection patients.
3. In terms of time: As shown in Figure 4, the infection time of patients is mainly concentrated in 22–32 weeks (June-August). The 24th, 25th, and 26th week is the HFMD epidemic period, and the number of infections reaches a large peak. There are also multiple occurrences in 36–48 weeks, reaching a small peak of infection around the 44th week. Therefore, the prevalence of HFMD is characterized by a strong seasonal infection. The relevant weather indicators can be used as one of the important factors in determining the prevalence of HFMD.
4. In term of age: As shown in Figure 5, infants and children aged 0–6 years of HFMD infection account for a considerable portion, accounting for about 95% of all infected people. Therefore, the number of children aged 0–6 in each region can be used as an important indicator to predict the prevalence of HFMD.

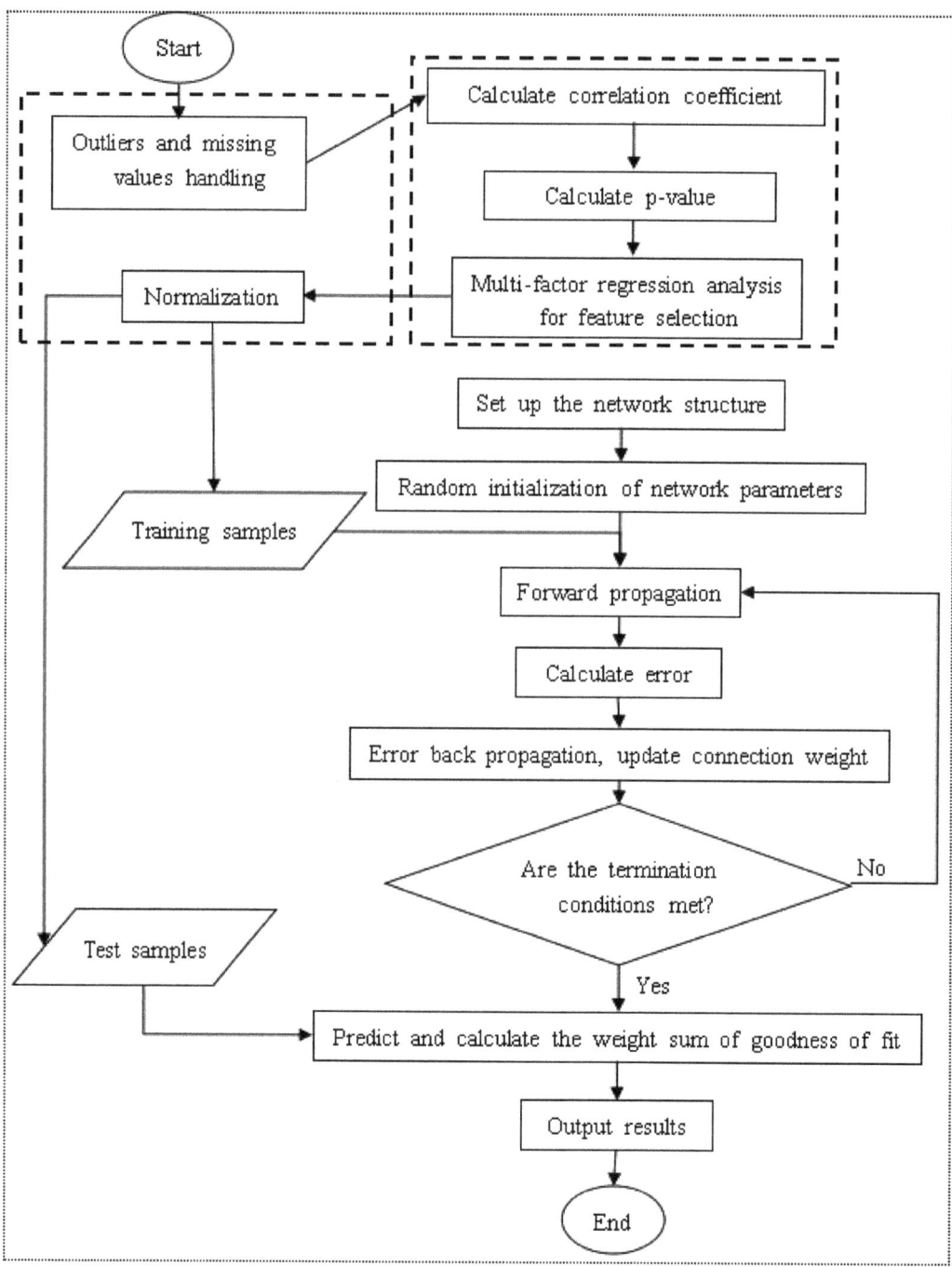

Figure 1. Flow chart of HFMD epidemic prediction model based on BP neural network.

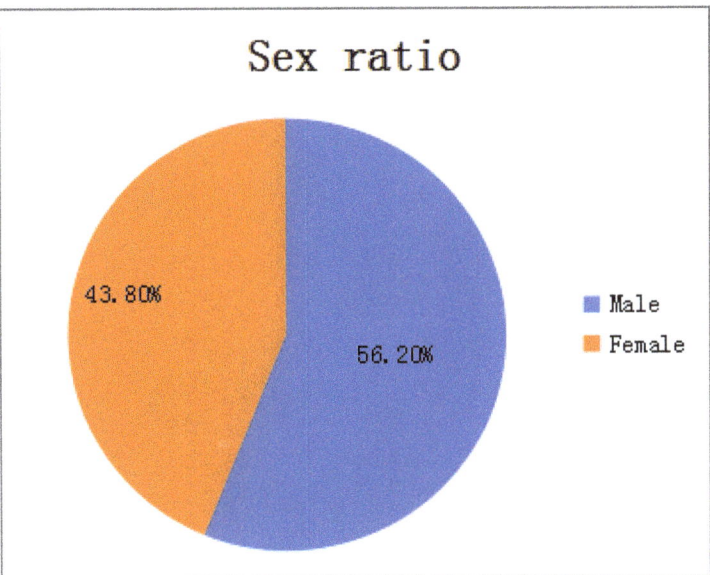

Figure 2. Sex ratio of HFMD patients.

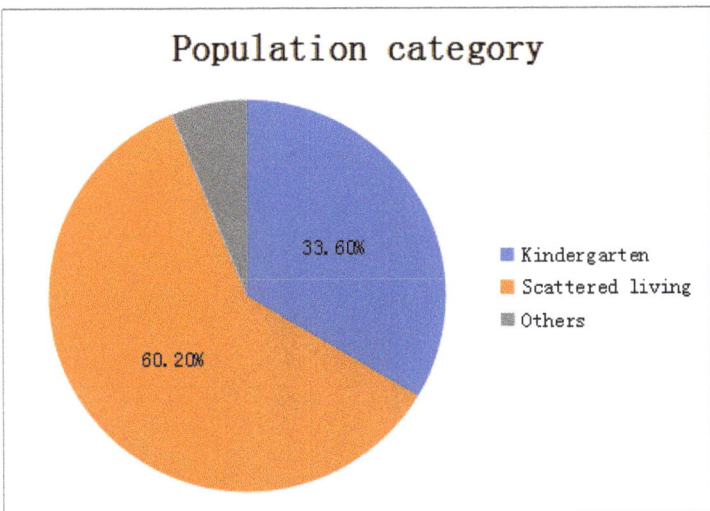

Figure 3. HFMD's proportion of each population category.

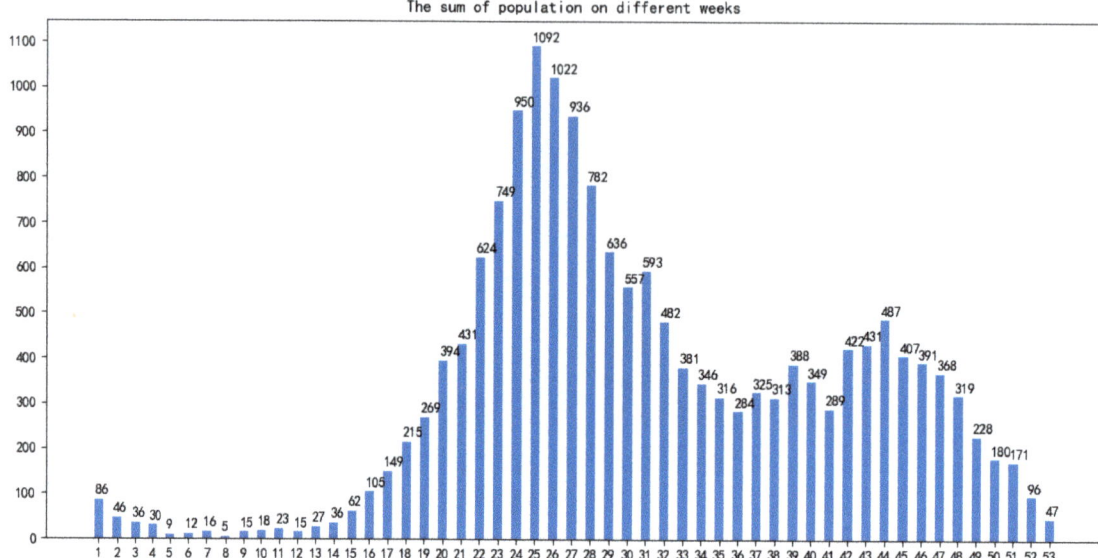

Figure 4. HFMD's proportion of each population category.

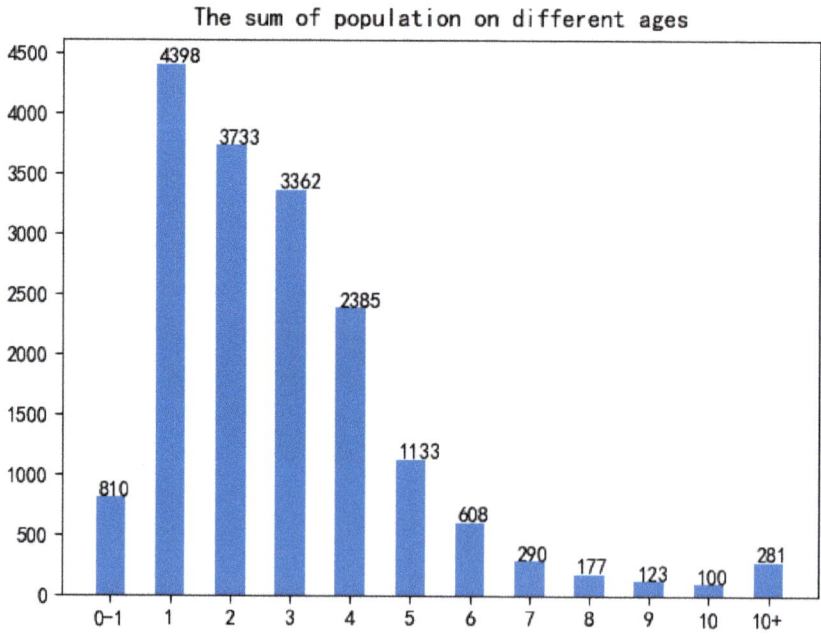

Figure 5. Age distribution of HFMD epidemic. the link (http://data.sheshiyuanyi.com/WeatherData/, accessed on 1 March 2020). x-axis is in years.

After the epidemic analysis of the original data, according to the number of cases per day in each district and county, the statistics are summarized, and only the date, area and statistical incidence in the original data file are retained.

Then, according to the results of epidemic analysis, the daily weather of each district and county was obtained. Due to different weather data sources and different ways of data acquisition, some weather data (maximum temperature, minimum temperature, wind level) need to be obtained from lishi.tianqi.com by web crawler; the other part of weather data (sunshine duration, air humidity, average air pressure) is obtained by file download. Because this part of the weather data only exists in the meteorological stations in the province and the data index is stable, the three weather data of 18 meteorological stations in Shanxi Province are downloaded from the http://data.sheshiyuanyi.com/WeatherData/, accessed on 1 March 2020, and the statistical areas are allocated according to the weather data of the nearest meteorological stations. Before the distribution, the nearest meteorological stations can be found by crawling the geographical location of the regions and meteorological stations, i.e., latitude and longitude data, and the three weather data of the nearest stations are allocated to the statistical areas; to consider the effect of the incubation period (usually 4 days) on the daily incidence of disease, the corresponding weather data of the day before 4 days were obtained, and the weather indexes such as maximum temperature, minimum temperature, wind grade, average sunshine duration, average air humidity and average air pressure were obtained in the same way.

Finally, according to the results of HFMD epidemic analysis, population data needs to be summarized, so the internal population data is calculated to count the number of children aged 0–6 in each region, and integrated into the data file generated in the previous step; at the same time, in order to consider the impact of the incidence of the day before the day on the day, the number of cases from the previous day is also included in the model characteristics to generate complete data for establishing the HFMD epidemic prediction model.

3.2. Data Preprocessing

The process of data preprocessing will greatly influence the result of data analysis [20].

3.2.1. Missing Value Processing

Among the data related to the factors affecting the spread of HFMD, the weather data or the population data of districts and counties on the day have some variable values missing, so appropriate methods must be used to deal with them. First of all, for variables whose values are not collected and most of the individuals whose variables are missing, the simple deletion method is used to directly delete variables or individual data, and will not be included in experimental research and data analysis. Then, the nearest neighbor padding method is used to fill the attributes with stable attribute values and small numerical variance. Finally, the mean value filling method is used to deal with the situation where a small part of the data is missing.

3.2.2. Outlier Handling

The regional weather data obtained by the web crawler is identified through outliers, and it is found that some data is abnormal, so the outliers need to be replaced or corrected. First, for univariate factors, define constraints that meet actual needs, and use the mean replacement method for variable outliers that do not meet the constraint definition. That is, when the value of a certain variable of a certain object is found to be abnormal, the average value of all other normal and non-missing values on the variable is calculated to replace the abnormal value. Secondly, for multiple variable factors, the order of the highest temperature and the lowest temperature often changes due to changes in the structure and content of the crawler page. Therefore, it is necessary to identify the individual data with the lowest temperature higher than the highest temperature, and exchange the two to make the data meet the constraints.

3.2.3. Data Standardization

The Z-score standardization method used in this paper. This paper also uses a simple downgrading standardization method, because the number of population plays a crucial role in the incidence of HFMD, and the magnitude of the difference between the number of population and the actual incidence of HFMD is large, which is not conducive to analysis. Therefore, the value of this variable is degraded.

3.3. Feature Selection

Through the data preprocessing process, we finally established the data table shown in Table 1.

Table 1. HFMD epidemiological research data sheet.

Variable Name	Basic Meaning of Data	Type of Data	Range
weekofyear	week of statistical time	discrete variable	1–53
addID	statistical area code	discrete variable	1401–1411
count	number of infections	integer variable	0–
last_count	number of infections in the previous week	integer variable	0–
highTem	average maximum temperature	continuous variable	0–39
lowTem	average minimum temperature	continuous variable	0–39
windLevel	average wind level	continuous variable	0–12
p_highTem	average maximum temperature before the incubation period	continuous variable	0–39
p_lowTem	average minimum temperature before incubation period	continuous variable	0–39
p_windLevel	average wind level before the incubation period	continuous variable	0–12
hTemDiff	maximum temperature difference	continuous variable	−15–15
lTemDiff	lowest temperature difference	continuous variable	−15–15
windLevDiff	wind power difference	continuous variable	−3–3
wet	average air humidity	continuous variable	0–100
sunshine	average sunshine duration	continuous variable	0–10
pressure	average air pressure	continuous variable	−2–2
p_wet	average air humidity before incubation period	continuous variable	0–100
p_sunshine	average sunshine duration before incubation period	continuous variable	0–10
p_pressure	average pressure before the incubation period	continuous variable	−2–2
wetDiff	average humidity difference	continuous variable	−100–100
sunDiff	average sunshine duration difference	continuous variable	−10–10
pressDiff	average air pressure difference	continuous variable	−5–5
Children	number of children under 6	integer variable	1–

When constructing the supervised learning model for the prediction of the number of HFMD cases, we maximized the fact that many a priori unknown related features (meteorological and demographic features) were incorporated into the learning objectives. So that the target problem (the number of HFMD cases) can be trained and learned more effectively. However, some of the related features are not very relevant to the learning goal, or even have no relationship. These features are usually called redundant features. When they are added to the learning task, problems such as poor learner performance and data disaster are likely to occur. Therefore, it is very necessary to select all features to greatly enhance the generalization ability of the prediction model. This paper uses a multivariate joint feature selection method based on correlation analysis.

In the study of the HFMD epidemic prediction model, three comprehensive feature selection algorithms including filtering, wrapping and embedding are used. Different methods are used in different training and learning stages, using filtering algorithms before training, using embedded algorithms during training, and using wrapped algorithms after training. In this way, the feature subset with the best performance is selected, the learner with the strongest generalization ability is selected, and the number of cases is predicted more accurately for scientific prevention and control.

The core of the embedded algorithm is to integrate the feature selection process into the model learning process, and the features are selected cleverly while learning, so the algorithm depends on the machine learning algorithm used. However, embedded algorithms are not used in the preprocessing of data in the early stage, and only used during model training.

The core of the wrapped algorithm is to directly use the evaluation index of the learner to reflect the pros and cons of the feature subset. The higher the accuracy of the learner, the better the feature subset. Therefore, it is necessary to repeatedly use different feature subsets to construct multiple learners until the best learner is obtained and the best feature subset is obtained.

The core of the filtering algorithm is to directly filter out undesirable features to filter out relatively good feature subsets. Then, without training the model, use an appropriate evaluation function to evaluate the pros and cons of the feature subset until the best evaluated feature subset is selected. Therefore, the feature selection of this method is independent of the target learner, and the advantage is that it is simple, efficient and fast.

Before the actual training of the learner, the filter method is usually used to select the features, and the dependency metric is used to evaluate the feature subset. At the same time, according to the results of the dependency measurement, the measurement threshold is set, and the features whose relevant indicators are greater than the threshold are selected, and further statistically significant tests are performed on them as a double standard for selecting features. At the same time, bivariate correlation analysis is difficult to escape the influence of confounding factors, so multiple linear regression analysis methods must be used to establish a regression model for the influencing factors and the number of hand, foot and mouth cases, and find the secondary confounding factors according to the partial regression coefficients. The previous filtering feature selection process is completed.

The selection process can be divided into the following steps:

1. Calculate the variance of all variables using a single variable analysis method;
2. Filter out attributes whose variance is greater than the variance threshold, and get a preliminary feature subset;
3. Using bivariate correlation analysis method, calculate the Pearson coefficient, Spearman coefficient, distance correlation coefficient and p-value of the independent variable and the dependent variable;
4. According to the correlation coefficient and statistical p-value results, select the features whose p-value is less than the significance level and the correlation coefficient is greater than the coefficient threshold to obtain a more accurate initial feature subset;
5. According to the feature subset selected by the variable analysis method, establish a multivariate joint regression model based on the multiple linear regression model, and obtain the partial regression coefficient, intercept and statistical p-value of the model;
6. According to the multiple regression parameter table, filter and select variables whose p value is less than the significance level, and obtain the feature subset in the linear model;
7. Then the k features with the largest nonlinear correlation coefficients in the initial feature subset, which do not exist in the linear model feature subset, are included in the nonlinear model feature subset.

3.4. Construction of HFMD Prediction Model

Commonly used machine learning regression prediction algorithms include multiple linear regression (LR), support vector regression (SVR), differential integrated moving average autoregressive models and BP neural networks [15] and so on. Through analysis, we will select BP neural network to construct an early prediction model for HFMD on big data.

After analysis of related factors, seven related variables were obtained. After these seven related variables are normalized by Min-Max, the training set and the test set are randomly selected according to the ratio of 7:3. Then input the training set into the prediction model to be established, and train and adjust the parameters in the model. After a series of training processes, a HFMD epidemic prediction model suitable for solving this problem is obtained. Then input the test set into the HFMD prevalence prediction model for prediction, obtain the prediction result, and compare the result with the expected output to evaluate the HFMD prevalence prediction model.

The structure of the HFMD prediction model based on the machine learning regression algorithm is shown in Figure 6. It includes six modules: data acquisition and summary, data preprocessing, influencing factor analysis, model learning, epidemic case number prediction, and model evaluation analysis. In the data acquisition and summary module, the meteorological factors and demographic factors data related to the HFMD epidemic are acquired in multiple ways, and the county daily data is summarized as city weekly data; the dirty data is mainly cleaned in the data preprocessing module; in the influencing factor analysis module, univariate, bivariate and multivariate joint analysis of the correlation between influencing factors and the number of popular populations are carried out, and the feature set of relevant HFMD epidemic influencing factors suitable for modeling is selected; in the process of model learning, the machine learning regression model is used to learn to obtain the optimal structure; in the HFMD epidemic case number prediction module, the test set is input into the model; in the model evaluation and analysis module, the learned optimal model is analyzed with different weights on the training set and the test set, and the relevant evaluation index values are obtained to judge the pros and cons of the model.

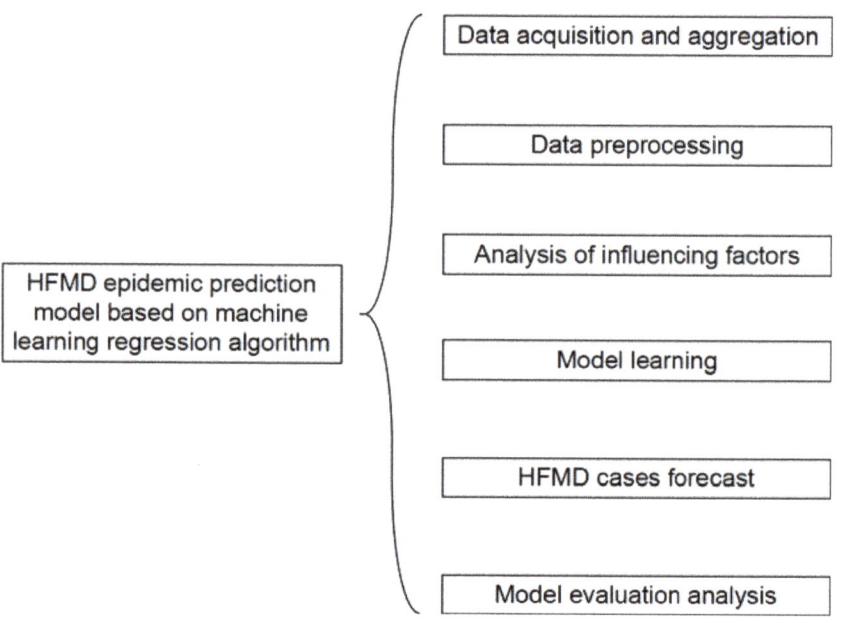

Figure 6. Structure diagram of HFMD epidemic prediction model based on machine learning regression algorithm.

Figure 7 shows the three-layer structure of the BP neural network used in this article. The number of neurons in each layer is m, k, and 1, respectively. The number of hidden layers and the number of neurons in each layer can be dynamically adjusted according to the training effect. However, the number of neurons in the first and last layers is fixed. The training process of BP neural network is realized by error feedback mechanism [16]. The activation function used is the relu function.

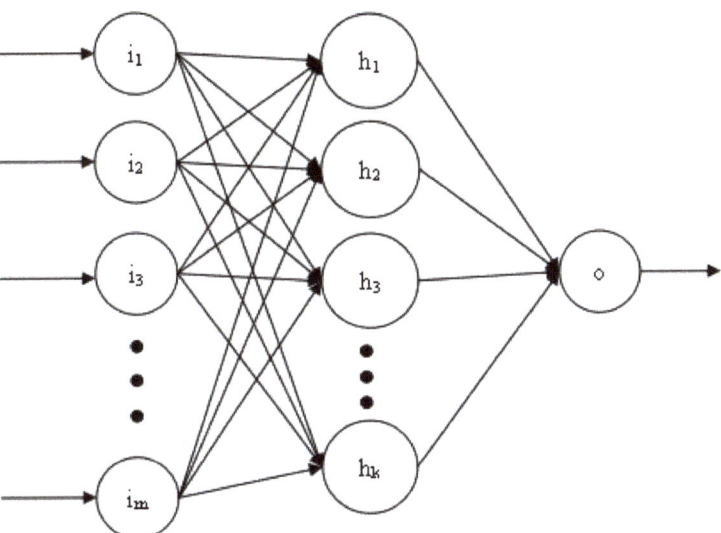

Figure 7. Three-layer single output BP neural network structure diagram.

The model training process is:
1. Establish the network structure according to the actual HFMD prediction problem. There is only one input layer and output layer, which contain the number of neurons as the feature number and 1, respectively. A hidden layer with k neurons is initially set. If the training result is not Ideally, the number of layers and the number of neurons on each layer can be dynamically changed, but not more than three hidden layers;
2. Initialize the hyperparameters in the network structure, including learning rate, training times, and connection weights. If the training results are not ideal, the hyperparameter values can also be dynamically adjusted;
3. Start to input training samples into the network, obtain the predicted value of each sample through the forward propagation process, and calculate the overall error between the output predicted value and the expected value;
4. If the error does not meet the condition or the training does not reach the number of generations, the error is propagated back to the input layer, and the connection weight is updated in the process;
5. If it is greater than the set number of generations, the training process is ended, the structure of the BP neural network is output, and the test data is evaluated according to relevant indicators;
6. If the test result does not reach a certain threshold, it is necessary to adjust the relevant hyperparameters or the number of hidden layers or the number of neurons in each hidden layer in the network, and repeat the above training process.

4. Neural Network Parameter Optimization Based on GA

In the training process of BP neural network, the gradient descent method and error feedback propagation mechanism are essentially used to dynamically update the connection weights, which also exposes the shortcomings of this training method [21]. First of all, there are strict requirements for model hyperparameters such as learning rate, too large or too small learning rate will affect the optimization effect; Secondly, if the number of training iterations is too large, the convergence efficiency is low when the error function gradually becomes flat in the later stage, and it is difficult to converge to a flat point if the number of generations is too small; Finally, it is because the training starts according to the initial set of random weights, looking for a smooth gradient and falling into a local minimum state, it is difficult to jump out to find the global minimum state. Therefore, in view of the above shortcomings, we use genetic algorithm (GA) to globally optimize the connection weights.

First determine the BP network structure, and encode the target individual with floating-point numbers. Arrange all the connection weights in the neural network in order to form the row vector $W_j = (w_1, w_2, \cdots, w_n)$ of individual j, which represents the genetic code of chromosome j in the population, The weight w_i of connection i in the network represents the genotype of gene i on the chromosome, and n represents the number of all connections in the neural network. In this model, if the number of neurons contained in the input layer, the first hidden layer, the second hidden layer, and the output layer are m, k, h, 1, respectively, then the number of genes n is calculated as in Equation (1).

$$n = m \times k + k \times h + h \tag{1}$$

Secondly, all individuals in the population must be initialized randomly. Each individual has a chromosome vector, which can be decoded back into a BP neural network model with floating-point numbers. Therefore, before learning, all individual vectors must be initialized with random real numbers in the range of $[-1, 1]$ to generate the first generation population.

Finally, it is necessary to calculate the fitness of all individuals, select individuals for genetic operations, including replication, crossover and mutation, to generate a new generation of populations [22]. In this paper, the fitness can be calculated directly from the average error of the individual on the sample. Therefore, select high fitness, i.e., individuals with small errors for retention, and select low fitness, i.e., individuals with large errors for elimination. Thus, individual neural networks with poor fit are discarded in the training process. Then, perform uniform mutation and arithmetic crossover operations on general individuals to obtain a new generation. After repeated training reaches the specified number of evolutions, the optimal model is obtained. Otherwise, it returns to the fitness calculation step to reiterate. The final individual is decoded to obtain all the connection weights in the neural network, which are used for actual prediction and quantitative evaluation indicators are obtained. Figure 8 is a detailed flowchart of the GA-BP HFMD prediction model.

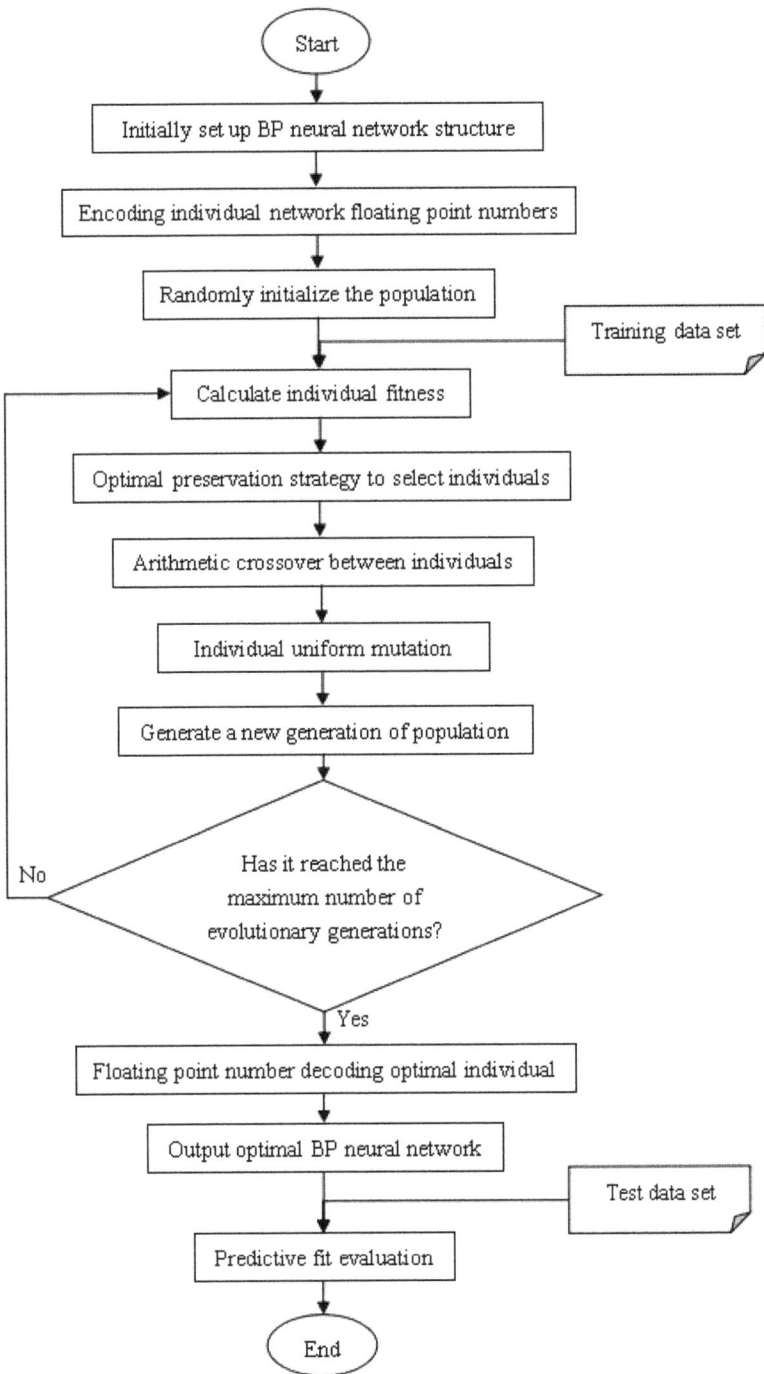

Figure 8. Flow chart of GA-BP HFMD epidemic prediction model.

5. Construction of HFMD Early-Warning Model Based on Big Data

The traditional HFMD epidemic warning model is mainly based on two major methods of time and space, namely the moving percentile prediction method and the spatial scanning statistical method. It also needs to use the repeated warning kicking algorithm to remove duplicates. The early-warning method is only based on historical data before and after the same period. It does not consider that the HFMD outbreak may be related to related weather and demographic factors. Blind warning and the warning process are cumbersome and wrong. There is a situation of blind warning every day and everywhere.

As there is no yet a complete and accurate early-warning mechanism for infectious diseases, HFMD epidemic early-warning methods based on adjustable parameters, moving percentiles and a combination of the two are proposed, mainly proposed different methods for the setting of HFMD early-warning threshold. The HFMD epidemic early-warning model is mainly based on the number of HFMD cases in the region generated by the above HFMD epidemic prediction model and the number of cases in the same period in history. That is, whether there will be an outbreak of HFMD epidemic in the early warning area, Or according to historical data in the same period, relevant health departments need to be warned to increase the vigilance of the HFMD epidemic in the region. The overall process of the model is shown in Figure 9.

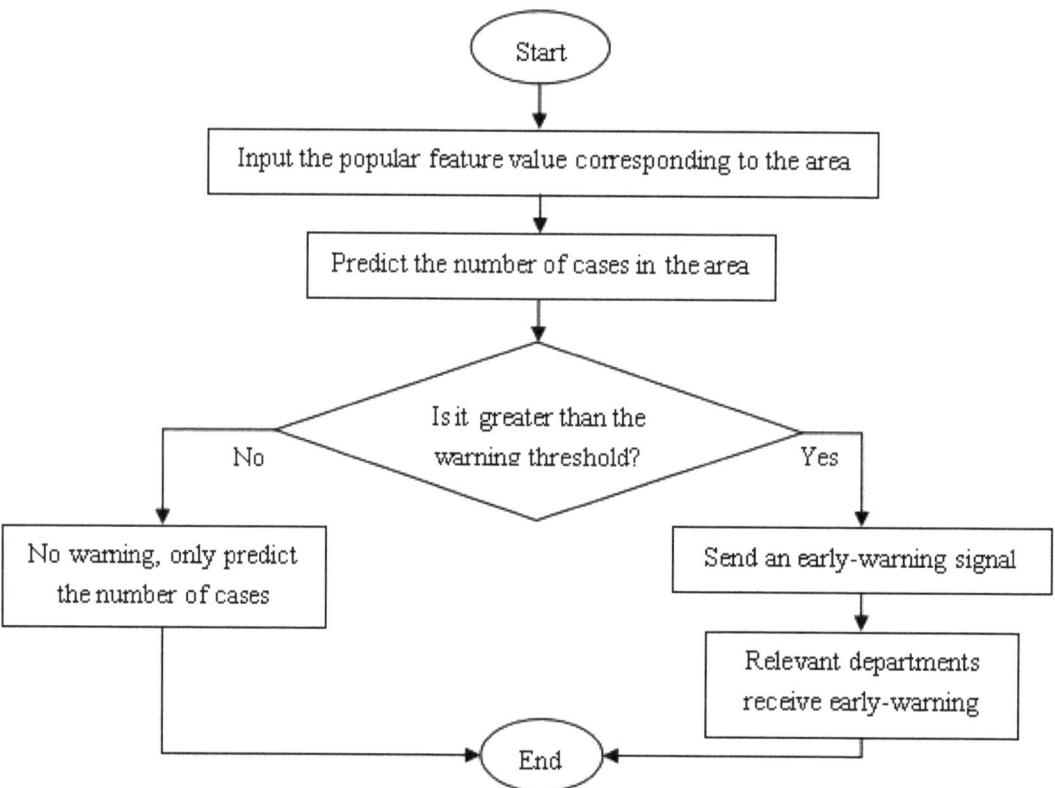

Figure 9. Flow chart of HFMD epidemic warning model.

5.1. HFMD Epidemic Warning Model Based on Adjustable Parameters

The parameters are adjustable, referring to different HFMD epidemic areas, according to the epidemic time of different seasons, the corresponding characteristic parameters in the HFMD prediction model can be dynamically adjusted according to the actual local conditions. The corresponding features can be obtained by the feature selection method, and the number of patients output by the feature parameters through the model is used as the early-warning threshold of HFMD infectious diseases. If the actual predicted value exceeds the early-warning threshold, the system will issue an early-warning signal. For example, when the minimum temperature, air humidity, the number of illnesses last week, the number of children aged 0–6, and the number of weeks are 24 degrees Celsius, 40%, 45 cases, 28 thousand people, and 16:00, through the HFMD epidemic prediction model, the incidence under this feature is obtained and used as the early-warning threshold. These characteristic values can be dynamically adjusted according to different regions and different times.

5.2. HFMD Epidemic Warning Model Based on Historical Percentile Method

First, establish a database of local historical cases of HFMD with the city as the unit, refer to the historical incidence of the same period in the past 3–5 years and two cycles before and after the same period. Like the forecast period, the general historical period is seven days. Then get the percentile (usually 80% after sorting from small to large) from the historical incidence as the early-warning threshold. When the predicted incidence in the statistical period is greater than this early-warning threshold, the system will automatically send an early-warning signal to relevant departments in the observation area within one day. For example, it is predicted that the weekly incidence of the area will reach 100. Among the nine incidence data of the same period and before and after the past three years, the incidence at the 80th percentile is 80. Then the system will send an early-warning signal to the relevant departments in the forecast area to remind the area that there may be an outbreak, or the need to strengthen prevention and control higher than the historical level.

5.3. HFMD Epidemic Warning Model Based on Threshold Comparison

Threshold comparison is to compare the two early-warning thresholds obtained by the above-mentioned parameter adjustable method and the historical percentile method, and use the smallest as the new early-warning threshold. The flow chart of the HFMD epidemic warning model based on threshold comparison is shown in Figure 10.

First, set the characteristic thresholds of the influencing factors of the HFMD epidemic, i.e., under the corresponding weather factors and demographic factors, the number of possible HFMD incidences is the number at risk of HFMD outbreaks, and these characteristic values are substituted into the HFMD prediction model to obtain the incidence number threshold.

Then, according to the local database of historical HFMD cases, calculate the 80th percentile number of cases in the same cycle and two swing cycles in the past three years, and use this value as another threshold for early-warning. This threshold is compared with the early-warning threshold obtained by parameter adjustment, and the minimum incidence threshold is used as the early-warning threshold of HFMD early-warning model.

Finally, the HFMD epidemic prediction model is used to predict the number of local cases. When the number of cases exceeds the early-warning threshold, the local health department will send an early-warning signal and take corresponding measures after verification. At the same time, it can feed back suggestions, continuously adjust the characteristic parameter thresholds, and improve the precise HFMD early-warning mechanism; When this incidence does not exceed the warning threshold, no warning signal is issued, only the number of HFMD infections that may occur in the local area.

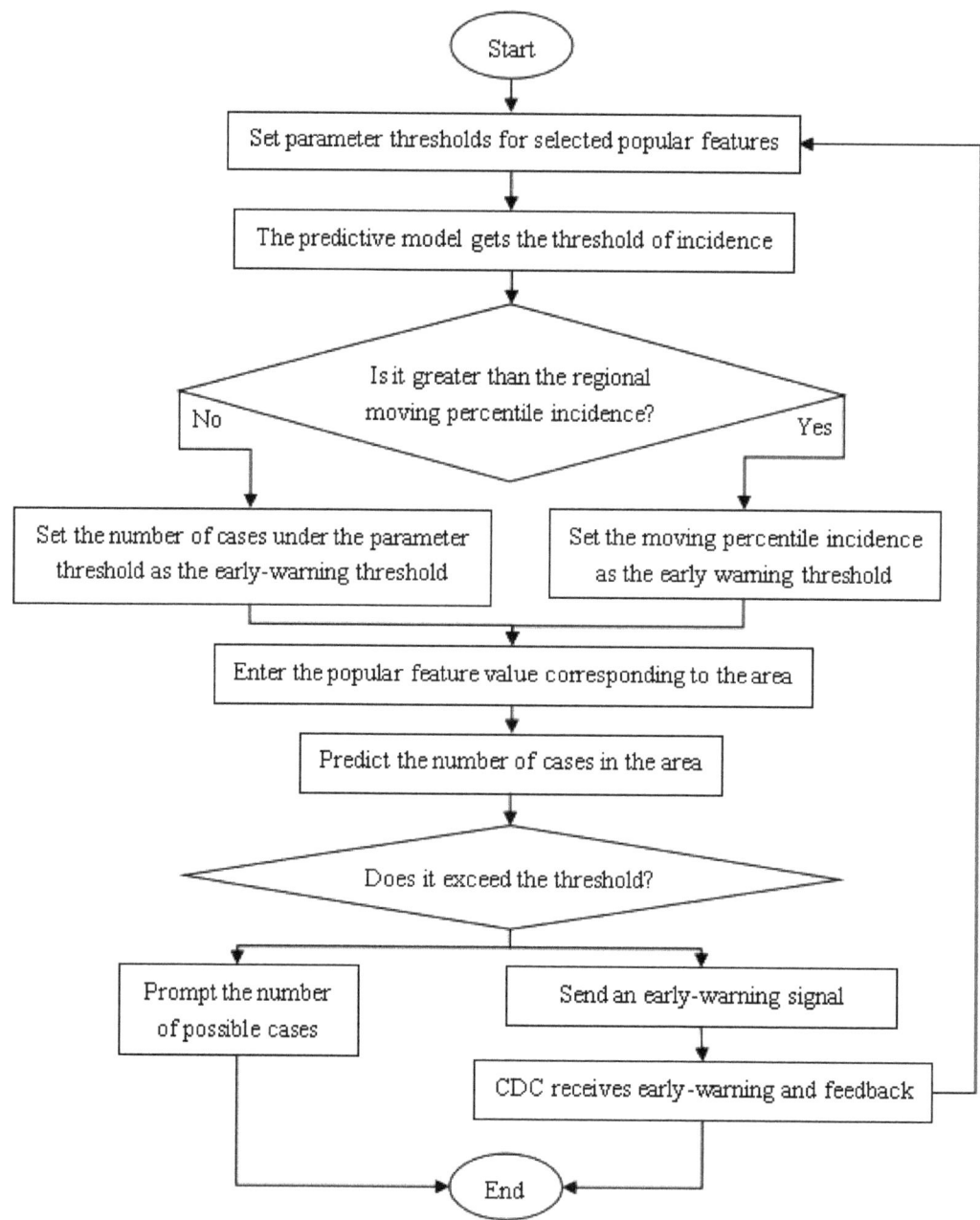

Figure 10. Flow chart of HFMD epidemic warning model based on threshold comparison.

6. Experiments

6.1. Predictive Model Evaluation Index

6.1.1. Goodness of Fit

Goodness of fit refers to the degree of fit of the regression model to the observations, and its measurement statistic is the coefficient of determination R^2. The value range of R^2 is [0, 1]. The larger the value in this range, the better the fitting effect of the regression equation to the training sample; on the contrary, the worse the fitting degree. When the goodness of fit is negative, It shows that the fitting effect of this regression model is too poor and has no practical significance. Suppose y is the value to be fitted, its mean value is $\bar{y}$, the fitted predicted value is rounded to $\hat{y}$, the total square sum (SST) is $\sum_{i=1}^{n}(y_i - \bar{y})^2$, the regression square sum (SSR) is $\sum_{i=1}^{n}(\hat{y}_i - \bar{y})^2$, and the residual square sum (SSE) is $\sum_{i=1}^{n}(y_i - \hat{y}_i)^2$, then $SST = SSR + SSE$, the calculation method of the determination coefficient is as follows:

$$R^2 = \frac{SSR}{SST} = 1 - \frac{SSE}{SST} \quad (2)$$

Generalization ability is an important indicator for detecting regression prediction performance. Therefore, when designing a regression model, it is necessary to consider not only the model's correct prediction of the required regression prediction object, but also the prediction effect of the model on the new data. The preprocessed data is divided into training data and test data in a ratio of 7:3. The evaluation index of the final model is the sum of the weights of the goodness of fit of the two, and the weight ratio is 3:7.

6.1.2. Mean Absolute Error

The mean absolute error (MAE) refers to the average of the absolute value of the difference between multiple predicted values and the true value. In the HFMD epidemic prediction model, the average absolute error indicates the degree of deviation between the number of HFMD cases predicted by the model and the number of true cases when the number of HFMD cases is predicted in different regions or at different times. The smaller MAE, the more accurate the mode. The larger MAE, the worse the predictive ability of the model. Therefore, the magnitude of the average absolute error MAE reflects the pros and cons of the model, and its calculation formula is as follows:

$$MAE = \frac{1}{n}\sum_{i=1}^{n}|y_i - y| \quad (3)$$

where, n represents the number of predictions, y_i represents the predicted value, and y represents the true value.

6.1.3. Accuracy within Error

Similar to the accuracy rate in the classification problem, in order to avoid the influence of interference factors, the accuracy rate within the error is introduced. The accuracy within error (AWE) refers to the ratio of the number of samples correctly fitted by the regression model obtained through training to the total number of training samples in the regression analysis process of predicting integer dependent variables within a certain error tolerance. To a certain extent, AWE explains the generalization ability of the regression model. The higher the AWE, the stronger the fitting ability of the model, and the lower AWE, indicating the weak fitting ability of the regression model, which ranges between 0 and 100%. The calculation formula of AWE is as follows:

$$AWE = \frac{n}{N} \times 100\% \quad (n := n + 1 \quad when \quad |f(X_i) - y_i| \leq error_{people}) \quad (4)$$

where n represents the number of samples correctly predicted by the regression, and N represents the total number of samples. When the absolute value of the error between the predicted value and the true value is less than the specified error range, add 1 to the number of correctly fitted samples n, until all samples are trained, and the final number of samples correctly predicted is obtained.

When predicting the number of HFMD cases, the number of cases of the dependent variable is an integer number. Therefore, the predicted value must be rounded up, and then the predicted value after processing is compared with the true value. If the difference between the two is within the allowable range of the number of errors, it is considered that the trained model predicts the sample correctly, otherwise it is considered that there is a large error in the sample prediction. According to the analysis of infectious disease researchers and the regression model, the number of errors is five, i.e., when the difference between the predicted value and the true value does not exceed five, it is determined that the model fits this sample correctly.

6.2. Early-Warning Model Evaluation Index

6.2.1. Warning Rate

The warning rate (WR) refers to the ratio of the number of samples that use the early warning model to send out early warning signals to the total number of samples, and its value is within the range of [0%, 100%]. Appropriate warning rate can reflect the difference of the model to different test data, and avoid the phenomenon of full warning and no warning. If the warning rate is too large or too small, it reflects the large error of the early warning model and the failure of correct warning.

6.2.2. Accuracy Rate

Accuracy rate (ACR) refers to the ratio of the number of samples with the same early warning results of the model to the test data and the real early-warning results to the total sample, reflecting the accuracy of the HFMD epidemic early-warning model, and its value range is Between [0, 1].

The higher the accuracy rate, the better the prediction ability of the early-warning model, and the lower the accuracy rate, the worse the prediction ability of the early-warning model. Therefore, the accuracy rate can truly reflect the prediction effect of the HFMD epidemic early-warning model.

6.3. Comparison of Different Prediction Time and Space Accuracy

To obtain a more accurate prediction model of the number of HFMD cases, the different temporal and spatial precisions were compared. From the finest time accuracy (day) and spatial accuracy (districts and counties) to a week and prefectures, respectively, linear regression, BP neural network and SVR are used to fit predictions. Because the average and variance of the number of cases in different time and space accuracy are very different, only the goodness of fit R^2 is used to compare the models. The experimental results are shown in Table 2, and the broken line graph is shown in Figure 11. With the expansion of time and space accuracy, the goodness of fit of the model doubles. At the same time, in the comparison of three different methods, the BP neural network prediction model has the largest R^2, so the city-level weekly prediction model based on the BP neural network has the highest accuracy.

Table 2. Experimental results of different time precision and spatial precision prediction.

Forecast Model Name	District/County, Daily Forecast	District/County, Weekly Forecast	City-Level, Weekly Forecast
LR	0.3914	0.7611	0.8983
BP-NN	0.3931	0.7613	0.8994
SVR	0.3041	0.7597	0.8948

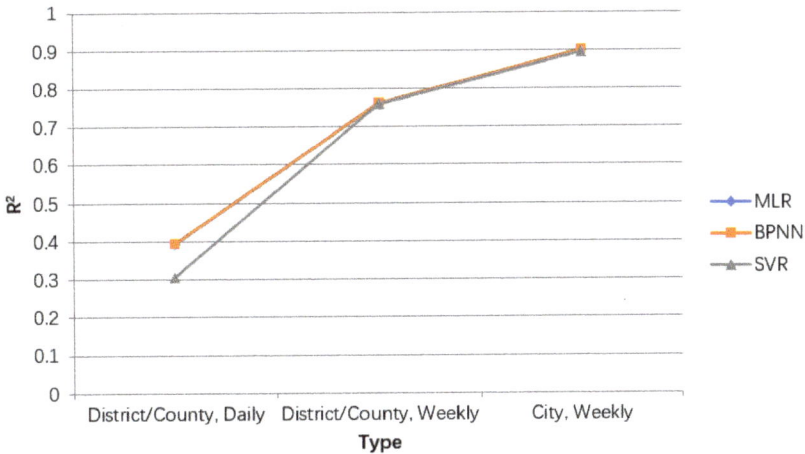

Figure 11. Comparison line chart of results of different prediction accuracy. The value represents results for R2, MAE/10, AWE for different parameters settings.

6.4. Comparative Analysis of Forecasting Models

In this paper, by training and forecasting numerical variables, based on the weekly incidence of HFMD in the city and the weekly weather data that affects the epidemic and the child population data, the relevant variable analysis of the influencing factors is carried out. After that, a multivariate joint feature selection method based on correlation analysis was used to screen out a subset of features suitable for building a linear model, including the weekly ordinal number of the statistical time, the incidence of the previous week, the weekly average air pressure, and the number of children aged 0–6. At the same time, a subset of features suitable for establishing a nonlinear model is obtained, including the weekly ordinal number of the statistical time, the incidence of the previous week, the weekly average air pressure, the weekly minimum temperature, the weekly air humidity, the wind level and the number of children aged 0–6. Three regression methods were used to establish a model to fit the weekly incidence. Under different evaluation indicators, the training results of each model are shown in Table 3 and Figure 12. The analysis shows that the R^2 of the BP neural network reaches the maximum and the MAE reaches the minimum. At the same time, when the prediction error does not exceed the MAE, the AWE reaches its maximum value. Therefore, the HFMD epidemic prediction model based on BP neural network performs best, and the fitting effect is relatively best.

Table 3. Training results of different machine learning regression algorithms.

Evaluation Index	LR	BP-NN	SVR
R^2	0.9193	0.9243	0.9142
MAE	8	7	7
AWE	58.94%	69.94%	63.85%

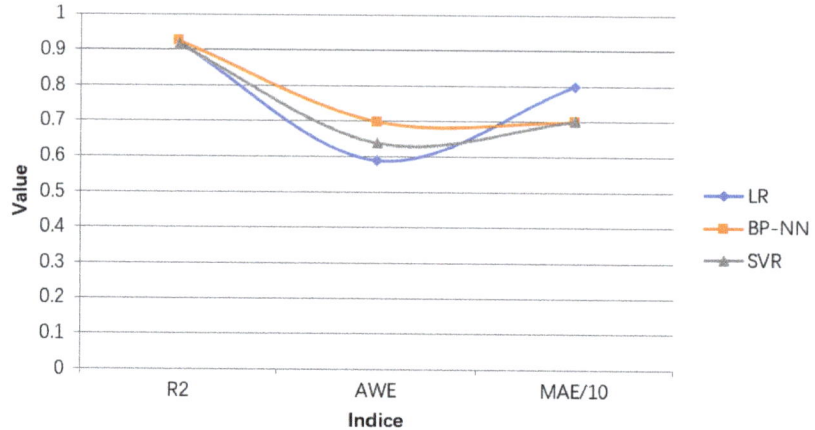

Figure 12. Line chart comparing the training results of different machine learning regression algorithms. The value represents results for R2, MAE/10, AWE for different parameters settings.

6.5. GA Tuning Parameter Analysis

When optimizing the connection weights of the BP neural network prediction model with a good fit effect, it is necessary to adjust and compare the hyperparameters such as the number of individuals in the population, the number of generations, the crossover and mutation probability in the genetic algorithm. Therefore, in this section, the hyperparameters in Table 4 are adjusted from the default values, and the optimal value is selected as the result of this test after three tests under the same conditions. It is used to evaluate the comparison results of R^2, MAE and AWE recording the changes of various hyperparameters, find the relevant hyperparameters of the model with the strongest generalization ability, and find the HFMD epidemic prediction model with the highest prediction accuracy based on these hyperparameters.

Table 4. Hyperparameters related to genetic algorithm in GA-BP neural network model.

Hyperparameter Name	Description	Default
Population size	number of individuals in the population	70
Number of generations	population evolution times	60
Mutation probability	probability of genetic mutation on individual chromosomes	0.1
Crossover probability	probability of genetic recombination on chromosomes of two individuals	0.9

6.5.1. Impact of the Number of Generations

The model evaluation results of adjusting the number of generations are shown in Table 5, and the line graph shown in Figure 13 is drawn accordingly.

According to Table 5 and Figure 13, when the number of generations reaches 90 times, the goodness of fit and the accuracy within error achieve the maximum value. When it is greater than or less than this value, these two indicators will become smaller and affect the prediction effect. At the same time, MAE reaches the minimum value, and increases whenever it is greater or less than this value. Therefore, the population evolution is iterated 90 times, and the model is optimal.

Table 5. Evaluation table for adjusting the number of generations of hyperparameters in GA-BP model.

Number of Generations	R^2	MAE	AWE
30	0.7933	13	0.3922
40	0.7916	12	0.4902
50	0.8538	10	0.5752
60	0.6798	17	0.2549
70	0.8622	10	0.5556
80	0.8539	10	0.5163
90	0.8992	8	0.5962
100	0.8328	11	0.5033
110	0.8209	12	0.4314
120	0.8628	11	0.4510

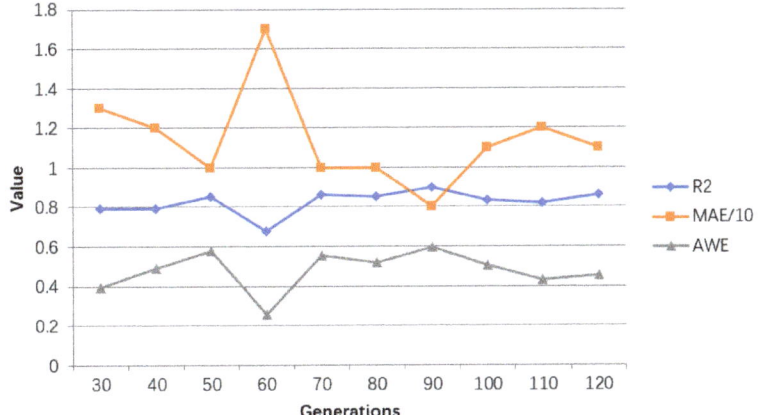

Figure 13. Line chart of adjustment results of hyperparameters in GA-BP model. The value represents results for R2, MAE/10, AWE for different parameters settings.

6.5.2. Effect of Population Size

The evaluation results of the model for adjusting the population size are shown in Table 6, and the line graph shown in Figure 14 is drawn accordingly.

Table 6. The population size adjustment evaluation table of the hyperparameters in the GA-BP model.

Population Size	R^2	MAE	AWE
10	−0.7920	35	0.2418
20	−0.1791	30	0.2353
30	0.6508	16	0.3203
40	0.6592	17	0.3072
50	0.7964	13	0.3856
60	0.9023	7	0.6053
70	0.8131	12	0.4575
80	0.7942	13	0.4379
90	0.7422	13	0.4575
100	0.8052	13	0.3856

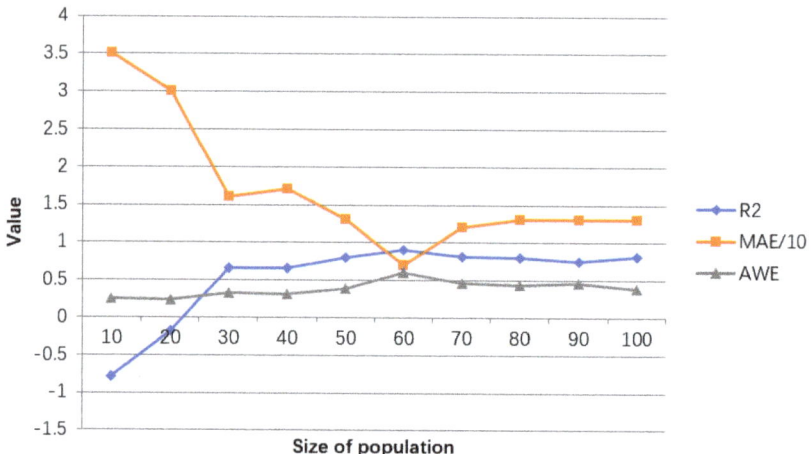

Figure 14. Line chart of adjustment results of hyperparameters in GA-BP model. The value represents results for R2, MAE/10, AWE for different parameters settings.

According to Table 6 and Figure 14, when the population size reaches 60, the goodness of fit and AWE take the maximum value. When it is greater than or less than 60, the value decreases. At the same time, MAE is the smallest, and when it is greater than or less than 60, its value will increase. Therefore, the model with a population size of 60 is optimal.

6.5.3. Impact of Crossover Probability

The model evaluation results for adjusting the cross probability are shown in Table 7, and the line graph shown in Figure 15 is drawn accordingly.

It can be obtained from Table 7 and Figure 15 that when the crossover probability reaches 0.8, the goodness of fit and AWE achieve the maximum value, while MAE is the smallest. When the crossover probability is not 0.8, the relevant index values are not ideal. Therefore, the GA model with a crossover probability of 0.8 performs best.

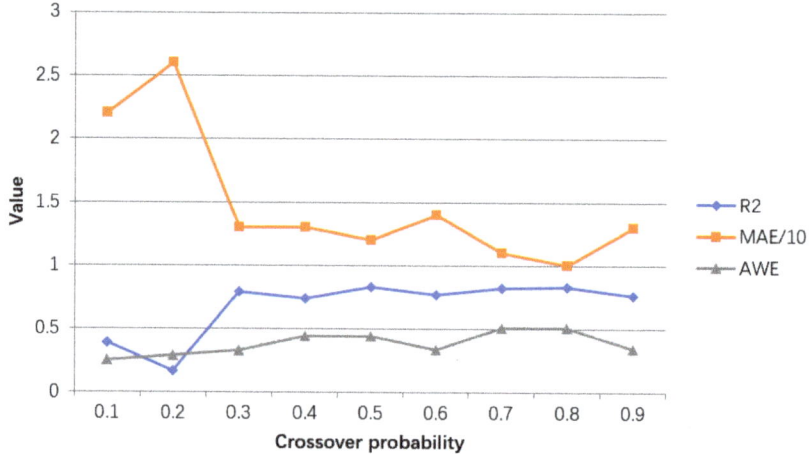

Figure 15. Line chart of the adjustment results of the crossover probability of the hyperparameters in the GA-BP model. The value represents results for R2, MAE/10, AWE for different parameters settings.

Table 7. Adjustment evaluation table of cross probability of hyperparameters in GA-BP model.

Crossover Probability	R^2	MAE	AWE
0.1	0.3900	22	0.2484
0.2	0.1680	26	0.2876
0.3	0.7922	13	0.3268
0.4	0.7411	13	0.4444
0.5	0.8301	12	0.4444
0.6	0.7688	14	0.3333
0.7	0.8258	11	0.5074
0.8	0.8341	10	0.5098
0.9	0.7635	13	0.3399

6.5.4. Impact of Gene Mutation Probability

The evaluation results of the model for regulating the probability of gene mutation are shown in Table 8, and the line graph shown in Figure 16 is drawn accordingly.

Table 8. Adjustment evaluation table of hyperparameter mutation probability in GA-BP model.

Mutation Probability	R^2	MAE	AWE
0.10	0.8270	11	0.4837
0.09	0.8194	12	0.4444
0.08	0.8036	13	0.3464
0.07	0.8053	13	0.3399
0.06	0.8137	12	0.3660
0.05	0.8400	11	0.4706
0.04	0.9256	9	0.7011
0.03	0.7796	12	0.4033
0.02	0.7484	14	0.3725
0.01	0.7643	13	0.4314

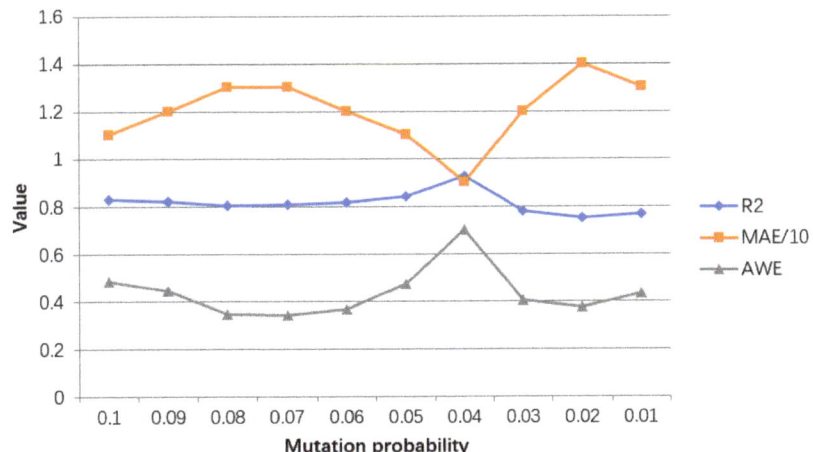

Figure 16. Line chart of adjustment results of hyperparameter mutation probability in GA-BP model. The value represents results for R2, MAE/10, AWE for different parameters settings.

It can be obtained from Table 8 and Figure 16 that when the mutation probability is 0.04, the goodness of fit and AWE reach a good result, the maximum value is selected, and MAE is minimum. Higher or lower than this probability will make the relevant index value worse. Therefore, the GA model with a mutation probability of 0.04 has the best performance and a better effect.

Through the adjustment and comparison of these four hyperparameters in GA, it is found that the individual population is 60, the number of evolutionary iterations is 90, the gene crossover probability is 0.8, and the gene mutation probability is 0.04. At this time, the neural network HFMD prevalence prediction model based on GA has the strongest generalization ability, the smallest error, and best results.

6.6. Comparative Analysis of Early-Warning Models

According to our experiment, we have built the GA-BP HFMD prediction model. We set the critical eigenvalue of HFMD outbreak and substitute the eigenvalue into the prediction model to obtain the first HFMD outbreak threshold. Then, the samples of test data were input into three early warning models, and the 80 percentile incidence of the region was calculated as the second HFMD outbreak threshold for the same period of 3 years and 2 weeks before and after the same period. Finally, the WR and ACR values of different warning models were counted, as shown in Table 9.

Table 9. Comparison of different early-warning models.

	Adjustable Parameters	Historical Percentile	Threshold Comparison
WR	4.13%	29.08%	32.02%
ACR	98.62%	85.46%	87.28%

According to the comparison, we could see that although warning model based on adjustable parameters has the best ACR, its WR is too small, so it is not generalized. Therefore, we conclude that the warning-model based on threshold comparison should be the optimal one.

7. Conclusions

This paper proposes a prediction and early-warning model for HFMD and the model uses big data. Data used in this paper are patient data and weather data. We can obtain a more accurate early-warning effect by constructing integrated prediction and early-warning model based on big data.

This paper constructs the prediction model by using GA to optimize the BP neural network. The best prediction accuracy could be gain as 92.56%. Then we explores the various construction methods of early-warning model. Through the comparison of experiment results, it is found that the early-warning model based on the comparison of threshold has the highest accuracy. And the optimal accuracy of the early-warning method is around 87.28%.There are still many parts that can be optimized in the research of this paper. For example, we would want to add more factors to enhance the accuracy of the prediction model. We will continue to study in depth accordingly.

Author Contributions: Conceptualization, X.W. and Y.W.; methodology, Y.W.; software, X.D.; validation, L.J.; formal analysis, M.W.; investigation, M.W.; resources, H.G.; data curation, X.L.; writing—original draft preparation, X.L.; writing—review and editing, X.Y.; visualization, X.L.; supervision, X.Y.; project administration, H.G.; funding acquisition, H.G., and X.Y. All authors have read and agreed to the published version of the manuscript.

Funding: This work is supported by the National Science and Technology Major Project of China under Grant No. 2018ZX10201-002, and the National Natural Science Foundation of China under Grant No. 91846303.

Institutional Review Board Statement: Not applicable.

Informed Consent Statement: Not applicable.

Data Availability Statement: Not applicable

Conflicts of Interest: The authors declare no conflict of interest.

References

1. Yang, R.; Hu, S.; Zen, X.; Peng, X. Advances in study on the prediction and alert models of hand foot and mouth disease. *Pract. Prev. Med.* **2015**, *22*, 1399–1402.
2. Liu, T.; Li, Q.; Qi, L.; Li, B.; Xia, Y.; Yang, L.; Zhao, H. Establishment of early warning model of hand, foot and mouth disease based on moving epidemic method in Chongqing. *Dis. Surveill.* **2020**, *35*, 1020–1024.
3. Nie, T.; Cui, J.; Ren, M.; Liu, F.; Sun, J.; Zhang, J.; Chang, Z. Applying moving epidemic interval to determine the threshold of hand, foot and mouth disease epidemic intensity in southern China. *Chin. J. Epidemiol.* **2020**, *41*, 1047–1053.
4. Zheng, G.; Cai, J. Application of multi-layer perceptron neural network in the prediction model of hand-foot-mouth disease. *Chin. J. PHM* **2020**, *36*, 67–73.
5. Yao, Y.; Huo, D.; Jia, L.; Wang, X. Early warning model of hand, foot and mouth disease and its application status. *Int. J. Virol.* **2018**, *25*, 136–139.
6. Cao, M.; Li, Q.; Hu, C. Overview on early outbreak detection system. *Chin. J. Epidemiol.* **2006**, *27*, 1005–1007.
7. Zhang, Z.; Chen, W.; Zhong, C. Aattempt at establishment and aplication of symptom monitoring system of hospital infectious disease. *Dis. Surveill.* **2008**, *23*, 67–69.
8. Hu, X.; Wu, H.; Qi, S.; Yan, S.; Ling, G.; Han, J. Overview of symptom surveillance and prewarning indicators systems. *Chin. Front. Health Quar.* **2012**, *35*, 212–216.
9. Yan, W.; Shi, L.; Ran, P.; Zhou, Y. Introduction to the U.S. early warning system. *Med. Soc.* **2006**, *19*, 19–21.
10. Zhang, H.; Wang, L.; Lai, S.; Li, Z.; Sun, Q.; Zhang, P. Surveillance and early warning systems of infectious disease in China. *Int. J. Health Plan. Manag.* **2017**, *32*, 329–338. [CrossRef] [PubMed]
11. Nie, S.; Huang, S. Research on the status quo of construction of infectious disease forecast and early warning system. *J. Pub. Health Prev. Med.* **2010**, *21*, 1–3.
12. Li, X.; Wang, J.; Yang, W.; Yan, S.; Li, Z.; Lai, S.; Liao, Y. The Effect Comparison of Spatial Scan Statistic Method Based on Different Parameters in Early Warning of Infectious Disease Outbreak. *Chin. J. Health Stat.* **2014**, *31*, 236–239.
13. Chen, X.; Zhang, Y.; Jin, Y.; Liu, F.; Wang, J.; Li, G.; Chen, S. Study of early detection for hand-foot-mouth diseases by moving percentile mothod in Baoji City. *Chin. J. Pub. Health Prev. Med.* **2015**, *31*, 34–36.
14. An, Q.; Zhou, Y.; Yao, W. Comparison of three methods for predicting the incidence of hand, foot and mouth disease in a city. *Chin. J. Health Stat.* **2011**, *28*, 314–315.
15. Yin, Y.; Jin, D.; He, Y.; Qiao, F.; Zhang, X.; Cui, L.; Tian, L.; Gao, Q. Relation between daily incidence of hand-foot-mouth disease and meteorological factors in Anshan City and the establishment of prediction model. *Guangxi Med J.* **2019**, *41*, 600–603.
16. Jing, Q.; Wu, Q.; Lu, Y.; Zhang, Z.; Yang, Z. Studies on early warning threshold of meteorological parameters related to the epidemic and outbreak of hand-foot-mouth disease. *Chin. Prev. Med.* **2019**, *20*, 579–583.
17. Liu, Y.; Liu, T.; Li, X. Application of SARIMA model and seasonal trend model to predict the incidence of hand, foot and mouth disease. *Jiangsu J. Prev. Med.* **2019**, *30*, 150–152.
18. Yang, X.; Chen, G.; Qian, Y.; Wang, Y.; Zhai, Y.; Fan, D.; Xu, Y. Prediction of Myopia in Adolescents through Machine Learning Methods. *Int. J. Environ. Res. Public Health* **2020**, *17*, 463. [CrossRef]
19. Peng, T.; Chen, X.; Wan, M.; Jin, L.; Wang, X.; Du, X.; Ge, H.; Yang, X. On Prediction of Hepatitis E through Ensemble Learning. *Int. J. Environ. Res. Public Health* **2021**, *18*, 159. [CrossRef]
20. Jiang, X.; Lai, S.; Zhong, J. Preliminary application of China infectious diseases automated-alert and response system in Quzhou city. *Chin. J. Health Lab. Technol.* **2012**, *22*, 2727–2729.
21. Chi, W. Forecasting stock index based on BP neural network algorithm. In Proceedings of the 2018 International Conference on Mechanical, Electronic, Control and Automation Engineering (MECAE 2018), Qingdao, China, 30–31 March 2018.
22. Ding, S.; Su, C.; Yu, J. An optimizing BP neural network algorithm based on genetic algorithm. *Artif. Intell. Rev.* **2011**, *36*, 153–162. [CrossRef]

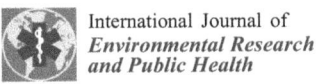

International Journal of
Environmental Research and Public Health

Article

Development and Validation of a Machine Learning Model Predicting Arteriovenous Fistula Failure in a Large Network of Dialysis Clinics

Ricardo Peralta [1], Mario Garbelli [2], Francesco Bellocchio [2], Pedro Ponce [1], Stefano Stuard [3], Maddalena Lodigiani [2], João Fazendeiro Matos [1], Raquel Ribeiro [4], Milind Nikam [5], Max Botler [6], Erik Schumacher [6], Diego Brancaccio [3] and Luca Neri [2,*]

1. NephroCare Portugal, Fresenius Medical Care Portugal, 1750-130 Lisboa, Portugal; ricardo.peralta@fmc-ag.com (R.P.); pedro.ponce@fmc-ag.com (P.P.); jfazendeiro.matos@fmc-ag.com (J.F.M.)
2. Clinical & Data Intelligence Systems-Advanced Analytics, Fresenius Medical Care, 26020 Vaiano Cremasco, Italy; mario.garbelli@fmc-ag.com (M.G.); francesco.bellocchio@fmc-ag.com (F.B.); maddalena.lodigiani@fmc-ag.com (M.L.)
3. Global Medical Office-Clinical & Therapeutic Governance Fresenius Medical Care, 61352 Bad Homburg, Germany; Stefano.stuard@fmc-ag.com (S.S.); diego.brancaccio@tiscali.it (D.B.)
4. Nursing Care, Care Operations EMEA, 61352 Bad Homburg, Germany; raquel.ribeiro@fmc-ag.com
5. Global Medical Office, Global Clinical Affairs, Medical Governance & Digital Health AP, Fresenius Medical Care, Singapore 307684, Singapore; Milind.Nikam@fmc-asia.com
6. Global Research & Development, Data Solutions, Fresenius Medical Care, 10117 Berlin, Germany; Max.botler@fmc-data-solutions.com (M.B.); erik.schumacher@fmc-data-solutions.com (E.S.)
* Correspondence: luca.neri@fmc-ag.com

Abstract: Background: Vascular access surveillance of dialysis patients is a challenging task for clinicians. We derived and validated an arteriovenous fistula failure model (AVF-FM) based on machine learning. **Methods:** The AVF-FM is an XG-Boost algorithm aimed at predicting AVF failure within three months among in-centre dialysis patients. The model was trained in the derivation set (70% of initial cohort) by exploiting the information routinely collected in the Nephrocare European Clinical Database (EuCliD®). Model performance was tested by concordance statistic and calibration charts in the remaining 30% of records. Features importance was computed using the SHAP method. **Results:** We included 13,369 patients, overall. The Area Under the ROC Curve (AUC-ROC) of AVF-FM was 0.80 (95% CI 0.79–0.81). Model calibration showed excellent representation of observed failure risk. Variables associated with the greatest impact on risk estimates were previous history of AVF complications, followed by access recirculation and other functional parameters including metrics describing temporal pattern of dialysis dose, blood flow, dynamic venous and arterial pressures. **Conclusions:** The AVF-FM achieved good discrimination and calibration properties by combining routinely collected clinical and sensor data that require no additional effort by healthcare staff. Therefore, it can potentially enable risk-based personalization of AVF surveillance strategies.

Keywords: machine learning; artificial intelligence; vascular access surveillance; arteriovenous fistula; end stage kidney disease; dialysis; kidney failure

1. Introduction

Arteriovenous fistula (AVF) represents the gold standard vascular access (VA) for haemodialysis (HD). Over time, AVFs may develop dysfunction and lower blood flow due to a series of biological changes that can lead to the formation of a stenosis and subsequent thrombosis. This event has a severe impact on the clinical status of dialysis patients; in the best scenario, endovascular and surgical interventions can restore a satisfactory AVF flow; if not, a central venous catheter (CVC) needs to be placed for interim dialysis access.

Considering the strong negative impact of AVF failure on patient survival, morbidity and quality of life, recent guidelines focused on potential strategies for AVF preservation.

The National Kidney Foundation's (NKF) (KDOQI) Guidelines [1], recommend AVF periodical physical examination (PE), or ultrasound evaluation as primary monitoring methods to detect access dysfunction. However, there is no evidence on the advantages to routine AVF surveillance by measuring intra access blood flow (Qa) [1,2] to improve access patency; nevertheless, its assessment should be considered [3,4].

The controversy concerning the best surveillance strategy to ascertain and evaluate venous stenoses has not yet been solved [5]. The rationale for surveillance is based on the hypothesis that progressive stenosis can be accurately detected by reduced Qa and increased venous pressure (VP) before VA thrombosis occurs [4,6].

Even though both Qa surveillance and ultrasound examination, coupled with preemptive correction of hemodynamically significantly reduces the risk of thrombosis and access loss [7–12], false positive tests would lead to unnecessary intervention procedures [13] which may ultimately promote further neointimal hyperplasia [14]. No current surveillance method is without pitfalls. Major concerns for Qa surveillance relate to low reproducibility in clinical practice which corresponds to a minimal detectable change as large as 25%, questionable cost-effectiveness as the sole surveillance strategy [15] and suboptimal inter-rater agreement across different measurement techniques [16]. Furthermore, the accuracy in identifying stenosis with Qa varies according to patient characteristics and location [15,17]. On the other hand, ultrasound examination requires significant operator training and skill, may not be readily available in all clinical contexts and may not yield conclusive indications for interventions [18,19]. Structured physical examination has been proposed as a convenient alternative monitoring method. The assessment of PE accuracy in detecting and locating AVF stenosis has shown mixed results; whereas few studies have shown acceptable accuracy in either the diagnosis of outflow and of inflow stenosis [20,21] compared with angiography; few others [22,23] reached opposite conclusions. In addition, a meta-analysis of randomized control trial (RCT) studies showed that blood flow measurement was superior in predicting outcomes [24–26]. Furthermore, PE is operator-dependent [27], and has limited long-term prediction power thus explaining why, in a large majority of the cases, many patients may need more frequent surveillance when assuming a rapid AVF deterioration. Taken together, the impact of PE alone on actual prevention of thrombosis is limited [28].

An excellent surveillance method should be quick, easy, accurate, non-invasive, non-operator-dependent and cost-effective. It is clear, that none of the existing methods can fulfil such expectations alone and a one-fits-all approach is not be able to adequately capture the diversity of AVF functional trajectories between and within patients.

In principle, an automatic triage system based on routinely recorded data requiring no additional effort by healthcare professionals may be used to personalize surveillance strategies based on expected risk stratification.

To this end, we sought to develop and validate a risk model based on the machine learning methods predicting the occurrence of AVF failure within three months.

2. Materials and Methods

2.1. General Description of the Arteriovenous Fistula Failure Model (AVF-FM)

The AVF Failure Model (AVF-FM) aims at predicting the occurrence of a composite AVF failure endpoint (see, Endpoint Definition below) within three months based on routinely recorded clinical information readily available in health information systems for dialysis patients.

The model is based on the XGBoost algorithm, an iterative method where, at each iteration, a new sub-model is added to correct the prediction error of the previous iteration. Each sub-model is an ensemble of decision trees. A decision tree can be roughly described as a flowchart-like structure in which each internal node represents a "discrimination test" on a given attribute (e.g., any clinical parameter or demographic characteristics); each branch of the decision tree represents the result of the discrimination test (i.e., passed or not), and each leaf node represent the probability of the outcome. This probability represents the prevalence of events occurring in each leaf in the training set.

The iterative process ends in accordance with a pre-specified stopping rule (e.g., maximum number of iterations or minimal acceptable average prediction error). The structure of the model is computed as a function optimization process combining the minimization of both training error and model complexity.

We selected XGBoost since it is characterized by a good prediction accuracy in a broad variety of problems coupled with short computational time. Furthermore, SHapley Additive exPlanations (SHAP) analysis [29] enables intuitive model interpretation through an accurate and efficient estimation of the contribution of each input variable to the risk.

2.2. AVF-FM Training

The AVF-FM was derived using the information collected in the European Clinical Database (EuCliD®, Fresenius Medical Care, Deutschland GmbH, Wendel, Germany), a large, multinational, database including in-centre dialysis patients [30].

We enrolled all HD/HDF adult patients in Italy, Spain, and Portugal with at least five treatments performed using AVF as vascular access, in the period January 2015–October 2019 and at least three months of follow-up. Furthermore, we considered only AVFs with more than three months of maturation. The unit of analysis for model development and testing was the patient-quarter. The final dataset included all eligible patient quarters (January, April, July and October) for each year. The ascertainment period for feature computation is represented in Figure 1. To ensure sufficient data completeness, we excluded patients with less than 90 days of ascertainment period before the index date for computation.

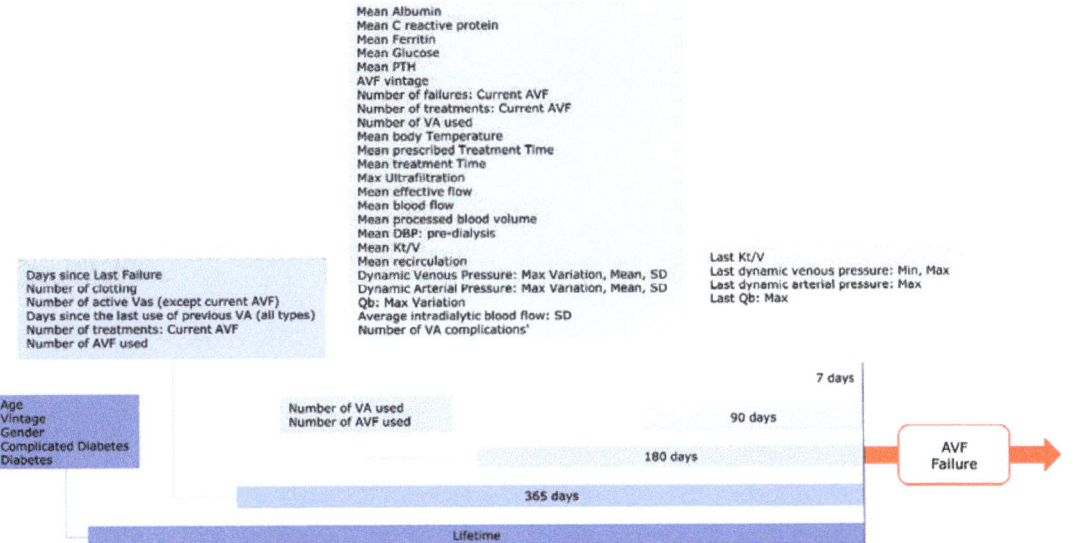

Figure 1. Study Design: the diagram represents the ascertainment period design for different groups of variables.

2.3. Measures

2.3.1. Endpoint Definition

We used a composite endpoint to define AVF failure. EuCliD® has a dedicated module for record AVF failure event. However, reporting in this module may be incomplete. In order reduce the impact of reporting bias, we used a set of proxy variables suggestive of AVF failure. Therefore, we considered as an AVF failure any switch to a different vascular access, the occurrence of procedures aimed at re-establishing AVF patency (e.g., angiography with percutaneous angioplasty, stent placement or surgical AVF revision) and hospitalization due to AVF complications. The exact operative definition of the endpoint variable is described in Supplementary Table S1.

2.3.2. Input Variables

The following classes of variables were considered for model input:
- Socio-demographic and anthropometric parameters;
- Biochemical parameters;
- Vital Signs;
- Dialysis Treatment parameters;
- AVF-related parameters;
- Comorbidities.

We ascertained diabetes by the occurrence of suggestive ICD10 codes according to the Charlson Comorbidity Index (CCI) definition [31]. Additionally, we extracted age, biological sex, dialysis vintage and number of patient's dialysis access.

2.3.3. Features Generation

We computed several metrics (minimum, maximum, average, standard deviation, slope) for continuous variables (e.g., dynamic venous and arterial needle pressure). Each metric was computed considering different time periods (e.g., last 7, 30, 90 days before index date).

2.3.4. Features Selection

All features have been included in the first model iteration (Supplementary Table S2). Features that provided trivial contribution to model prediction based on feature importance statistics were excluded from the following training iterations. The final model included a total of 46 features derived from 28 variables (Table 1).

Table 1. Patients Characteristics.

Variables	Values
Socio-Demographics, vital signs and Comorbidities	
Age (years), median (IQR)	70 (58–78)
Male, n (%)	8971 (67.1)
Body temperature, median (IQR)	36.1 (35.9–36.3)
Renal Replacement Therapy Vintage (months), median (IQR)	17.3 (5.3–59.3)
AVF vintage (months), median (IQR)	9.3 (3.7–42.7)
Diabetes mellitus, n (%)	4959 (37.1)
Complicated Diabetes, n (%)	4238 (31.7)
Biochemical parameters	
Albumin (g/dL), mean (IQR)	3.9 (3.6–4.1)
C-reactive protein (mg/L), mean (IQR)	5.1 (2.1–12)
Ferritin (ng/mL), median (IQR)	391 (204–615)
Glucose (mg/dL), median (IQR)	113 (94–152)
PTH (pg/mL), median (IQR)	245 (143–392)
HD treatment parameters	
Treatment time (min), median (IQR)	240 (239–242)
Ultrafiltration (L), median (IQR)	3.3 (2.8–4)
Effective blood flow (mL/min), median (IQR)	397 (357–428)
Effective processed blood volume (L), median (IQR)	95.7 (85.1–103.9)
Kt/V, mean (SD)	1.8 (0.4)
Recirculation, median (IQR)	13.9 (11.4–17.7)
Characteristics of AVF in use	
Days since the last use of previous vascular access, median (IQR)	74 (38–115)
Number of vascular accesses used in the past 6 months, mean (SD)	1.3 (0.5)
Number of treatments with AVF in the past 6 months, mean (SD)	88.6 (56.3)

Table 1. Cont.

Variables	Values
AVF hemodynamic properties	
Dynamic venous pressure: Mean (mmHg), median (IQR)	182 (165–202)
Dynamic arterial pressure: Mean (mmHg), median (IQR)	−200 (−216–−181)
AVF failure history and previous adverse events	
Number of failures: current AVF, mean (SD)	0.6 (1.5)
Days since the last failure, mean (SD)	168 (88.6)
Number of previous thrombosis, mean (SD)	0.4 (1)
Other active vascular access, mean (SD)	0.4 (0.7)
History of vascular access complications, mean (SD)	0.5 (1.4)

All variables were included in the AVF Failure Model. IQR, interquartile range; SD, standard deviation; AVF, arteriovenous fistula.

2.3.5. Missing Variables Handling

Missing values for the input variables are automatically managed by XGBoost, so no data manipulation was required. The algorithm has proven greater accuracy compared to the standard statistical sample or model based missing data handling methods, as well as other machine learning techniques such as random forest or Bayesian ridge methods. A detailed explanation of how XGboost handles missing variables for a wide range of missingness patterns is beyond the scope of the manuscript and it has been thoroughly described in previous technical publications [32]

2.4. Statistical Analysis and Model Performance Evaluation

Model derivation was conducted in a randomly selected partition representing 70% of the original dataset. The final set of variables was obtained as the result of backward stepwise feature selection [33]. Model performance and calibration have been evaluated in the remaining 30% of patients. Model performance was evaluated by concordance statistic and calibration charts. Discrimination was quantified by calculating the area under the receiver operating characteristic curve (ROC AUC) Calibration was visually inspected by plotting observed outcomes incidence by predicted risk score. To evaluate model stability, both training and test has been repeated over 30 random resampling. All statistics are reported as pooled estimates (inverse variance method) and 95% confidence intervals of metrics obtained in the 30 resampling exercises obtained by fixed effect meta-analysis. The importance of input variables for risk prediction was computed using SHAP method. All analysis was performed with Python version 3.7.10, MetaXL® and SAS 9.4®.

3. Results

3.1. Derivation & Test Dataset

The final dataset consisted of 13,369 patients, which provided 113,592 patients-quarters. AVF failure incidence density was 6.6 events/100 patient-quarters or 26.4 events/100 patient years. The AVF failure incidence density in the test set was 6.38 (95% CI: 6.33–6.43). A breakdown of AVF failure events by type is reported in supplementary Table S3. Baseline characteristics of participants are shown in Table 1.

3.2. Discrimination and Calibration in the Validation Sample

The final model had a very good discrimination accuracy. The Area Under the ROC Curve (AUC-ROC) for the AVF-FM was 0.80 (95% CI 0.79–0.81). Model calibration showed excellent representation of observed failure risk (Figure 2).

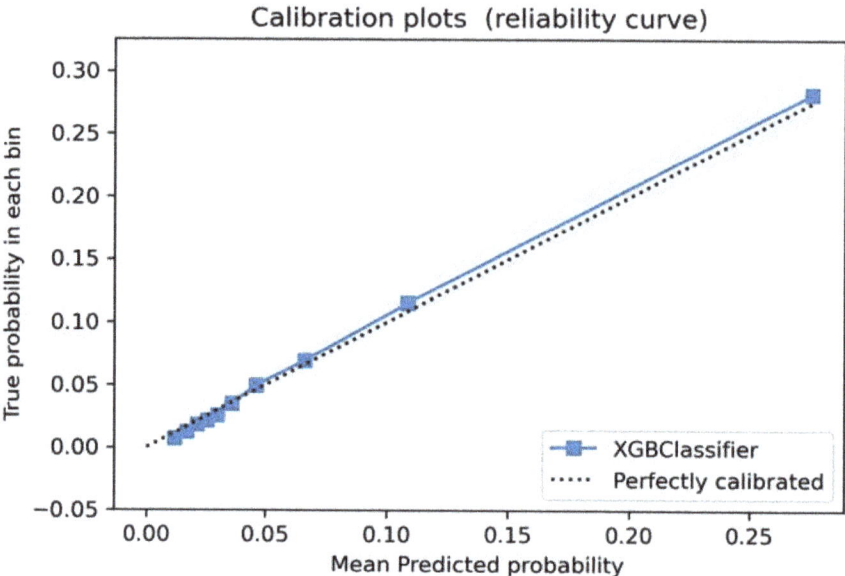

Figure 2. Calibration Plot. The calibration plot represents the relationship between predicted probabilities and observed frequency of events in the test dataset. The shaded band represents the 95% confidence interval of the calibration curve. The dotted line represents perfect calibration. The observed calibration curve overlaps with the perfect calibration line over the whole predicted probability distribution.

Based on model calibration we established three thresholds identifying 4 risk classes: prevalence and observed event incidence for each risk group is summarized in Table 2.

Table 2. Arteriovenous fistula risk score classes.

Risk Class	Prevalence (%)	AVF Failure Risk *	Risk Rate Ratio
Low	45.0 (95% CI: 44.9–45.1)	1.61 (95% CI: 1.57–1.64)	Ref.
Moderate	38.9 (95% CI: 38.8–39.0)	5.29 (95% CI: 5.22–5.36)	3.29 (95% CI: 3.2–3.38)
High	15.7 (95% CI: 15.7–15.8)	21.46 (95% CI: 21.23–21.68)	13.37 (95% CI: 13.04–13.72)
Very high	0.4 (95% CI: 0.3–0.4)	65.76 (95% CI: 63.16–68.45)	41.18 (95% CI: 39.29–43.17)

Risk classes are defined based on three action thresholds of the AVF-FM risk score. Prevalence of each risk class, event rates and risk ratios were estimated in 30 test set obtained as random partition of the original cohort with a 70–30 split. Figures represent pooled estimates (inverse variance method) from 30 random samplings of the of the original cohort. Source figures for each random sampling is reported in Supplementary Table S4. * The AVF Failure Risk is the Positive Predictive Value (events/100 patient-quarters) computed for patients classified in a given risk class; that is PPV = P (Failure | Class). Note: AVF, Arteriovenous fistula.

3.3. Feature Analysis

The 20 most important data features contributing to performance of AVF failure risk score model, are shown in Figures 3 and 4. Previous history of AVF complications occurred on the vascular access under consideration was the most impactful variable, followed by recirculation and other functional parameters including metrics describing temporal pattern of spKt/V, blood pump flow (Qb), dynamic venous and arterial pressures. Furthermore, AVF vintage, diastolic blood pressure, serum albumin and C-reactive protein were ranked among the top-20 risk contributors.

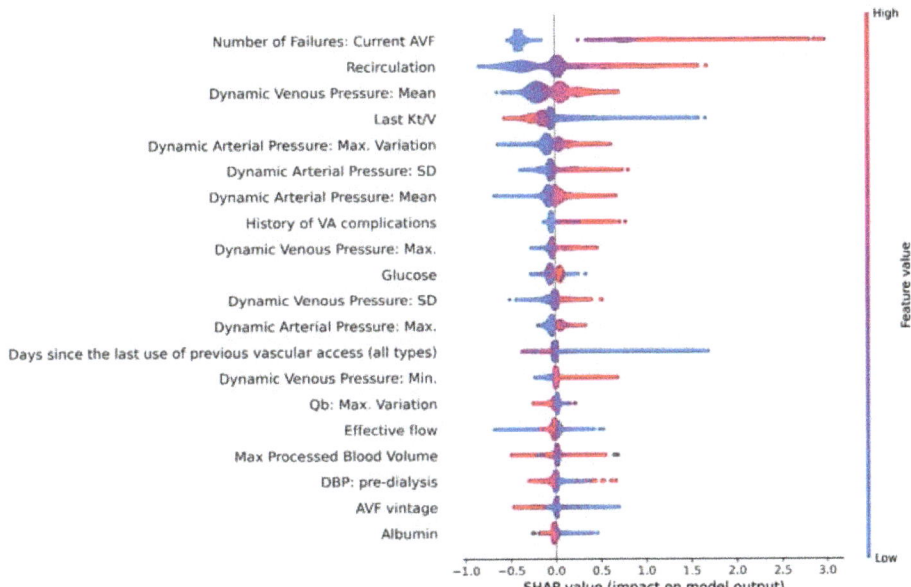

Figure 3. Shapley additive explanations (SHAP) plot showing relative feature importance. Each dot represents one individual subject from the test dataset. Colour Coding: the red colour represents higher value of the variable; the blue colour represents a lower value of the variable. The X axis represent the impact of variables on risk in terms of SHAP values. Positive values suggest direct correlations between risk factors and the occurrence of AVF failures. Negative values suggest inverse correlation between risk factors and the occurrence of AVF failures. Note: AVF, arteriovenous fistula; DBP, diastolic blood pressure; SD, standard deviation; Qb, blood pump flow.

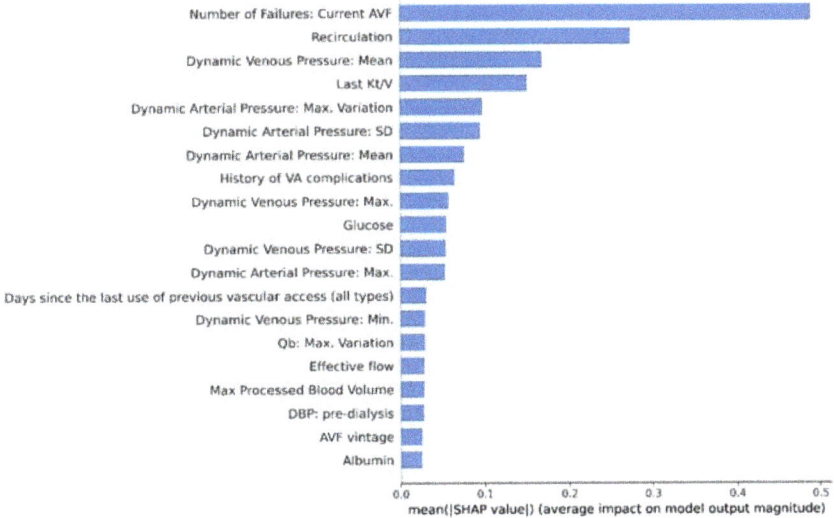

Figure 4. Variable Importance plot. Mean SHAP values represent variable importance plot for the top 20 features in the final model Notes: AVF, arteriovenous fistula; DBP, diastolic blood pressure; SD, standard deviation; Qb, blood pump flow.

4. Discussion

The wide scale implementation of electronic health record technology has led to an important and unprecedented accumulation of clinical data, and patient information is immediately accessible to computer systems. We exploited the wealth of information stored in the EuCliD® system to derive a machine-learning algorithm for the prediction of AVF failure within three months.

The model showed good discrimination and excellent calibration. To enhance the interpretation and usability of risk estimates yielded by the model we selected three thresholds identifying four distinct risk classes. The largest group was represented by very low risk patients for whom the expected incidence of the composite AVF failure endpoint was remarkably lower than the observed incidence in the whole target population. On the other side of the spectrum there is a small group of patients accounting for less than 1% of the target population with extremely high risk of clinically significant AVF disfunctions within three months. This risk classification can be used to design personalized clinical management workflows. For example, routine monitoring using dialysis parameters and physical examination may suffice for the very low risk group, thus reducing the costs, resource requirements and importantly, unnecessary interventions. Conversely, the very high-risk patient group may be candidate for a more intensive surveillance and clinical review protocol to rule out conditions deserving immediate interventions. In-between, we found two risk classes with moderate and high risk of AVF failure, respectively. For both such classes, the optimal surveillance strategy could be designed to suit the needs and resources of the local clinic, regions, or larger geography. Importantly, accurate risk estimation makes the process of AVF surveillance optimization transparent and reproducible.

Feature analysis disclosed key information to inspect model functioning and enhance score interpretation. Among the 46 input variables, the main contribution to model performance was the past history of failures for the AVF in use, a condition associated with both constitutional proneness to thrombosis and increased AVF vulnerability due to previous surgical interventions aimed at re-establishing patency [34]. In fact, AVF stenosis are one of the most common reasons for repeated endovascular or surgical intervention and are a well-known problem in AV access maintenance. The high re-intervention rate observed (i.e., 2.46 ± 1.40 procedures/patient/year) [35], clearly explains the importance of past history of failure events as a key variable for our model.

One important finding of our study was that the majority of the 15 most important variables in the model were represented by metrics tapping functional parameters of the AVF under examination, namely recirculation rate, dynamic arterial and venous access pressures, effective blood flow and spKt/V. Access recirculation was the second most important contributing feature to risk estimates in our model. The measurement of access recirculation has been used as a non-invasive method based by ultrasound dilution technique (or dilutional-based method) to determine access blood flow (Qa) [36], and stenosis identification. A high degree of access recirculation is one of the factors more importance to identify AVF inflow problems among HD patients and was routinely used for screening of stenosis in 64% from facilities in northern Italy [37]. Access recirculation and poor HD adequacy assessed by spKt/V, may help indicate AV access dysfunction [1]. A recent study by Robert et al. [38] concluded that routine measurements of spKt/V was a quick and straightforward method for early detection of hemodynamically significant AV fistula stenosis.

Similarly, hemodynamic metrics representing the trajectory of dynamic venous and arterial pressures in the dialysis access circuit along time were strong contributors of risk estimates. Alteration of metrics representing the temporal profile of dynamic venous and arterial pressures suggest a high predictive risk of AVF failure. Abnormal dynamic arterial pressure (DAP) may be suggestive of access inflow problems while alterations of dynamic venous pressure (DVP) is associated with outflow stenosis. The incidence of inflow stenosis in patients with AVF from the cases referred to interventional facilities can reach rates of 40% with significant effects in reducing dialysis blood pump flow (Qb) [39]; therefore, combining several AVF dysfunction predictors during the same surveillance evaluation is of paramount importance.

Of note, all such measures are automatically recorded by sensors installed on HD machines and have been used, alone or in conjunction for AVF monitoring [1]. The great advantage of such metrics over routine access flow measurement (Qa) relates to their continuous, effortless availability, since they are measured without any interruption in the patient's dialysis process, and without time-consuming procedures. Despite Qa has been shown to outperform each of these functional parameters taken alone, this is the first study showing the potential of their combined use for AVF functional assessment. Given that Qa may be consistently available for a minority of patient, we did not include it in the input matrix for model generation. Whether the combination of our risk estimates and Qa provides additional predictive power in selected patients is a matter of further research.

Furthermore, given the strong dependency of risk estimates on AVF functional parameters, our model is sensitive to their changes in AVF and can be used to track risk trajectories over time without any additional data collection burden to the healthcare staff.

Our study has several strengths. The large sample size gathered from multiple dialysis centres across several countries ensured capturing wide diversity in clinical practice and case-mix, two necessary pre-condition for reproducibility and generalizability in machine learning. Additionally, we could leverage on a wide array of clinical variables to characterize patients' health status including laboratory test results, socio-demographic information, medication, dialysis treatment parameters, comorbidities and data continuously recorded by the dialysis machine during each dialysis session. The evidence regarding risk factors associated with AVF patency loss is still limited. Most studies have small sample size, and a limited set of variables was available [40]. On the contrary, we were able to evaluate the association of AVF patency loss with over 100 clinical parameters and their temporal dynamics, an unprecedented wealth of information. One additional benefit of XGBoost-based algorithm is their inherent explainability, which ensures transparency in clinical decision making. For each patient the model produces SHAP metrics which represent the importance of clinical parameters on risk estimates, allowing independent assessment by the attending physician.

On the other hand, we should acknowledge some limitations as well. Our endpoint definition is a composite outcome including thrombosis, switch to another vascular access, interventions aimed at re-establishing patency in outpatient setting and day hospital admission related to intervention to re-establish patency of the AVF. Despite our operational definition is consistent with the endpoint criteria for AVF patency loss described in the *Recommended standards for reports dealing with arteriovenous hemodialysis accesses* issued by the International Society of Vascular Surgery [41], we rely on data reported by healthcare professionals in clinical practice. Therefore, we cannot rule out the possibility that information bias affected our results. Additionally, our definition reflects medical treatment decision and therefore we cannot exclude that inappropriate surgical intervention have been conducted. This may be reflected in our risk estimates (A detailed description of the endpoint definition is reported Supplementary Table S2). Furthermore, all patients included in our analysis received treatment in the NephroCare network. Despite the multicentre, cross-country design of the study, whether the accuracy and calibration of the AVF-FM can be replicated in centres outside the NephroCare network is a matter of further research.

5. Conclusions

The fundamental principle for performing routine vascular access monitoring and surveillance is timely identification and correction of significant stenosis, thus prolonging patency. Current monitoring and surveillance methods remain operator dependent, may be inefficient and may potentially lead to unnecessary interventions.

The AVF Failure Model has shown promising discrimination performance by combining routinely collected clinical as well as sensor data; therefore, the AVF Failure Model can potentially enable risk-based personalization of AVF surveillance strategies. Whether the use of the AVF Failure Model in clinical practice would translate in more efficient care and prolonged access survival is a matter of further clinical testing.

Supplementary Materials: The following are available online at https://www.mdpi.com/article/10.3390/ijerph182312355/s1, Supplementary Table S1: Detailed description of the endpoint definition; Supplementary Table S2: All variables included in the first training iteration; Supplementary Table S3: breakdown of AVF Failure causes in our study; Supplementary Table S4: Distribution of AVF-FM risk classes in 30 re-samplings of the test set.

Author Contributions: The first draft of the manuscript was written by R.P. and M.G. M.G. also contributed to data management, data analysis, model development, and approved the final version of the manuscript. L.N. contributed to the study concept and design, model development, interpretation of results, manuscript drafting and oversaw the conduct of the study. F.B. contributed to study concept and design, model development, interpretation of results, manuscript drafting, and approved the final version of the manuscript. M.L. contributed to model development, interpretation of results and approved the final version of the manuscript. D.B. Contributed to study concept, interpretation of results and approved the final version of the manuscript. P.P., S.S., J.F.M., R.R., M.N., M.B., E.S. contributed to interpretation of results and approved the final version of the manuscript. All authors have read and agreed to the published version of the manuscript.

Funding: This research received no external funding. DB received consulting fees from FMC gmbh in the past 3 years. All remaining authors are full time employees at FMC.

Institutional Review Board Statement: The analysis has been conducted in accordance with the declaration of Helsinki. The analysis has been conducted to inform a continuous quality improvement program of health care practice. The Institutional Review Board of FMC-Nephrocare Portugal has confirmed that the study adheres to ethical standards and retrospectively approved the study protocol on 11 October 2021 (see Supplementary Material: Ethics Committee Approval).

Informed Consent Statement: All patients included in the study consented their data be used in pseudo-anonymized form for continuous quality improvement and scientific research at their registration to dialysis centers belonging to the Nephrocare network.

Data Availability Statement: The datasets used and/or analysed during the current study are personal health information obtained during provision of healthcare services and cannot be shared to protect their confidentiality in compliance with GDPR regulation.

Conflicts of Interest: D.B. received consulting fees from FMC in the past 3 years. R.P., M.G., L.N., F.B., M.L., P.P., S.S., M.B., E.S., M.N., J.F.M., R.R. are full time employees at FMC.

References

1. Lok, C.E.; Huber, T.S.; Lee, T.; Shenoy, S.; Yevzlin, A.S.; Abreo, K.; Allon, M.; Asif, A.; Astor, B.C.; Glickman, M.H.; et al. KDOQI Clinical Practice Guideline for Vascular Access: 2019 Update. *Am. J. Kidney Dis.* **2020**, *75*, S1–S164. [CrossRef] [PubMed]
2. Gallieni, M.; Hollenbeck, M.; Inston, N.; Kumwenda, M.; Powell, S.; Tordoir, J.; Al Shakarchi, J.; Berger, P.; Bolignano, D.; Cassidy, D.; et al. Clinical practice guideline on peri- and postoperative care of arteriovenous fistulas and grafts for haemodialysis in adults. *Nephrol. Dial. Transplant.* **2019**, *34* (Suppl. 2), II1–II42. [CrossRef] [PubMed]
3. Ibeas, J.; Roca-Tey, R.; Vallespín, J.; Moreno, T.; Moñux, G.; Martí-Monrós, A. por la Guía Clínica Española del Acceso Vascular para Hemodiálisis. Spanish Clinical Guidelines on Vascular Access for Haemodialysis. *Nefrología* **2017**, *37*, 1–193. [CrossRef] [PubMed]
4. Schmidli, J.; Widmer, M.K.; Basile, C.; de Donato, G.; Gallieni, M.; Gibbons, C.P.; Haage, P.; Hamilton, G.; Hedin, U.; Kamper, L.; et al. Editor's Choice—Vascular Access: 2018 Clinical Practice Guidelines of the European Society for Vascular Surgery (ESVS). *Eur. J. Vasc. Endovasc. Surg.* **2018**, *55*, 757–818. [CrossRef] [PubMed]
5. Paulson, W.D.; Moist, L.; Lok, C.E. Vascular access surveillance: An ongoing controversy. *Kidney Int.* **2012**, *81*, 132–142. [CrossRef]
6. Schmidli, J.; Widmer, M.K.; Basile, C.; de Donato, G.; Gallieni, M.; Gibbons, C.P.; Haage, P.; Hamilton, G.; Hedin, U.; Kamper, L.; et al. How to Carry out Monthly Blood Flow Surveillance of Fistula in Large-Scale Hemodialysis Units: A Cross-Sectional Study. *J. Vasc. Access* **2021**, *22*, 75–80.
7. Aragoncillo, I.; Amézquita, Y.; Caldés, S.; Abad, S.; Vega, A.; Cirugeda, A.; Moratilla, C.; Ibeas, J.; Roca-Tey, R.; Fernández, C.; et al. The impact of access blood flow surveillance on reduction of thrombosis in native arteriovenous fistula: A randomized clinical trial. *J. Vasc. Access.* **2016**, *17*, 13–19. [CrossRef]

8. Hwang, S.D.; Lee, J.H.; Lee, S.W.; Kim, J.K.; Kim, M.J.; Song, J.H. Comparison of ultrasound scan blood flow measurement versus other forms of surveillance in the thrombosis rate of hemodialysis access: A systemic review and meta-analysis. *Medicine* **2018**, *97*, e11194. [CrossRef]
9. Tessitore, N.; Poli, A. Pro: Vascular access surveillance in mature fistulas: Is it worthwhile? *Nephrol. Dial. Transplant.* **2019**, *34*, 1102–1106. [CrossRef]
10. Salman, L.; Rizvi, A.; Contreras, G.; Manning, C.; Feustel, P.J.; Machado, I.; Briones, P.L.; Jamal, A.; Bateman, N.; Martinez, L.; et al. A Multicenter Randomized Clinical Trial of Hemodialysis Access Blood Flow Surveillance Compared to Standard of Care: The Hemodialysis Access Surveillance Evaluation (HASE) Study. *Kidney Int. Rep.* **2020**, *5*, 1937–1944. [CrossRef]
11. Raimann, J.G.; Waldron, L.; Koh, E.; Miller, G.A.; Sor, M.H.; Gray, R.J.; Kotanko, P. Meta-analysis and commentary: Preemptive correction of arteriovenous access stenosis. *Hemodial. Int.* **2018**, *22*, 279–280. [CrossRef] [PubMed]
12. Ravani, P.; Quinn, R.R.; Oliver, M.J.; Karsanji, D.J.; James, M.T.; Macrae, J.M.; Palmer, S.C.; Strippoli, G.F. Pre-emptive correction for haemodialysis arteriovenous access stenosis. *Cochrane Database Syst. Rev.* **2016**, *2016*, CD010709. [CrossRef] [PubMed]
13. Ram, S.J.; Nassar, R.; Work, J.; Abreo, K.; Dossabhoy, N.R.; Paulson, W.D. Risk of Hemodialysis Graft Thrombosis: Analysis of Monthly Flow Surveillance. *Am. J. Kidney Dis.* **2008**, *52*, 930–938. [CrossRef] [PubMed]
14. Chang, C.J.; Ko, P.J.; Hsu, L.A.; Ko, Y.S.; Ko, Y.L.; Chen, C.F.; Huang, C.C.; Hsu, T.S.; Lee, Y.S.; Pang, J.H. Highly Increased Cell Proliferation Activity in the Restenotic Hemodialysis Vascular Access after Percutaneous Transluminal Angioplasty: Implication in Prevention of Restenosis. *Am. J. Kidney Dis.* **2004**, *43*, 74–84. [CrossRef] [PubMed]
15. Tessitore, N.; Bedogna, V.; Verlato, G.; Poli, A. The rise and fall of access blood flow surveillance in arteriovenous fistulas. *Semin. Dial.* **2014**, *27*, 108–118. [CrossRef]
16. Eloot, S.; Dhondt, A.; Hoeben, H.; Vanholder, R. Comparison of different methods to assess fistula flow. *Blood Purif.* **2010**, *30*, 89–95. [CrossRef] [PubMed]
17. Tessitore, N.; Bedogna, V.; Verlato, G.; Poli, A. Clinical access assessment. *J. Vasc. Access.* **2014**, *15* (Suppl. 7), S20–S27. [CrossRef]
18. Ćosović, A.; van der Kleij, F.G.; Callenbach, P.M.; Hoekstra, M.C.; Hissink, R.J.; van den Berg, M. The diagnostic value of duplex ultrasound in detecting the presence and location of a stenosis in an autologous arteriovenous fistula. *J. Vasc. Access* **2019**, *21*, 217–222. [CrossRef]
19. Nalesso, F.; Garzotto, F.; Petrucci, I.; Samoni, S.; Virzì, G.M.; Gregori, D.; Meola, M.; Ronco, C. Standardized Protocol for Hemodialysis Vascular Access Assessment: The Role of Ultrasound and ColorDoppler. *Blood Purif.* **2018**, *45*, 260–269. [CrossRef]
20. Leon, C.; Asif, A. Physical examination of arteriovenous fistulae by a renal fellow: Does it compare favorably to an experienced interventionalist? *Semin. Dial.* **2008**, *21*, 557–560. [CrossRef]
21. Coentrão, L.; Faria, B.; Pestana, M. Physical examination of dysfunctional arteriovenous fistulae by non-interventionalists: A skill worth teaching. *Nephrol. Dial. Transplant.* **2012**, *27*, 1993–1996. [CrossRef] [PubMed]
22. Asif, A.; Leon, C.; Orozco-Vargas, L.C.; Krishnamurthy, G.; Choi, K.L.; Mercado, C.; Merrill, D.; Thomas, I.; Salman, L.; Artikov, S.; et al. Accuracy of physical examination in the detection of arteriovenous fistula stenosis. *Clin. J. Am. Soc. Nephrol.* **2007**, *2*, 1191–1194. [CrossRef] [PubMed]
23. Campos, R.P.; Chula, D.C.; Perreto, S.; Riella, M.C.; Do Nascimento, M.M. Accuracy of physical examination and intra-access pressure in the detection of stenosis in hemodialysis arteriovenous fistula. *Semin. Dial.* **2008**, *21*, 269–273. [CrossRef] [PubMed]
24. Tonelli, M.; James, M.; Wiebe, N.; Jindal, K.; Hemmelgarn, B.; Kidney, A. Ultrasound Monitoring to Detect Access Stenosis in Hemodialysis Patients: A Systematic Review. *Am. J. Kidney Dis.* **2008**, *51*, 630–640. [CrossRef]
25. Tessitore, N.; Lipari, G.; Poli, A.; Bedogna, V.; Baggio, E.; Loschiavo, C.; Mansueto, G.; Lupo, A. Can blood flow surveillance and pre-emptive repair of subclinical stenosis prolong the useful life of arteriovenous fistulae? A randomized controlled study. *Nephrol. Dial. Transplant.* **2004**, *19*, 2325–2333. [CrossRef]
26. Polkinghorne, K.R.; Lau, K.K.P.; Saunder, A.; Atkins, R.C.; Kerr, P.G. Does monthly native arteriovenous fistula blood-flow surveillance detect significant stenosis—A randomized controlled trial. *Nephrol. Dial. Transplant.* **2006**, *19*, 2498–2506. [CrossRef]
27. Jackson, V.E.; Hurst, H.; Mitra, S. Structured physical assessment of arteriovenous fistulae in haemodialysis access surveillance: A missed opportunity? *J. Vasc. Access* **2018**, *19*, 221–229. [CrossRef]
28. Abreo, K.; Amin, B.M.; Abreo, A.P. Physical examination of the hemodialysis arteriovenous fistula to detect early dysfunction. *J. Vasc. Access.* **2018**, *20*, 7–11. [CrossRef]
29. Lundberg, S.M.; Lee, S. A Unified Approach to Interpreting Model Predictions. In Proceedings of the 31st Conference on Neural Information Processing Systems (NIPS 2017), Long Beach, CA, USA, 4 December 2017; pp. 1–10.
30. Stopper, A.; Amato, C.; Gioberge, S.; Giordana, G.; Marcelli, D.; Gatti, E. Managing complexity at dialysis service centers across Europe. *Blood Purif.* **2006**, *25*, 77–89. [CrossRef]
31. Quan, H.; Sundararajan, V.; Halfon, P.; Fong, A.; Burnand, B.; Luthi, J.C.; Saunders, L.D.; Beck, C.A.; Feasby, T.E.; Ghali, W.A. Coding algorithms for defining comorbidities in ICD-9-CM and ICD-10 administrative data. *Med. Care* **2005**, *43*, 1130–1139. [CrossRef]
32. Rusdah, D.A.; Murfi, H. XGBoost in handling missing values for life insurance risk prediction. *SN Appl. Sci.* **2020**, *2*, 1336. [CrossRef]
33. Tanaka, K.; Kurita, T.; Meyer, F.; Berthouze, L.; Kawabe, T. Stepwise feature selection by cross validation for EEG-based brain computer interface. In Proceedings of the 2006 IEEE International Joint Conference on Neural Network Proceedings, Vancouver, BC, Canada, 16–21 July 2006; pp. 4672–4677. [CrossRef]

34. Turmel-Rodrigues, L.; Pengloan, J.; Baudin, S.; Testou, D.; Abaza, M.; Dahdah, G.; Mouton, A.; Blanchard, D. Treatment of stenosis and thrombosis in haemodialysis fistulas and grafts by interventional radiology. *Nephrol. Dial. Transplant.* **2000**, *15*, 2029–2036. [CrossRef] [PubMed]
35. Balamuthusamy, S.; Reddi, A.L.; Madhrira, M.H.; Sankarapandian, B.; Nguyen, P.; Vallurupalli, A.; Gabbard, W.; Jalandhara, N.; Yurvati, A. Clinical predictors of recurrent stenosis and need for re-intervention in the cephalic arch in patients with brachiocephalic AV fistulas. *J. Vasc. Access.* **2017**, *18*, 319–324. [CrossRef] [PubMed]
36. Depner, T.A.; Krivitski, N.M.; MacGibbon, D. Hemodialysis Access Recirculation Measured by Ultrasound Dilution. *ASAIO J.* **1995**, *41*, M749–M753. [CrossRef] [PubMed]
37. Tessitore, N.; Bedogna, V.; Poli, A.; Impedovo, A.; Antonucci, F.; Teodori, T.; Lupo, A. Practice patterns in the management of arteriovenous fistula stenosis: A northern Italian survey. *J. Nephrol.* **2006**, *19*, 200–204. [PubMed]
38. Ekart, R.; Varda, L.; Vodošek Hojs, N.; Dvoršak, B.; Piko, N.; Bevc, S.; Hojs, R. Early Detection of Arteriovenous Fistula Stenosis in Hemodialysis Patients through Routine Measurements of Dialysis Dose (Kt/V). *Blood Purif.* **2021**, 1–8. [CrossRef]
39. Asif, A.; Gadalean, F.N.; Merrill, D.; Cherla, G.; Cipleu, C.D.; Epstein, D.L.; Roth, D. Inflow stenosis in arteriovenous fistulas and grafts: A multicenter, prospective study. *Kidney Int.* **2005**, *67*, 1986–1992. [CrossRef]
40. Stirbu, O.; Gadalean, F.; Pitea, I.V.; Ciobanu, G.; Schiller, A.; Grosu, I.; Nes, A.; Bratescu, R.; Olariu, N.; Timar, B.; et al. C-reactive protein as a prognostic risk factor for loss of arteriovenous fistula patency in hemodialyzed patients. *J. Vasc. Surg.* **2019**, *70*, 208–215. [CrossRef]
41. Sidawy, A.N.; Gray, R.; Besarab, A.; Henry, M.; Ascher, E.; Silva, M., Jr.; Miller, A.; Scher, L.; Trerotola, S.; Gregory, R.T.; et al. Recommended standards for reports dealing with arteriovenous hemodialysis accesses. *J. Vasc. Surg.* **2002**, *35*, 603–610. [CrossRef]

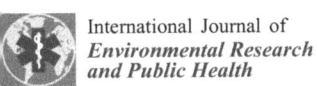
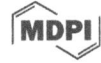

Article

Validation of a Novel Predictive Algorithm for Kidney Failure in Patients Suffering from Chronic Kidney Disease: The Prognostic Reasoning System for Chronic Kidney Disease (PROGRES-CKD)

Francesco Bellocchio [1,*], Caterina Lonati [2], Jasmine Ion Titapiccolo [1], Jennifer Nadal [3], Heike Meiselbach [4], Matthias Schmid [3], Barbara Baerthlein [5], Ulrich Tschulena [6], Markus Schneider [3], Ulla T. Schultheiss [7,8], Carlo Barbieri [6], Christoph Moore [6], Sonja Steppan [6], Kai-Uwe Eckardt [4,9], Stefano Stuard [6] and Luca Neri [1]

1 Clinical & Data Intelligence Systems-Advanced Analytics, Fresenius Medical Care Deutschland GmbH, 26020 Vaiano Cremasco, Italy; Jasmine.IonTitapiccolo@fmc-ag.com (J.I.T.); luca.neri@fmc-ag.com (L.N.)
2 Center for Preclinical Research, Fondazione IRCCS Ca' Granda Ospedale Maggiore Policlinico, 20122 Milan, Italy; caterina.lonati@gmail.com
3 Department of Medical Biometry, Informatics, and Epidemiology (IMBIE), Faculty of Medicine, University of Bonn, 53113 Bonn, Germany; Jennifer.Nadal@ukbonn.de (J.N.); matthias.schmid@imbie.uni-bonn.de (M.S.); markus.schneider@extern.uk-erlangen.de (M.S.)
4 Department of Nephrology and Hypertension, Friedrich-Alexander University of Erlangen-Nürnberg, 91054 Erlangen, Germany; Heike.Meiselbach@uk-erlangen.de (H.M.); kai-uwe.eckardt@charite.de (K.-U.E.)
5 Medical Centre for Information and Communication Technology (MIK), University Hospital Erlangen, 91054 Erlangen, Germany; Barbara.Baerthlein@uk-erlangen.de
6 Fresenius Medical Care, Deutschland GmbH, 61352 Bad Homburg, Germany; Ulrich.Tschulena@fmc-ag.com (U.T.); carlo.barbieri@fmc-ag.com (C.B.); Christoph.Moore@fmc-ag.com (C.M.); Sonja.Steppan@fmc-ag.com (S.S.); Stefano.stuard@fmc-ag.com (S.S.)
7 Institute of Genetic Epidemiology, Faculty of Medicine and Medical Center, University of Freiburg, 79085 Freiburg, Germany; ulla.schultheiss@uniklinik-freiburg.de
8 Department of Medicine IV–Nephrology and Primary Care, Faculty of Medicine and Medical Center, University of Freiburg, 79085 Freiburg, Germany
9 Department of Nephrology and Medical Intensive Care, Charité Universitätsmedizin Berlin, 10117 Berlin, Germany
* Correspondence: francesco.bellocchio@fmc-ag.com

Abstract: Current equation-based risk stratification algorithms for kidney failure (KF) may have limited applicability in real world settings, where missing information may impede their computation for a large share of patients, hampering one from taking full advantage of the wealth of information collected in electronic health records. To overcome such limitations, we trained and validated the Prognostic Reasoning System for Chronic Kidney Disease (PROGRES-CKD), a novel algorithm predicting end-stage kidney disease (ESKD). PROGRES-CKD is a naïve Bayes classifier predicting ESKD onset within 6 and 24 months in adult, stage 3-to-5 CKD patients. PROGRES-CKD trained on 17,775 CKD patients treated in the Fresenius Medical Care (FMC) NephroCare network. The algorithm was validated in a second independent FMC cohort ($n = 6760$) and in the German Chronic Kidney Disease (GCKD) study cohort ($n = 4058$). We contrasted PROGRES-CKD accuracy against the performance of the Kidney Failure Risk Equation (KFRE). Discrimination accuracy in the validation cohorts was excellent for both short-term (stage 4–5 CKD, FMC: AUC = 0.90, 95%CI 0.88–0.91; GCKD: AUC = 0.91, 95% CI 0.86–0.97) and long-term (stage 3–5 CKD, FMC: AUC = 0.85, 95%CI 0.83–0.88; GCKD: AUC = 0.85, 95%CI 0.83–0.88) forecasting horizons. The performance of PROGRES-CKD was non-inferior to KFRE for the 24-month horizon and proved more accurate for the 6-month horizon forecast in both validation cohorts. In the real world setting captured in the FMC validation cohort, PROGRES-CKD was computable for all patients, whereas KFRE could be computed for complete cases only (i.e., 30% and 16% of the cohort in 6- and 24-month horizons). PROGRES-CKD accurately predicts KF onset among CKD patients. Contrary to equation-based scores, PROGRES-CKD extends to patients with incomplete data and allows explicit assessment of prediction robustness in case of missing values. PROGRES-CKD may efficiently assist physicians' prognostic reasoning in real-life applications.

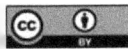

Keywords: chronic kidney disease (CKD); end-stage kidney disease (ESKD); kidney replacement therapy (KRT); risk prediction; artificial intelligence; machine learning; naïve Bayes classifiers; precision medicine

1. Introduction

Multiple behavioral and pharmacological interventions have proven effective in reducing the burden of risk factors for chronic kidney disease (CKD) progression [1–4]. Furthermore, timely transition management (i.e., vascular access creation and training) for patients needing Kidney Replacement Therapy (KRT) is associated with prolonged survival and reduced complication rates once on dialysis, while delayed referrals are associated with increased morbidity, mortality, and healthcare costs [5], as well as worse patient quality of life [6]. Therefore, early identification of high risk patients is an essential prerequisite of personalized clinical decision making [7–9].

Several prediction models were developed to assist physicians in forecasting CKD progression [10]. However, most of them have not been consistently implemented in clinical practice [9,11,12]. Indeed, the majority of published risk scores lack external validation [11,13,14], leading to suboptimal discrimination in external populations [12] and limited generalizability to clinical settings [11]. One prominent exception is represented by the Kidney Failure Risk Equations (KFREs) developed by Tangri and colleagues [15], which showed stable discrimination in different validation studies [16–18]. However, KFREs do not provide short-term forecasts, are not calculable for patients with incomplete data, and need re-calibration when applied to CKD populations with risk factor distributions departing from those of the original derivation dataset.

To overcome such limitations, we developed the Prognostic Reasoning System for Chronic Kidney Disease (PROGRES-CKD), a risk score application for adult patients suffering from CKD stages 3–5. PROGRES-CKD is based on a naïve Bayes Classifier (NBC) algorithm and it was trained on a large-multinational clinical dataset, reflecting real-world clinical practice. The application includes PROGRES-CKD-6 for 6-month forecasting and PROGRES-CKD-24 for 24-month forecasting.

In the present study, we reported the training and validation of both PROGRES-CKD-6 and PROGRES-CKD-24 in two independent samples of CKD patients: the FMC NephroCare cohort (European Clinical Database, EuCliD®, [19,20]) and the German Chronic Kidney Disease (GCKD) study cohort [21]. Moreover, we compared the PROGRES-CKD discrimination accuracy and suitability for clinical practice against the KFREs equations.

2. Materials and Methods

In reporting PROGRES-CKD training and validation studies we adhered to the Transparent reporting of a multivariable prediction model for individual prognosis or diagnosis (TRIPOD) statement [22] and to the Guidelines for Developing and Reporting Machine Learning Predictive Models in Biomedical Research [23].

2.1. Description of Naïve Bayes Classifiers

All PROGRES-CKD models are NBCs. NBCs are probabilistic models based on application of the Bayes' theorem. The basic assumption of NBCs is conditional independence of predictors given the outcome. NBCs are represented through directed acyclic graphs (Figure 1). NBCs have been previously used in medical applications for diagnostic and prognostic reasoning in several therapeutic areas [24,25]. In fact, once derived and validated, NBCs generate metrics informing medical prognostic reasoning. First, they generate a risk score representing the expected incidence of a disease/event given a vector of known patient characteristics. Furthermore, NBCs can be used to generate value of information (VOI) statistics and impact metrics. VOI statistics represent the reduction in uncertainty (i.e., entropy) in the outcome variable that would be obtained had the value of missing variables been observed instead [26]. Therefore, it can be used to prioritize additional diagnostic testing or biomarker assays for patients with incomplete medical records. Third, NBCs can provide impact metrics (i.e., Normalized Likelihood (NL) [27]) for each observed variable. Impact metrics can be interpreted as the magnitude of association of different subsets of evidence on the outcome variable.

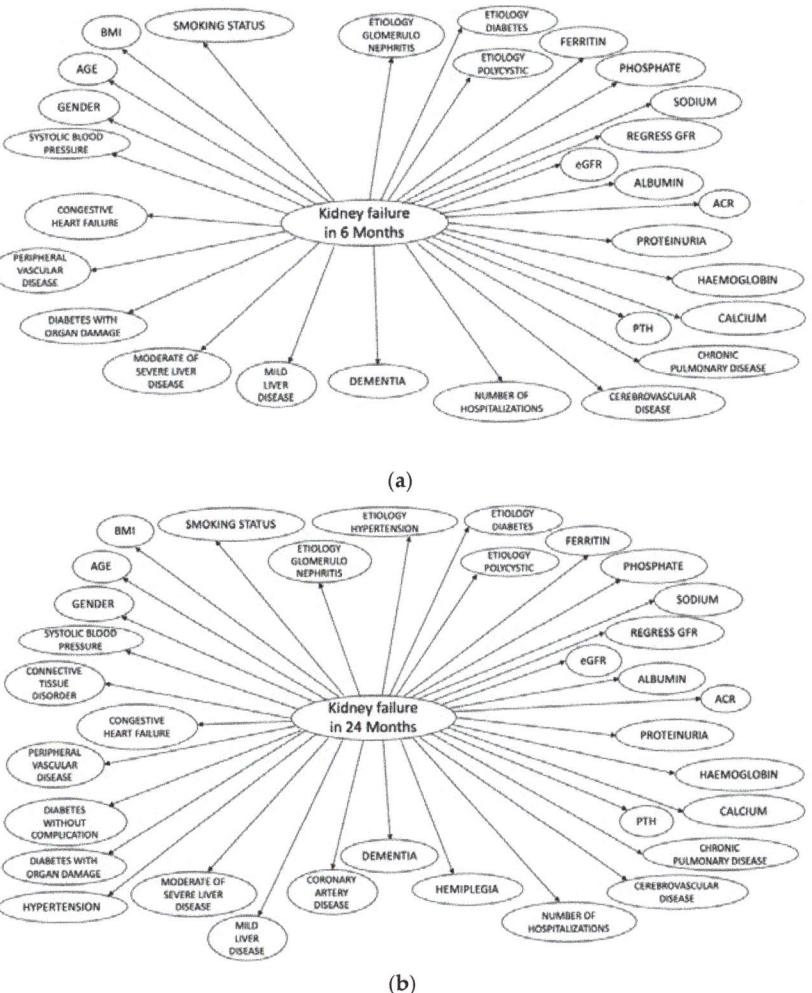

Figure 1. The Bayesian Network structure of PROGRES-CKD. (**a**) PROGRESS-CKD-6; (**b**) PROGRESS-CKD-24.

2.2. PROGRES-CKD Training

In this application of NBCs, we aimed at developing a model to predict the risk of KRT initiation within 6 and 24 months. The risk score is anchored at 0.00 = no risk at all to 1.00 = certainty of failure within the prediction horizons.

We derived model weights for the PROGRES-CKD by a data-driven algorithm, exploiting the wealth of information collected in the European Clinical Database (EuCliD®, Fresenius Medical Care Deutschland GmbH, Bad Homburg, Germany), a large, multinational, database of CKD patients. All nephrology clinics belonging to the Fresenius Medical Care (FMC) NephroCare network confer data collected for healthcare practice into this centralized data-repository. EuCliD® is a fully codified database recording clinical, laboratory, socio-demographic, treatment and prescription data for each medical encounter [19,20]. Information is collected by healthcare professionals either manually or by means of interfaces to existing local data managing systems.

All non-dialysis dependent, stage 3–5 CKD patients receiving care in outpatient renal clinics belonging to the NephroCare network from 2017 to 2018 were screened for eligibility. We enrolled only patients who received at least one outpatient visit and one serum creatinine (s-cr) assessment. The endpoints of interest were KRT initiation within 6 and 24 months. We excluded patients dying before reaching the endpoint or before the end-of-follow-up (i.e., 6 or 24 months, depending on endpoint of interest). Overall, 22,535 subjects met the inclusion criteria. This initial dataset was randomly partitioned into 2 analytical samples: development (70%, n = 17,775), and validation (30%, n = 6760). The derivation of NBC weights was obtained with Hugin 8.5.

2.3. Measures

2.3.1. Endpoint Definition

The primary endpoint was KRT initiation within 6 and 24 months. Outcome definition does not include episodes of dialysis treatment for acute and transient kidney derangement.

We defined patients as "lost to follow" when no additional s-cr assessments after end of follow-up date and no dialysis-dependence onset notes were present in the clinical records.

2.3.2. Input Variables

A list of all the variables included in the final model is provided in Table 1. The final model for the 6-month forecast incorporates 28 independent variables, while the model for the 24-month forecast includes 34 variables.

Table 1. Variables included in PROGRES-CKD models.

Group	Variable	PROGRES-CKD-6 n = 28	PROGRES-CKD-24 n = 34
Demographics and anthropometrics			
	Age	X	X
	Gender	X	X
	BMI, Kg/m^2	X	X
	Smoking status	X	X
Kidney function			
	Albumin, g/dL	X	X
	Albumin Creatinine Ratio (ACR), mg/mmol **	X	X
	Calcium, mg/dL	X	X
	eGFR, (ml/min/173 m^2)	X	X
	regressGFR *	X	X
	Hemoglobin, g/dL	X	X
	Phosphate, mg/dL	X	X
	Urine protein, g/24 h	X	X
	Parathyroid hormone, ng/L	X	X
	Sodium, mmol/L	X	X
	Ferritin, microg/L	X	X
Etiology of kidney disease			
	Diabetes	X	X
	Hypertension		X
	Glomerulonephritis	X	X
	Polycystic	X	X

Table 1. Cont.

Group	Variable	PROGRES-CKD-6 $n = 28$	PROGRES-CKD-24 $n = 34$
Comorbidities			
	Cerebrovascular disease	X	X
	Chronic Pulmonary Disease	X	X
	Congestive heart failure	X	X
	Connective tissue disorder		X
	Coronary artery disease		X
	Dementia	X	X
	Diabetes with organ damage	X	X
	Diabetes without complications		X
	Hemiplegia		X
	Hypertension		X
	Mild liver disease	X	X
	Moderate or severe liver disease	X	X
	Peripheral vascular disease	X	X
Other			
	Number of hospitalizations	X	X
	Systolic blood pressure	X	X

* Slope of linear regression of eGFR values over the last 12 months. ** Urine Protein-Creatinine Ratio was converted to ACR by ACR = Urin protein*PCR (Urine protein = 0.6) (please, see the Supplementary Material for the conversion table).

We assessed demographic, anthropometric, and lifestyle variables at index visit; blood biomarkers were collected and averaged over 12 months before index date (i.e., during the ascertainment period); their slope (i.e., change rate) was likewise calculated. Lifetime occurrence of comorbidities was evaluated by abstracting ICD10 codes [28] from outpatient medical records (Supplementary Material). Finally, etiologies of kidney disease were also noted.

2.3.3. Definition of CKD Stages

GFR was estimated in adults using the 2009 CKD-EPI creatinine equation [29]. Patients are classified into one of the following GFR categories: (1) G1 normal or high, GFR: $\geq$90 mL/min/1.73 m^2; (2) G2 mildly decreased, GFR: 60–89 mL/min/1.73 m^2; (3) G3a mildly to moderately decreased, GFR: 45–59; (4) G3b moderately to severely decreased, GFR: 30–44; (5) G4 severely decreased, GFR: 15–29; (6) G5 kidney failure, GFR: <15.3.

2.4. Design and Setting of PROGRES-CKD Validation Studies

For the validation study we randomly selected one visit from patients' histories (index date) before occurrence of study endpoint. All information collected before the index data was used as an input variable for the model. Patients dying before reaching the endpoint or before the end-of-follow-up (i.e., 6 or 24 months, depending on endpoint of interest) were excluded.

Based on this general design setting, we validated PROGRES-CKD models in two independent cohorts.

2.4.1. Study A

The first validation study was performed in the testing cohort derived from 30% partitioning of the clinical data abstracted from the FMC NephroCare cohort.

2.4.2. Study B

A second analysis evaluated PROGRES-CKD performance using data from the German CKD study [21]. Briefly, the GCKD study is an ongoing prospective observational national study that recruited 5217 patients with CKD of various etiologies. The enrolment period started in July 2011 and ended in 2012. Patient recruitment and follow-up is organized through a network of academic nephrology centers collaborating with practicing nephrologists throughout Germany. The main study endpoints were mortality, decline in kidney function, and cardiovascular events. At the time of recruitment, patients were under nephrological care and showed either eGFR of 30–60 mL/min/1.73 m^2 or overt urin protein in the presence of an eGFR > 60 mL/min/1.73 m^2. In our validation analysis, only patients subjected to serum creatinine evaluation at baseline and followed for at least 2 years were considered.

2.4.3. Study C

We conducted an impact study assessing concordance of nephrologists' and PROGRES-CKD-24 ratings of risk. Four experts were asked to forecast KRT initiation risk for 78 CKD patients based on their demographic, anthropometric, and clinical data. These patients were randomly selected from the FMC NephroCare cohort and had complete clinical history up to 24 months after the index date. Information related to all input variables used by the model were extracted from existing clinical records. Information extracts for each patient were collected in real-world clinical practice by physicians during outpatient visits. Doctors were asked to rate KRT risk on a 10-point rating scale anchored at 1 (risk is negligible, almost no patient with these characteristics would require RRT within 2 years), 5 (about 50% of patients with these characteristics would require RRT within 2 years) and 10 (almost 100% patients with these characteristics would require RRT within 2 years). Risk ratings provided by the physicians were then compared to scores obtained from PROGRES-CKD-24 for the same patients. Comparative analysis included accuracy, sensitivity, and specificity based on score cut-off that maximized Youden's Index. Thereafter, we investigated the potential impact of using risk scores provided by either experts or PROGRES-CKD-24 in referring patterns to intensified healthcare prevention programs aimed at delaying CKD progression. We simulated the use of risk estimates on a large, hypothetical CKD population of stage 3–5 CKD patients (n = 10,000), assuming an ESRD incidence within 24 months of 4.6% (i.e., n = 460 expected ESKD cases) and an intervention effect size of 1.5 (i.e., patients in the standard of care arm would face 50% higher risk of ESKD compared to those allocated in the intensified healthcare program). The intervention effect size was estimated based on expert opinion and several intensified intervention programs reported in diabetic and non-diabetic CKD [30–32].

2.5. Statistical Analysis

We computed the cumulative incidence and the incidence density of KRT initiation events in the study population and their 95% confidence intervals based on the Poisson distribution.

Since PROGRES-CKD models are NBCs, no data manipulation was required to explicitly handle missing variables.

Model performance was evaluated by concordance statistic and calibration charts in the FMC NephroCare and the GCKD cohorts. Discrimination was quantified by calculating the area under the receiver operating characteristic curve (ROC AUC) [33]. An AUC >0.70 was considered acceptable. Calibration was visually inspected by plotting observed outcome incidence by quintiles of the risk score [34].

A further analysis investigated non-inferiority (defined as ΔAUC < 0.05) of both PROGRES-CKD-6 and PROGRES-CKD-24 relative to the KFREs [15] calibrated for the European population [16]. Briefly, Tangri's models were developed using Cox proportional hazards regression methods in stage 3–5 CKD patients. In the present study, the following Tangri's equations were used: (1) 4 Variables (4VAR), includes Age, Gender, eGFR, and Albumin-Creatinine Ratio (ACR); (2) 6 Variables (6VAR), includes Age, Gender, eGFR, ACR, Diabetes, and Hypertension. We could not apply the 8 Variables (8VAR) equation given the lack of serum bicarbonate assessments in both study cohorts. Non-inferiority was assessed by checking whether a one-sided confidence interval of the AUC remained entirely above the non-inferiority threshold (0.05). In case non-inferiority was achieved, we evaluated superiority of PROGRES-CKD compared to benchmark models; superiority was set at $\Delta AUC \geq 0.05$. Given the sequential nature of testing in a fixed order method approach, type I error is not inflated by multiple testing. Superiority was tested with the DeLong non-parametric approach [35]. Statistical significance was claimed at $\alpha < 0.05$.

For study C, the following accuracy parameters were considered: Sensitivity, Specificity, Positive Predictive Value (PPV), and False Omission Rate (FOR). We also calculated the number needed to treat (NNT) in order to avoid 1 KRT event as the reciprocal of the absolute risk difference between the hypothetical prevention program and standard of care for all patients:

$$NNT = (\#patients\ int\ tr/[(\#patients\ int\ tr*PPV) - ((\#patients\ int\ tr*PPV)/(effect-size))]$$

Model training was performed using Hugin Explorer. All analyses for the validation study were performed with SAS 9.4®.

3. Results

3.1. Cohort Characteristics

Table 2 reports baseline demographic and clinical data of the whole FMC NephroCare cohort. Among 22,535 non-dialysis-dependent stage 3–5 CKD patients, 18,504 and 9407 patients had 6 and 24 months of follow-up, respectively. KRT events were 801 within 6 months (8.66 events/100 person-year) and 1817 within 24 months (9.66 events/100 person-year). On the other hand, KRT events in the validation sample (derived from 30% partitioning of the whole FMC cohort) were 248 (2.24 events/100 person-year) and 537 (9.36 events/100 person-year) within 6 and 24 months, respectively.

Table 2. Baseline characteristics of patients from the FMC NephroCare and GCKD cohorts.

	FMC Cohort		GCKD Cohort	
Variable	n	Mean ± SD or Median (IQR) or n (%)	n	Mean ± SD or Median (IQR) or n (%)
Stage 3	11,965	11,965 (53.1%)	3593	3593 (88.54%)
Stage 4	8026	8026 (35.62%)	460	460 (11.34%)
Stage 5	2544	2544 (11.29%)	5	5 (0.12%)
Age (year)	22,535	72.15 ± 11.7	4058	62.12 ± 10.50
BMI (kg/cm^2)	21,655	30.63 ± 10.92	4015	30.03 ± 5.91
eGFR ((mL/min/1.73 m^2)	22,535	31.93 ± 13.4	4058	41.92 ± 9.76
Albumin (g/dL)	19,004	4.19 ± 0.4	4055	3.85 ± 0.42
Ferritin (μg/L)	7303	222.18 ± 260.98	1044	200.48 ± 196.11
Hemoglobin (g/dL)	21,916	12.65 ± 1.83	3978	13.49 ± 1.69
Phosphate (mg/dL)	20,362	3.65 ± 0.74	4058	3.45 ± 0.64
Calcium (mg/dL)	20,686	9.36 ± 0.73	4058	9.07 ± 0.63
Sodium (mmol/L)	20,612	140.17 ± 3.16	4057	139.70 ± 3.14
PTH (ng/L)	9466	131.84 ± 150.12	0	-
ACR (mg/mmol)	90	138.67 ± 568.28	3999	393.63 ± 888.48
Proteinuria (g/24 h)	8780	3.58 ± 150.29	0	-
Systolic (mmHg)	17,963	137.33 ± 18.41	4030	140.27 ± 20.53
CRP (mg/L)	13,468	4.23 (7.63)	4056	2.41 (4.27)
Glucose (mg/dL)	19,499	126.45 ± 48.59	0	-
HDL Cholesterol (mg/dL)	7074	48.3 ± 16.74	4051	50.72 ± 17.35
LDL Cholesterol (mg/dL)	7084	107.59 ± 219.29	4051	116.33 ± 42.93
Triglyceride (mg/dL)	15,191	142.77 (95.72)	4050	173.38 (126.45)
hsTNT (ng/L)	0	-	3976	13 (11)
Uric Acid (mg/dL)	20,273	6.68 ± 1.61	4058	7.40 ± 1.92

Table 2. Cont.

		FMC Cohort		GCKD Cohort	
Variable	n	Mean ± SD or Median (IQR) or n (%)	n	Mean ± SD or Median (IQR) or n (%)
---	---	---	---	---
Gender (M)	22,535	11,349 (50.36%)	4058	2510 (61.85%)
Etiology Diabetes	22,535	3614 (16.04%)	4058	666 (16.41%)
Etiology Polycystic	22,535	477 (2.12%)	4058	157 (3.87%)
Etiology Hypertension	22,535	5281 (23.43%)	4058	1011 (24.91%)
Etiology Glomerulonephrite	22,535	987 (4.38%)	4058	623 (15.35%)
Smoking status: ex-smoker	3502	3502 (15.54%)	1819	1819 (44.96%)
Smoking status: no smoker	10,066	10,066 (44.67%)	1649	1649 (40.76%)
Smoking status: smoker	2274	2274 (10.09%)	578	578 (14.29%)
Alcohol: abuse	8636	8636 (38.32%)	771	771 (19.10%)
Alcohol: moderate	0	0 (0%)	3265	3265 (80.90%)
Alcohol: abstinence	6984	6984 (30.99%)	0	0 (%)
Peripheral Vascular Disease	22,535	1875 (8.32%)	4058	424 (10.45%)
Coronary Artery Disease	22,535	4336 (19.24%)	4058	908 (22.38%)
Congestive Heart Failure	22,535	1887 (8.37%)	4058	776 (19.12%)
Cerebrovascular Disease	22,535	1876 (8.32%)	4058	472 (10.52%)
Connective Tissue Disorder	22,535	399 (1.77%)	0	-
Cancer	22,535	2469 (10.96%)	4058	532 (13.11%)
Diabetes	22,535	9021 (40.03%)	4058	1545 (38.07%)
Anemia	22,535	9800 (43.49%)	4058	1057 (26.05%)
Hypertension	22,535	17,871 (79.3%)	4058	3951 (97.36%)
Atrial Fibrillation	22,535	2337 (10.37%)	4058	876 (21.59%)
Diabetes Without Complications (CCI)	22,535	3013 (13.37%)	4058	1545 (38.07%)
Chronic Pulmonary Disease (CCI)	22,535	1618 (7.18%)	4058	285 (7.02%)
Psychiatric Disease	22,535	177 (0.79%)	0	-
Liver Disease	22,535	987 (4.38%)	0	-
RRT in 24 months	9407	1817 (19.32%)	3684	80 (2.17%)
RRT in 6 months	18,504	801 (4.33%)	3888	11 (0.28%)

A second validation study was performed using data from the GCKD study. As shown in Table 2, a total of 4058 stage 3–5 CKD patients were included, of whom 3888 and 3687 subjects had 6 and 24 months of follow-up, respectively. RRT events were 11 within 6 months (0.5 events/100 person-year) and 80 (1.1 events/100 person-year) within 24 months.

Early CKD stages were predominantly represented in the GCKD study, whereas patients in stage 5 CKD were mostly enrolled in the FMC NephroCare cohort. Loss to follow-up within 6 months was 4031 (17.9%) and 170 (4.2%) participants, while loss to follow-up in 24 months was 13,128 (58.3%) and 371 (9.1%) participants in the FMC NephroCare and GCKD cohorts, respectively.

3.2. Model Discrimination in the Training and Validation Dataset from the FMC NephroCare Cohort

In the development dataset, AUC of PROGRES-CKD-6 was 0.88 (95%CI 0.86–0.89) in stage 4–5 patients, while AUC of PROGRES-CKD-24 was 0.86 (95%CI 0.85–0.87) in stage 3–5 patients.

External validation was performed in an independent sample of patients treated in the FMC NephroCare cohort. Analysis indicated a good discriminative ability for both PROGRES-CKD-6 and PROGRES-CKD-24 models, with a concordance statistic of 0.90 (95%CI 0.88–0.91, stage 4–5) and 0.85 (95%CI 0.83–0.88, stage 3–5), respectively.

Calibration of predicted versus observed risk is represented in Figure 2.

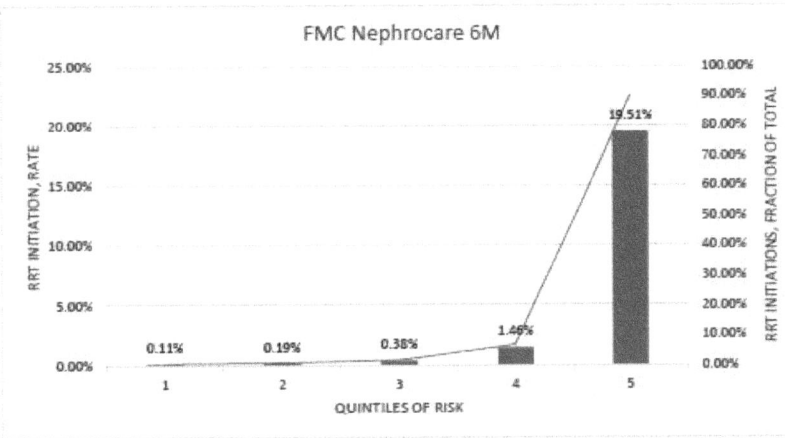

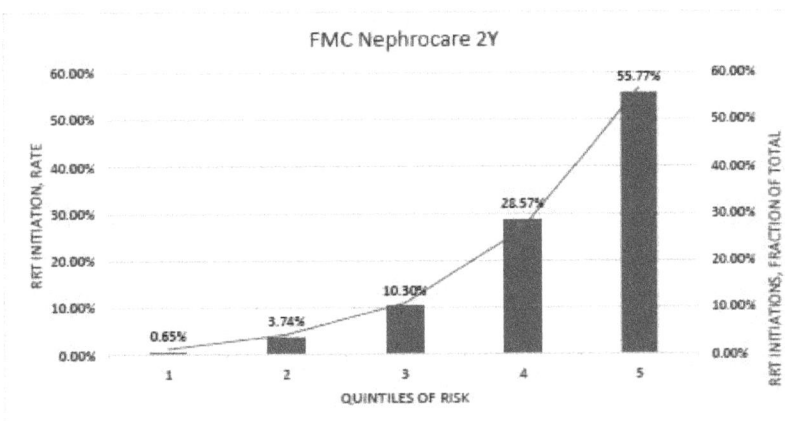

Figure 2. Calibration of (**A**) PROGRES-CKD-6, and (**B**) PROGRES-CKD-24 in the FMC cohort. Bar graph denotes the incidence of RRT initiation events observed in each quintile of risk (left axis); line graph denotes the fraction of RRT initiation events in each quintile with respect to the total number of RRT initiation events (right axis). Endpoint horizons: 6 months for PROGRES-CKD-6; 24 months for PROGRES-CKD-24.

3.3. Model Discrimination in the GCKD Cohort

PROGRES-CKD models showed a good discrimination accuracy in the GCKD dataset (PROGRES-CKD-6, CKD stages 4–5, AUC = 0.91 (95%CI 0.86–0.97); PROGRES-CKD-24, CKD stage 3–5, AUC = 0.85 (95%CI 0.83–0.88)).

Evaluation of ratios of observed risk across quintiles of predicted risk indicated that the model best discriminated low and high-risk patients compared to those classified in the central quintile or risk score distribution (Figure 3).

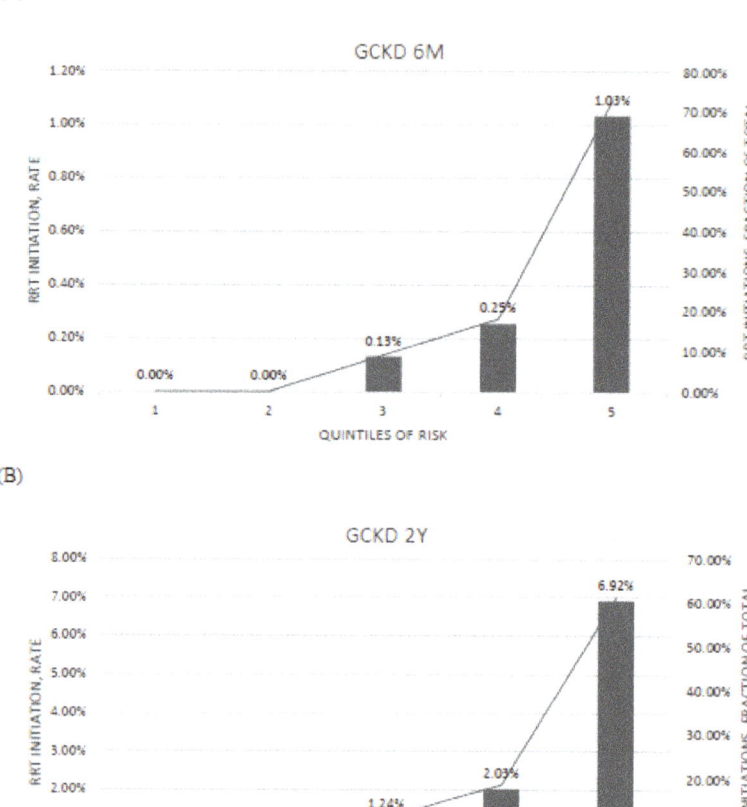

Figure 3. Calibration of (**A**) PROGRES-CKD-6, and (**B**) PROGRES-CKD-24 in the GCKD cohort. Bar graph denotes the incidence of RRT initiation events observed in each quintile of risk (left axis); line graph denotes the fraction of RRT initiation events in each quintile with respect to the total number of RRT initiation events (right axis). Endpoint horizons: 6 months for PROGRES-CKD-6; 24 months for PROGRES-CKD-24.

3.4. Comparison with KFRE Performance

Table 3 shows the comparison in discrimination accuracy between PROGRES-CKD and KFREs equations. Since KFREs equations are computable only for complete information cases, patients with missing data were listwise deleted from this analysis. Given the large amount of missing information for ACR, we converted timed proteinuria assays (proteinuria g/24 h) into ACR when available. The conversion was based on a published correspondence table (Supplementary Material).

Table 3. Comparison between discrimination ability of (A) PROGRES-CKD-6 and (B) PROGRES-CKD-24 and that of Tangri's Kidney Failure Risk Equations (KFREs) in the FMC and the GCKD cohort. The two scores were computed considering only complete cases (column "Effective sample size"), while patients with missing data were not included in the analysis. Endpoint horizons: 6 months for PROGRES-CKD-6; 24 months for PROGRES-CKD-24. Imputation method: Listwise. Non-inferiority was defined as AUC < 0.05, while superiority was set at ΔAUC ≥ 0.05. * Delta AUC: AUC of Tangri's KFRE–AUC of PROGRES-CKD model.

Model	Validation Cohort	Comparator Model	AUC PROGRES-CKD	Delta AUC *	p-Value	Effective Sample Size
PROGRES-CKD-6						
	FMC NephroCare					
		4VAR	0.90	−0.012	0.3255	927
		6VAR	0.90	−0.016	0.2220	927
	GCKD					
		4VAR	0.91	−0.146	0.0016	459
		6VAR	0.91	−0.149	0.0013	459
PROGRES-CKD-24						
	FMC NephroCare					
		4VAR	0.87	0.020	0.0483	1081
		6VAR	0.87	0.018	0.0888	1081
	GCKD					
		4VAR	0.85	0.030	0.0105	3999
		6VAR	0.85	0.027	0.0246	3999

Based on the superiority test criteria, the discrimination accuracy of PROGRES-CKD-6 was greater than KFRE equations for short term RRT risk among stage 4–5 CKD patients (Table 3). PROGRES-CKD-24 discrimination was not inferior to that of the gold standard algorithms (Table 3).

3.5. Potential Impact Simulation

A potential impact study compared the risk of KRT estimated by nephrologists with those calculated by PROGRES-CKD-24 and investigated the potential incremental efficiency of using PROGRES-CKD compared to physicians' assessments to inform referral to an intensified multidisciplinary prevention program to delay progression to ESKD.

Table 4 reports ratings of CKD progression risks provided by either physicians or the prediction model. In the evaluation sample, 25 patients required KRT within 2 years, while 53 patients did not reach the study endpoint. PROGRES-CKD-24 had excellent discrimination within this dataset (AUC = 0.96), while experts' ratings demonstrated good discrimination (average AUC = 0.79), with average sensitivity = 0.64 and average specificity = 0.85 at the optimal cut-off point (score > 6). Therefore, experts were less discriminative of endpoint occurrence compared to PROGRES-CKD-24 (ΔM-E = 0.17, p = 0.005). The correlation of physicians' ratings with PROGRES-CKD-24 ratings was moderate (r = 0.50, p < 0.01); furthermore, experts showed different abilities to discriminate patients' risk. (Table 4).

Table 4. PROGRES-CKD-24 and Experts' ratings of CKD progression risk.

		Experts			
	PROGRES-CKD-24	Expert 1	Expert 2	Expert 3	Expert 4
AUC	0.96	0.84	0.72	0.86	0.76
Sensitivity	0.76	0.80	0.50	0.75	0.60
Specificity	0.96	0.84	0.89	1.00	0.82

Figure 4 shows the results of our impact simulation. Based on the experts' ratings (PPV = 17%; FOR = 2%), n = 1725 (17.3%) patients would be assigned to the high-risk category, while n = 8275 (82.8%) would be recommended to the standard care program (Figure 4, panel A). Based on the assumptions set for the simulation exercise (i.e., ESKD overall incidence without intervention: 2.3 events/100 patient-years; ESKD risk is reduced by 50% in the intensified intervention group) there would be 362 ESKD events overall.

Therefore, in this scenario, physicians' referral to the intensified program would delay 98 ESKD cases (i.e., an Overall Program Effect Size of 1.27). The number of patients needed to treat would be NNT = 18 (Figure 4, panel D). Conversely, risk stratification by PROGRES-CKD-24 (PPV = 48%; FOR = 1.2%) leads to referral of n = 732 (0.73%) patients to intensified intervention (Figure 4, panel B). In this case, 117 ESRD events would be prevented, i.e., an Overall Program Effect Size of 1.36. The number needed to treat would be NNT = 6 (Figure 4, panel D). Finally, under a hypothetical risk averse policy that would refer all stage 3 CKD patients to the intensified program, 153 ESRD events would be prevented with NNT = 65 (Figure 4, panel C).

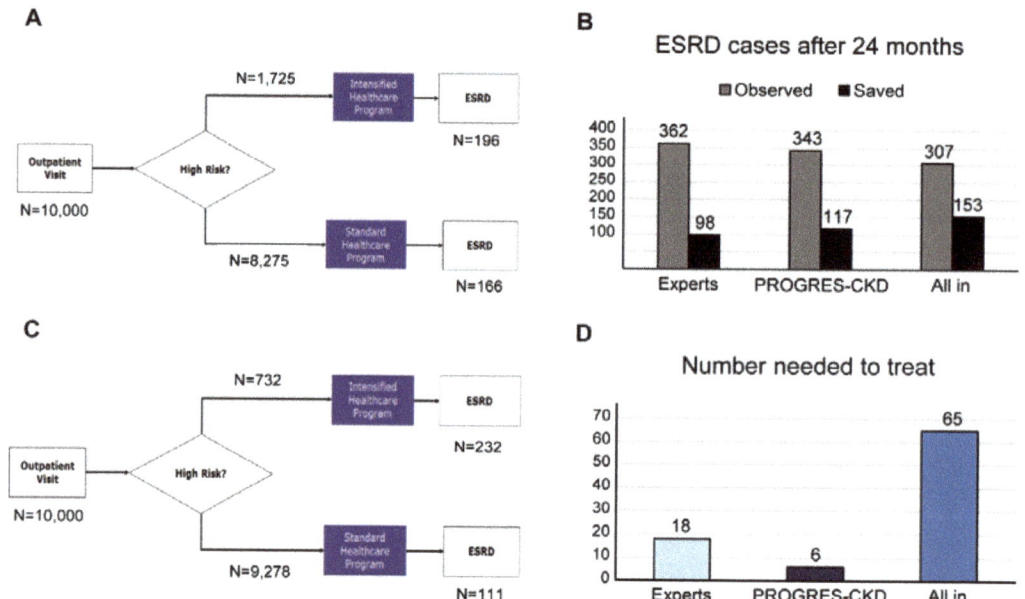

Figure 4. Potential impact simulation of PROGRES-CKD-24 implementation in a hypothetical CKD cohort. Flowcharts showing patients' referral to intensified intervention programs based on (**A**) experts' ratings, and (**B**) PROGRES-CKD scores; (**C**) Number of ESKD events within 24 months: both observed and saved cases are shown; D) Number of patients needed to treat to save 1 patient; "all-in strategy" involves referral of all stage 3 patients to the intensified healthcare program. Abbreviations: ESKD, end-stage kidney disease; NNT, Number needed to treat.

4. Discussion

The present study reports the derivation and validation of the PROGRES-CKD algorithm in two independent cohorts of non-dialysis dependent CKD patients. Discrimination accuracy of PROGRES-CKD was excellent for both the short-term prediction horizon (6 months) and the long-term prediction horizon (24 months).

Of note is the fact that PROGRES-CKD-6 and PROGRES-CKD-24 had reproducible discrimination accuracy in both validation studies. The FMC NephroCare cohort included real-world clinical data of stage 3–5 CKD patients from 15 countries (Europe, South-America, Africa), while the GCKD study is a prospective CKD cohort study recruiting a wider range of NDD-CKD patients with moderate GFR impairment in Germany [21]. Given the substantial differences between the two cohorts in geographical area of recruitment (international vs. national), inclusion/exclusion criteria, and data collection strategies (real-world vs. pre-specified protocol), the observed consistency in discrimination and calibration corroborates the generalizability of PROGRES-CKD across different CKD subpopulations and clinical settings.

To further characterize PROGRES-CKD accuracy, we compared its discrimination performance against KFREs which were extensively validated in different CKD patient populations [11,17,18] and are routinely used in clinical practice. PROGRES-CKD was as accurate as KFREs for 24-month prediction in both validation cohorts and more accurate for 6-month forecasting in the GCKD study. Even though the two algorithms showed comparable performance in long-term prediction, the KFRE risk score could not be computed in a vast share of patients of the FMC NephroCare cohort because of missing information of key input variables (Figure 5). Conversely, PROGRES-CKD was available for all patients due to accurate handling of missing variables inherent to naïve Bayes classifiers (Figure 5) [36]. In fact, PROGRES-CKD potentially incorporates input from as many as 32 clinical parameters, yet its prediction can be computed with any subset of information. Therefore, PROGRES-CKD performance remained stable even for patients with many missing parameters representative of a real-world clinical practice setting. Furthermore, by assessment of VOI metrics, PROGRES-CKD allows the graphical representation of the uncertainty around prediction due to missing data. Given that VOI metrics are calculated for each missing clinical parameter within the patient's health records, they can be used to rank the potential prognostic benefit of additional diagnostic testing or biomarker assays for patients with incomplete medical data. These peculiar features of PROGRES-CKD significantly increase its clinical usability in that they enable to address the problem of missing predictors in real-world data [17] by exploiting the full wealth of information collected in routine clinical practice.

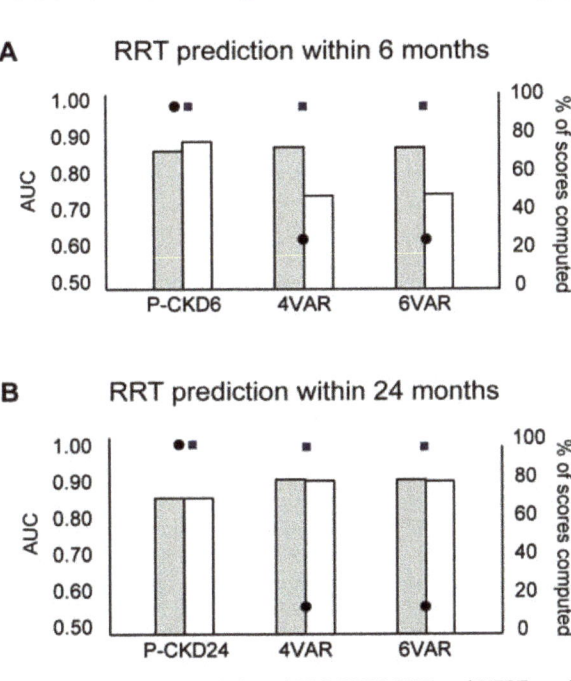

Figure 5. Discrimination ability of PROGRES-CKD and KFREs and percentage of computed scores by each prediction tool. Only cases with complete medical information were included in this analysis. (**A**) RRT prediction within 6 months; (**B**) RRT prediction within 24 months. Bars denote AUC (left y-axis), while dots denote the percentage of computed scores on the total number of recruited patients in each cohort (right y-axis). Abbreviations: P-CKD6, PROGRES-CKD-6; P-CKD24, PROGRES-CKD-24; 4VAR, KFRE 4 variables; 6VAR, KFRE 6 variables.

One additional advantage of NBCs such as PROGRES-CKD over traditional equation-based prediction tools rest in their ability to generate personalized, patient-specific impact metrics representing the relative contribution of each predictor to a patient's risk. Impact metrics can be used to estimate the potential impact of interventions addressing modifiable risk factors. This has important implications for patient care, since there can be considerable heterogeneity in underlying diseases, demographics, co-morbidities, and risk for progression among CKD patients and, consequently, optimal intervention strategies might deviate between patients with the same overall risk estimate depending on their individual high impact risk parameters. Therefore, both VOI and impact metrics could help physicians within their decision-making processes in tailoring interventions according to each individual patient's needs and characteristics [37]. Adoption of a more personalized clinical approach would lead not only to improved CKD clinical management (targeted diagnostic and treatment investigations with minimum adverse events and maximum efficacy, and consequently increased adherence to treatment), but it could also contribute towards optimizing the utilization of healthcare resources. In fact, ranking clinical parameters by their impact on risk score computation helps physicians' reasoning on priority and enables strategic and rational formulation of therapeutic plans considering both patient/disease-related factors and resource availability.

One specification of PROGRES-CKD allows the identification of patients whose kidney function is more likely to deteriorate within 6 months, a feature enabling timely referral to vascular access creation services and transition management [38,39]. The potential advantages of accurate short-term progression are two-fold. Patients starting on chronic dialysis with an arteriovenous fistula (AVF) rather than catheter have improved clinical outcomes in terms of survival, hospitalization, and complications [40]. On the other hand, inappropriate AVF creation in stage 4 and 5 patients who do not rapidly progress to KF is associated with complications and premature loss of patency [38].

Accurate risk prediction is a challenging task for physicians in real-world clinical practice, due to a number of disease, clinician, and organization related factors, including: inherent heterogeneity and variability in CKD progression rates [41,42], incomplete information, unrecognized case ambiguity, overconfidence leading to reduced analytical scrutiny, wrong perception of average population risk, over-generalization, fatigue, working overload, aging, altered affect impairing executive memory, switch of analytic scrutiny, and inexperience [43–48]. Therefore, readily available risk scores which prove to be accurate, generalizable to a wide array of CKD subpopulations and settings, and robust to missing data patterns observed in real-life applications may considerably assist clinical decision making, particularly when providing the opportunity to simulate the impact of interventions to individual patient cases.

In order to estimate the potential impact of improved prognostication around CKD progression on process outcomes, clinical outcomes, and costs [38,49], we conducted a simplified simulation using PROGRES-CKD as a patient stratification system for referral to intensified prevention programs for non-dialysis dependent (NDD)-CKD patients. In our simulation, risk estimates provided by either PROGRES-CKD or nephrology experts were used to stratify CKD patients. Subjects assigned to the "high-risk" category are referred to an intensified healthcare program aimed at reducing the risk of CKD progression. Our analysis suggested that PROGRES-CKD-driven referral to the intensified program would be more effective and largely more efficient than referral patterns determined by both healthcare expert risk assessment and an "all-in strategy" (i.e., all patients are referred to the intensified healthcare program when they reach stage 3 CKD). Therefore, personalized, risk-based referral may improve the efficiency of healthcare systems by enhancing the appropriateness of resource allocation in terms of direct expenditures and staff utilization. Personalized referral, however, is not just a matter of mere efficiency. In fact, inappropriate referral to the intensified intervention would involve unnecessary medicalization with greater risks of adverse events, impoverishment of quality of life even in people with a very low risk of progression, increased rate of therapeutic fatigue, and reduced adherence.

Conversely, accurate and reliable patient stratification helps physicians and healthcare providers balance individual patient needs with overall resource utilization, ultimately leading to more effective care for both the individual patient and the population [50].

5. Limitations

Validation of risk score should be considered a continuous process of generalization tests rather than a single experiment. While the performance of PROGRES-CKD was stable in both well-conducted longitudinal cohort studies (i.e., GCKD) and historical cohorts of real-life practice (i.e., FMC NephroCare), evidence concerning PROGRES-CKD robustness with real-world-representing clinical practices outside FMC NephroCare is still missing. For this reason, PROGRES-CKD undergoes a periodical process of performance monitoring while external cohorts for validation exercises are actively sought for.

6. Conclusions

The Prognostic Reasoning System for CKD patients (PROGRES-CKD) demonstrated excellent discrimination accuracy in two independent cohorts of NDD-CKD patients. The underlying models provide accurate prediction for both 24 and 6 months KRT risk. Contrary to traditional equation-based algorithms which cannot be applied to a large proportion of patients with incomplete data, PROGRES-CKD extends to all patients and allows explicit assessment of prediction robustness in case of missing values for key risk factors. Furthermore, PROGRES-CKD enhances prognostic reasoning by providing patient-specific impact metrics representing the relative contribution of each predictor to a patient's risk and can be used to estimate the potential impact of tailored interventions in addressing individual and modifiable risk factors. While PROGRES-CKD-24 may contribute to efficient and effective referral to intensified prevention programs for NDD-CKD patients, prediction of short-term outcomes (PROGRES-CKD-6) can be a key enabler of timely AVF creation and transition management. Given these results, both PROGRES-CKD algorithms reported here have the potential to advance current standards in routine CKD risk estimation, patient stratification, and individualizing interventions.

Supplementary Materials: The following supplements are available online at https://www.mdpi.com/article/10.3390/ijerph182312649/s1, Supplementary Table S1. List of ICD10 codes used to abstract comorbidity variables; Supplementary Table S2. Urin protein Conversion table; Supplementary results. Case study; Supplementary Figure S1. Graphical output of PROGRES-CKD.

Author Contributions: F.B. contributed to study concept, design, statistical analysis, interpretation of results, manuscript drafting, and approved the final version of the manuscript; C.L., performed literature search, contributed to interpretation of results, drafted the first version of the manuscript, and approved the final version of the manuscript; J.I.T. contributed to interpretation of results and drafted the first version of the manuscript and approved the final version of the manuscript; J.N. contributed to data acquisition, interpretation of results, and reviewed and approved the final version of the manuscript; H.M. contributed to data acquisition, interpretation of results, and reviewed and approved the final version of the manuscript; M.S. (Matthias Schmid) contributed to data acquisition, interpretation of results, and reviewed and approved the final version of the manuscript; B.B. contributed to data acquisition, interpretation of results, and reviewed and approved the final version of the manuscript; U.T. performed literature search, project conceptualization and project administration, and reviewed and approved the final version of the manuscript; M.S. (Markus Schneider), contributed to data acquisition, interpretation of results, and reviewed and approved the final version of the manuscript; U.T.S. contributed to data acquisition, interpretation of results, and reviewed and approved the final version of the manuscript; C.B. contributed to study concept, interpretation of results, and approved the final version of the manuscript; C.M. contributed to interpretation of results, and approved the final version of the manuscript; S.S. (Sonja Steppan) contributed to interpretation of results, and approved the final version of the manuscript; K.-U.E. contributed to data acquisition, interpretation of results, and reviewed and approved the final version of the manuscript; S.S. (Stefano Stuard) contributed to interpretation of results, and reviewed and approved the final version of the manuscript; L.N., contributed to study concept, design, statistical analysis, interpretation of results, manuscript drafting, and approved the final version of the manuscript. All authors have read and agreed to the published version of the manuscript. Authors confirm that they had full access to all the data in the study and accept responsibility of submission for publication.

Funding: This research was funded by Fresenius Medical Care Deutschland GmbH.

Institutional Review Board Statement: The study was approved by the ethics committees of all participating institutions and registered in the national registry for clinical studies (DRKS 00003971).

Informed Consent Statement: No patients' personal information has been used for the present study since all input data for modeling were aggregated statistics.

Data Availability Statement: We are unable to share the raw clinical data of the FMC NephroCare because data sharing would violate the terms and conditions under which Fresenius Medical Care acquired the data. Data from the GCKD study are not publicly available. External collaborators with a specific research proposal can access deidentified participant data only after review and approval of their proposal by the steering committee.

Acknowledgments: The GCKD study was supported by the German Ministry of Education and Research (Bundesministerium für Bildung und Forschung, FKZ 01ER 0804, 01ER 0818, 01ER 0819, 01ER 0820, and 01ER 0821), KfH Foundation for Preventive Medicine, Innovative Medicines Initiative 2 Joint Undertaking (BEAt-DKD, grant number 115974), and corporate sponsors (www.gckd.org).

Conflicts of Interest: The results presented in this paper have not been published previously in whole or part, except in abstract format. L.N., J.I.T., F.B., S.S. (Sonja Steppan), S.S. (Stefano Stuard), C.M., C.B., U.T. are full time employees at Fresenius Medical Care. C.L. provided medical writing services on behalf of Fresenius Medical Care. H.M. reports grants from KfH Foundation of Preventive Medicine, and grants from German ministry of Education and Research. M.S. (Matthias Schmid) reports grants from Fresenius Medical Care during the conduct of the study. B.B. reports grants from the Federal Ministry of Education and Research (Bundesministerium für Bildung und Forschung (www.bmbf.de), FKZ 01ER 0804, 01ER 0818, 01ER 0819, 01ER 0820 und 01ER 0821), and grants from Foundation for Preventive Medicine of the KfH (Kuratorium für Heimdialyse und Nierentransplantation e.V.–Stiftung Präventivmedizin; www.kfh-stiftung-praeventivmedizin.de). MSchneider reports grants from Fresenius Medical Care outside the submitted work. K.-U.E. reports grants from: Astra Zeneca, Bayer, Fresenius Medical Care, Vifor, and Amgen during the conduct of the study; personal fees from Akebia, Astellas, Astra Zeneca, Bayer, and Boehringer Ingelheim; and grants from Genzyme, Shire, and Vifor outside the submitted work. J.N. has no conflicts of interest to disclose. U.T.S. has no conflicts of interest to disclose.

References

1. Peng, S.; He, J.; Huang, J.; Lun, L.; Zeng, J.; Zeng, S.; Zhang, L.; Liu, X.; Wu, Y. Self-management interventions for chronic kidney disease: A systematic review and meta-analysis. *BMC Nephrol.* **2019**, *20*, 142. [CrossRef] [PubMed]
2. Navaneethan, S.D.; Shao, J.; Buysse, J.; Bushinsky, D.A. Effects of treatment of metabolic acidosis in CKD: A systematic review and meta-analysis. *Clin. J. Am. Soc. Nephrol.* **2019**, *14*, 1011–1120. [CrossRef] [PubMed]
3. Heerspink, H.J.L.; Greene, T.; Tighiouart, H.; Gansevoort, R.T.; Coresh, J.; Simon, A.L.; Chan, T.M.; Hou, F.F.; Lewis, J.B.; Locatelli, F.; et al. Change in albuminuria as a surrogate endpoint for progression of kidney disease: A meta-analysis of treatment effects in randomised clinical trials. *Lancet Diabetes Endocrinol.* **2019**, *7*, 128–139. [CrossRef]
4. Inker, L.A.; Heerspink, H.J.L.; Tighiouart, H.; Levey, A.S.; Coresh, J.; Gansevoort, R.T.; Simon, A.L.; Ying, J.; Beck, G.J.; Wanner, C.; et al. GFR slope as a surrogate end point for kidney disease progression in clinical trials: A meta-analysis of treatment effects of randomized controlled trials. *J. Am. Soc. Nephrol.* **2019**, *30*, 1735–1745. [CrossRef] [PubMed]
5. Campbell, G.A.; Bolton, W.K. Referral and comanagement of the patient with CKD. *Adv. Chronic Kidney Dis.* **2011**, *18*, 420–427. [CrossRef] [PubMed]
6. Levin, A. Consequences of late referral on patient outcomes. *Nephrol. Dial. Transplant.* **2000**, *15*, 8–13. [CrossRef] [PubMed]
7. Bartmańska, M.; Więcek, A. Chronic kidney disease and the aging population. *G. Ital. Nefrol.* **2014**, *36*, 1–5. [CrossRef]
8. Fedewa, S.A.; McClellan, W.M.; Judd, S.; Gutiérrez, O.M.; Crews, D.C. The association between race and income on risk of mortality in patients with moderate chronic kidney disease. *BMC Nephrol.* **2014**, *15*, 136. [CrossRef]
9. Kadatz, M.J.; Lee, E.S.; Levin, A. Predicting Progression in CKD: Perspectives and Precautions. *Am. J. Kidney Dis.* **2016**, *67*, 779–786. [CrossRef]
10. Tangri, N.; Kitsios, G.D.; Inker, L.A.; Griffith, J.; Naimark, D.M.; Walker, S.; Rigatto, C.; Uhlig, K.; Kent, D.M.; Levey, A.S. Risk prediction models for patients with chronic kidney disease a systematic review. *Ann. Intern. Med.* **2013**, *158*, 596–603. [CrossRef]

11. Ramspek, C.L.; de Jong, Y.; Dekker, F.W.; van Diepen, M. Towards the best kidney failure prediction tool: A systematic review and selection aid. *Nephrol. Dial. Transplant.* **2020**, *35*, 1527–1538. [CrossRef]
12. Dekker, F.W.; Ramspek, C.L.; Van Diepen, M. Con: Most clinical risk scores are useless. *Nephrol. Dial. Transplant.* **2017**, *32*, 752–755. [CrossRef]
13. Echouffo-Tcheugui, J.B.; Kengne, A.P. Risk Models to Predict Chronic Kidney Disease and Its Progression: A Systematic Review. *PLoS Med.* **2012**, *9*, e1001344. [CrossRef]
14. Collins, G.S.; Omar, O.; Shanyinde, M.; Yu, L.M. A systematic review finds prediction models for chronic kidney disease were poorly reported and often developed using inappropriate methods. *J. Clin. Epidemiol.* **2013**, *66*, 268–277. [CrossRef]
15. Tangri, N.; Stevens, L.A.; Griffith, J.; Tighiouart, H.; Djurdjev, O.; Naimark, D.; Levin, A.; Levey, A.S. A Predictive Model for Progression of Chronic Kidney Disease to Kidney Failure. *JAMA* **2011**, *305*, 1553–1559. [CrossRef]
16. Tangri, N.; Grams, M.E.; Levey, A.S.; Coresh, J.; Appel, L.J.; Astor, B.C.; Chodick, G.; Collins, A.J.; Djurdjev, O.; Raina Elley, C.; et al. Multinational Assessment of Accuracy of Equations for Predicting Risk of Kidney Failure ameta-analysis. *JAMA* **2016**, *315*, 164–174. [CrossRef]
17. Van Rijn, M.H.C.; van de Luijtgaarden, M.; van Zuilen, A.D.; Blankestijn, P.J.; Wetzels, J.F.M.; Debray, T.P.; Brand, J.A.J.G.V.D. Prognostic models for chronic kidney disease: A systematic review and external validation. *Nephrol. Dial. Transplant.* **2021**, *36*, 1837–1850. [CrossRef]
18. Kang, M.W.; Tangri, N.; Kim, Y.C.; An, J.N.; Lee, J.; Li, L.; Oh, Y.K.; Kim, D.K.; Joo, K.W.; Kim, Y.S.; et al. An independent validation of the kidney failure risk equation in an Asian population. *Sci. Rep.* **2020**, *10*, 1–10. [CrossRef]
19. Steil, H.; Amato, C.; Carioni, C.; Kirchgessner, J.; Marcelli, D.; Mitteregger, A.; Moscardo, V.; Orlandini, G.; Gatti, E. EuCliD®—A Medical Registry. *Methods Inf. Med.* **2004**, *43*, 83–88.
20. Merello Godino, J.I.; Rentero, R.; Orlandini, G.; Marcelli, D.; Ronco, C. Results from EuCliD® (European Clinical Dialysis Database): Impact of shifting treatment modality. *Int. J. Artif. Organs* **2002**, *25*, 1049–1060. [CrossRef]
21. Eckardt, K.U.; Bärthlein, B.; Seema, B.A.; Beck, A.; Busch, M.; Eitner, F.; Ekici, A.B.; Floege, J.; Gefeller, O.; Haller, H.; et al. The German Chronic Kidney Disease (GCKD) study: Design and methods. *Nephrol. Dial. Transplant.* **2011**, *27*, 1454–1460. [CrossRef] [PubMed]
22. Collins, G.S.; Reitsma, J.B.; Altman, D.G.; Moons, K.G.M. Transparent reporting of a multivariable prediction model for individual prognosis or diagnosis (TRIPOD): The TRIPOD statement. *BMJ* **2014**, *350*, g7594. [CrossRef] [PubMed]
23. Luo, W.; Phung, D.; Tran, T.; Gupta, S.; Rana, S.; Karmakar, C.; Shilton, A.; Yearwood, J.; Dimitrova, N.; Ho, T.B.; et al. Guidelines for developing and reporting machine learning predictive models in biomedical research: A multidisciplinary view. *J. Med. Internet Res.* **2016**, *18*, e323. [CrossRef] [PubMed]
24. McNally, R.J.; Heeren, A.; Robinaugh, D.J. A Bayesian network analysis of posttraumatic stress disorder symptoms in adults reporting childhood sexual abuse. *Eur. J. Psychotraumatol.* **2017**, *8*, 1341276. [CrossRef]
25. Khan, S.; Ghalib, M.R. A naive-bayes approach for disease diagnosis with analysis of disease type and symptoms. *Int. J. Appl. Eng. Res.* **2015**, *10*, 29005–29014.
26. Constantinou, A.C.; Yet, B.; Fenton, N.; Neil, M.; Marsh, W. Value of information analysis for interventional and counterfactual Bayesian networks in forensic medical sciences. *Artif. Intell. Med.* **2016**, *66*, 41–52. [CrossRef]
27. Kjærulff, U.B.; Madsen, A.L. *Bayesian Networks and Influence Diagrams: A Guide to Construction and Analysis*; Springer: New York, NY, USA, 2013.
28. Quan, H.; Sundararajan, V.; Halfon, P.; Fong, A.; Burnand, B.; Luthi, J.C.; Saunders, L.D.; Beck, C.A.; Feasby, T.E.; Ghali, W.A. Coding Algorithms for Defining Comorbidities in ICD-9-CM and ICD-10 Administrative Data. *Med. Care* **2005**, *43*, 1130–1139. [CrossRef]
29. Levey, A.S.; Stevens, L.A.; Schmid, C.H.; Zhang, Y.L.; Castro, A.F., III; Feldman, H.I.; Kusek, J.W.; Eggers, P.; Van Lente, F.; Greene, T.; et al. A New Equation to Estimate Glomerular Filtration Rate. *Ann. Intern. Med.* **2009**, *150*, 604–612. [CrossRef]
30. Oellgaard, J.; Gæde, P.; Rossing, P.; Persson, F.; Parving, H.-H.; Pedersen, O. Intensified multifactorial intervention in type 2 diabetics with microalbuminuria leads to long-term renal benefits. *Kidney Int.* **2017**, *91*, 982–988. [CrossRef]
31. Fogelfeld, L.; Hart, P.; Miernik, J.; Ko, J.; Calvin, D.; Tahsin, B.; Adhami, A.; Mehrotra, R.; Fogg, L. Combined diabetes-renal multifactorial intervention in patients with advanced diabetic nephropathy: Proof-of-concept. *J. Diabetes Its Complicat.* **2017**, *31*, 624–630. [CrossRef]
32. Peeters, M.J.; Van Zuilen, A.D.; Brand, J.A.J.G.V.D.; Bots, M.L.; Van Buren, M.; Dam, M.A.G.J.T.; Kaasjager, K.A.H.; Ligtenberg, G.; Sijpkens, Y.W.J.; Sluiter, H.E.; et al. Nurse Practitioner Care Improves Renal Outcome in Patients with CKD. *J. Am. Soc. Nephrol.* **2013**, *25*, 390–398. [CrossRef]
33. Linden, A. Measuring diagnostic and predictive accuracy in disease management: An introduction to receiver operating characteristic (ROC) analysis. *J. Eval. Clin. Pract.* **2006**, *12*, 132–139. [CrossRef]
34. Steyerberg, E.W.; Vickers, A.J.; Cook, N.R.; Gerds, T.; Gonen, M.; Obuchowski, N.; Pencina, M.J.; Kattan, M.W. Assessing the performance of prediction models: A framework for traditional and novel measures. *Epidemiology* **2010**, *21*, 128–138. [CrossRef]
35. Delong, E.R.; Delong, D.M.; Clarke-Pearson, D.L. Comparing the Areas under Two or More Correlated Receiver Operating Characteristic Curves: A Nonparametric Approach. *Biometrics* **1988**, *44*, 837–845. [CrossRef]
36. Nielsen, T.D.; Jensen, F.V. *Bayesian Networks and Decision Graphs*; Springer: New York, NY, USA, 2009.

37. Sun, L.; Zou, L.-X.; Chen, M.-J. Make Precision Medicine Work for Chronic Kidney Disease. *Med. Princ. Pract.* **2016**, *26*, 101–107. [CrossRef]
38. Lerner, B.; Desrochers, S.; Tangri, N. Risk Prediction Models in CKD. *Semin. Nephrol.* **2017**, *37*, 144–150. [CrossRef]
39. Bargman, J.M. Timing of Initiation of RRT and Modality Selection. *Clin. J. Am. Soc. Nephrol.* **2015**, *10*, 1072–1077. [CrossRef]
40. Allon, M. Vascular access for hemodialysis patients: New data should guide decision making. *Clin. J. Am. Soc. Nephrol.* **2019**, *14*, 954–961. [CrossRef]
41. Webster, A.C.; Nagler, E.V.; Morton, R.L.; Masson, P. Chronic Kidney Disease. *Lancet* **2017**, *389*, 1238–1252. [CrossRef]
42. Levey, A.S.; Coresh, J. Chronic kidney disease. *Lancet* **2012**, *379*, 165–180. [CrossRef]
43. Jacoby, L.L.; McElree, B.; Trainham, T.N. Automatic influences as accessibility bias in memory and Stroop tasks: Toward a formal model. In *Attention and Performance XVII: Cognitive Regulation of Performance: Interaction of Theory and Application*; Elsevier: Amsterdam, The Netherlands, 1999; pp. 461–486.
44. Qin, S.; Hermans, E.J.; van Marle, H.J.F.; Luo, J.; Fernández, G. Acute Psychological Stress Reduces Working Memory-Related Activity in the Dorsolateral Prefrontal Cortex. *Biol. Psychiatry* **2009**, *66*, 25–32. [CrossRef]
45. Eva, K.W.; Norman, G.R. Heuristics and biases—A biased perspective on clinical reasoning. *Med. Educ.* **2005**, *39*, 870–872. [CrossRef]
46. Mumford, A.D.; Banning, A.P. Minimising delays to thrombolysis in patients developing acute myocardial infarction in hospital. *Postgrad. Med. J.* **1997**, *73*, 491–495. [CrossRef]
47. Croskerry, P.; Norman, G. Overconfidence in Clinical Decision Making. *Am. J. Med.* **2008**, *121*, 24–29. [CrossRef] [PubMed]
48. Croskerry, P. A Universal Model of Diagnostic Reasoning. *Acad. Med.* **2009**, *84*, 1022–1028. [CrossRef] [PubMed]
49. Moons, K.G.M.; Kengne, A.P.; Grobbee, D.E.; Royston, P.; Vergouwe, Y.; Altman, D.G.; Woodward, M. Risk prediction models: II. External validation, model updating, and impact assessment. *Heart* **2012**, *98*, 691–698. [CrossRef] [PubMed]
50. Moosa, M.R.; Maree, J.D.; Chirehwa, M.T.; Benatar, S.R. Use of the "accountability for reasonableness" approach to improve fairness in accessing dialysis in a middle-income country. *PLoS ONE* **2016**, *11*, e0164201.

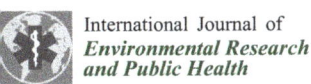

Article

Improved Machine Learning-Based Predictive Models for Breast Cancer Diagnosis

Abdur Rasool [1,2,†], Chayut Bunterngchit [1,3,†], Luo Tiejian [1,*], Md. Ruhul Islam [4], Qiang Qu [2] and Qingshan Jiang [2,*]

1. University of Chinese Academy of Sciences, Beijing 101408, China; rasool@siat.ac.cn (A.R.); chayutb@ia.ac.cn (C.B.)
2. Shenzhen Key Lab for High Performance Data Mining, Shenzhen Institute of Advanced Technology, Chinese Academy of Sciences, Shenzhen 518055, China; qiang@siat.ac.cn
3. State Key Laboratory of Management and Control for Complex Systems, Institute of Automation, Chinese Academy of Sciences, Beijing 100190, China
4. Department of Electrical Engineering and Computer Science, University of Stavanger, 4044 Stavanger, Norway; mr.islam@stud.uis.no
* Correspondence: tjluo@ucas.ac.cn (L.T.); qs.jiang@siat.ac.cn (Q.J.); Tel.: +86-137-0127-2380 (L.T.); +86-755-8639-2340 (Q.J.)
† These authors contributed equally to this work.

Abstract: Breast cancer death rates are higher than any other cancer in American women. Machine learning-based predictive models promise earlier detection techniques for breast cancer diagnosis. However, making an evaluation for models that efficiently diagnose cancer is still challenging. In this work, we proposed data exploratory techniques (DET) and developed four different predictive models to improve breast cancer diagnostic accuracy. Prior to models, four-layered essential DET, e.g., feature distribution, correlation, elimination, and hyperparameter optimization, were deep-dived to identify the robust feature classification into malignant and benign classes. These proposed techniques and classifiers were implemented on the Wisconsin Diagnostic Breast Cancer (WDBC) and Breast Cancer Coimbra Dataset (BCCD) datasets. Standard performance metrics, including confusion matrices and K-fold cross-validation techniques, were applied to assess each classifier's efficiency and training time. The models' diagnostic capability improved with our DET, i.e., polynomial SVM gained 99.3%, LR with 98.06%, KNN acquired 97.35%, and EC achieved 97.61% accuracy with the WDBC dataset. We also compared our significant results with previous studies in terms of accuracy. The implementation procedure and findings can guide physicians to adopt an effective model for a practical understanding and prognosis of breast cancer tumors.

Keywords: machine learning models; data exploratory techniques; breast cancer diagnosis; tumors classification

1. Introduction

Breast cancer (BC) is the world's leading cause of death in women after lung cancer, with approximately 2,261,419 new cases and 684,996 new deaths in 2020 [1]. In the United States, 281,550 new cases were diagnosed with breast cancer, and 43,600 deaths were reported in the females during 2021 [2]. Breast cancer is a type of cancer that originates from breast tissue, most generally from the internal layer of the milk conduit or the lobules that provide milk to the milk conduit. Cancer cells arise from natural cells due to modification or mutation of deoxyribonucleic acid (DNA) and ribonucleic acid (RNA). These modifications or mutations may occur spontaneously as a result of the increase in entropy, or they may be triggered by other factors. For example, electromagnetic radiation (X-rays, microwaves, ultraviolet-rays, gamma-rays, et cetera), nuclear radiation, bacteria, viruses, fungi, parasites, chemicals in the air, heat, food, water, free radicals, mechanical cell-level injury, evolution, and aging of DNA and RNA [3]. In general, benign and malignant are two classes of tumors. Although benign is not life-threatening and cancerous, it may boost the chances of breast cancer risk. In contrast, malignant is more alarming and cancerous tumors. A study performed breast cancer detection and reported 20% of women died due to malignant tumors [4].

These studies emphasize the diagnosis of tumors, and recently, it is a trending biomedical issue. The researchers are employing data mining (DM) and machine learning (ML) technologies for breast cancer prediction [5]. Classifier-based prediction models on DM and ML can limit the diagnosis errors and enhance the efficiency of a cancer diagnosis. DM is an extensive combination of different approaches to discover hidden knowledge and information from large-scale datasets that are difficult to analyze directly. It has been broadly used in the implementation of the prediction system for various diseases, such as heart disease [6], lung cancer [7], and thyroid cancer [8]. DM and ML techniques have been embedded for diagnosing breast cancer with computer-aided systems [9], and fuzzy-genetics [10]. The results of these studies successfully classify the features into two types of tumors by the evaluation of classifier and predicting the incoming tumor based on previous data.

In the literature, a research study proved that breast cancer prediction with machine learning classifiers in the early phases does not just increase the survival chances but can control the diffusion of cancerous cells in the body [11]. For instance, a study used the support vector machine (SVM) based method for breast cancer diagnosis and achieved practical results in prediction [12]. Similarly, Furey et al. [13] also employed SVM for cancer tissue classification with a linear kernel and attained a 93.4% accuracy. Later, this work was extended by Zheng et al. (2014) by delivering a K-SVM hybrid model for Wisconsin Diagnostic Breast Cancer (WDBC) dataset classification and acquiring 97% accuracy [14]. Meanwhile, some other researchers worked on different classifiers, such as Seddik et al. (2015), who proposed a method based on tumor variables for a binary logistic model to diagnose breast cancer WDBC data and secure good results [15]. Likewise, Mert et al. used a k-nearest neighbor (KNN) classifier to predict breast cancer by designing a feature reduction method with independent component analysis. It distributed the features with reduced one feature (1C) and 30 features and computed the performance, and attained 91% accuracy [16].

Apart from these advantageous accuracies with different classifiers and methods, these studies mentioned above have not considered the data exploratory techniques, which enable the data mining techniques to be more robust to acquire efficient performance. Due to the absence of such essential techniques, various studies [16–19] face the accuracy limitation of ML classifiers. Meanwhile, the confusion matrices misdiagnosed the malignant and benign classes in those studies due to the incorrect prediction of true negative and false negative matrices. Another defect was found in those previous studies that used criteria to assess the feature training with nonlinear classification. However, the performance of model execution time increases rapidly with the number of features [20]. As a result, the prediction model becomes slower, affecting the diagnosis accuracy. In contrast, the model's accuracy and time complexity are critical issues for the data analyst and physician. These problems, as mentioned above, and findings motivated us to pursue a new study for breast cancer diagnosis by proposing data mining techniques with different machine learning models.

In this research, four different prediction models were formulated with four machine learning algorithms (SVM, KNN, logistic regression (LR), and ensemble classifier (EC)) to deal with a massive volume of tumor features for the extraction of essential information for the diagnosis of breast cancer. The objective was to explore an accurate and efficient prediction model for tumor classification by using data mining techniques. It proposes four-layered significant data exploratory techniques (DET), including feature distribution, elimination, and constructing a hyperparameter for the practical analysis of Wisconsin Diagnostic Breast Cancer (WDBC) and Breast Cancer Coimbra Dataset (BCCD). These techniques enabled the machine learning predictive models to improve accuracy and enhance diagnostic efficiency. In the absence of these techniques, we observed some literature suffers from accuracy limitations. Although image data are more reasonable for breast cancer detection, we have not considered them in this work due to the targeted WDBC and BCCD datasets to apply the intelligent ML classifiers. It presents a framework by integrating DET and predictive models to explore the implementation method for breast cancer diagnosis. The tumor features can be presented in many details, which produces redundant information. Such features lead to tedious outcomes due to high computation times. As a result, our fundamental goal was not only to investigate the effective predictive model with attainable accuracy but also one with time complexity for the cancer diagnosis. The deliberation of time efficiency will enable our models to extract and mine vital information from a vast dataset by finding correlations and eliminating the features. The results presented satisfactory accuracy for the breast cancer diagnosis with the lowest computation time, which signifies the quality of our study as compared to others. This work will enable a data analyst to apply an intelligent machine learning model to analyze breast cancer data. Likewise, a physician would diagnose breast cancer precisely by the tumor classification. As the dataset is available publicly, we uploaded our code on GitHub (https://github.com/abdul-rasool/Improved-machine-learning-based-Predictive-Models-for-Breast-Cancer-Diagnosis (accessed on 11 November 2021)) to assist data analysts and physicians in further advancement and apply it in real-time. As summarized, the following are the significant contributions of this study:

- We investigated four prediction models (SVM, LR, KNN, and EC) with the WDBC and BCCD breast cancer datasets, which reached the next level of quality by diagnosing the tumor and classifying it into benign and malignant.
- It proposes four-layered data exploratory techniques before implementing four ML classifiers as prediction models. These techniques enable the predictive models to acquire peak accuracies for breast cancer diagnosis.
- We set up experiments to validate the models' prediction and classification accuracy with regard to time complexity and deliver comparative analysis with state-of-the-art studies and various evaluation matrices.

The rest of the article is organized as follows: Section 2 expands on the literature reviews; Section 3 explains the preliminary part for the introduction of proposed prediction models; Section 4 introduces the proposed methodology; Section 5 deals with the evaluation of the results; Section 6 deliberates the discussion, and Section 7 provides the conclusion.

2. Related Work

Breast cancer disease causes a massive number of deaths in the world. After the traditional cancer detection methods, the latest technologies enable experts with numerous adaptive methods to discover breast cancer in women. Along with the new technologies, various data science (DS) techniques assist in cancer-based data collection and evaluation to predict this deadly disease. Machine learning algorithms have been successfully applied to cancer-based data analysis among these DS technologies. For example, research [21] was conducted to prove that these machine learning algorithms can improve diagnostic accuracy. It turns out that a 79.97% diagnostic accuracy was achieved by an expert physician. However, 91.1% correct predictions were attained with machine learning.

In the last couple of decades, machine learning applications in the medical field have gradually increased. However, the data collected from the patients and evaluation by the medical expert are the essential factors for diagnosis. The machine learning classifiers have aided in minimizing human errors and delivered prompt analysis of medical data with greater depth [22]. There are several machine learning classifiers for data modeling and prediction; in our work, we employed support vector machine (SVM), logistic regression (LR), k-nearest neighbor (KNN), and ensemble classifier (EC) for breast cancer prediction.

In previous studies, SVM was a widely implemented machine learning algorithm in the diagnosis domain of breast cancer due to its highest prediction accuracy. For instance, Furey et al. (2000) presented SVM with a linear kernel for cancer tissue diagnosis and reached acceptable accuracy [13]. Similarly, Polat et al. (2007) used the least square SVM for breast cancer prediction to eliminate redundant features and secured a 98.53% accuracy. It was suggested that least square SVM assisted in model training with linear equations [23]. However, his method did not deliver the feature selection process. The author [24] delivered a distributed database for multi-active features to integrate different technologies. In 2010, Prasad and Jain et al. [25] proposed a heuristic model for feature subset to train the SVM classifier. It classifies the breast cancer data into two different classes with 91.7% accuracy. However, this accuracy can be adequately improved if the author employs the feature eradication method to get rid of the noise data.

Similarly, Zheng et al. (2014) proposed a hybrid model combining K-mean and SVM classifiers. This model objective was to diagnose the tumor features from the Wisconsin Diagnostic Breast Cancer (WDBC) dataset by employing the feature selection and extraction method. A K-mean classifier was employed to identify the benign and malignant tumor patterns. The generated patterns are computed and considered as new patterns for the training of the SVM model. Then, SVM is executed for the prediction of incoming tumors. The employment of their hybrid model improved the accuracy to 97%. However, the data exploratory techniques are the fundamental tasks for the data preparation, which have not been adequately addressed to train the proposed model [14].

Apart from the SVM, Lim and Sohn et al. (2013) performed logistic regression (LR) with optimal parameters on the Wisconsin Original Breast Cancer (WOBC) and WDBC datasets. It achieved 97.8% sufficient accuracy for the WOBC dataset and 93.8% accuracy for the WDBC dataset with optimized feature sets [26]. Similarly, Seddik et al. (2015) presented a binary logistic model for the diagnosis of breast cancer data based on variables with tumor image characteristics. The proposed model classifies the WDBC data into malignant and benign and accomplished the 98% average classification accuracy. This regression model found that area, texture, concavity, and symmetry are significant WDBC features [15].

Previous literature reviews found numerous studies based on the SVM model for breast cancer detection; however, few were based on others. For example, A. Mert et al. (2015) delivered a feature reduction method with independent component analysis to predict breast cancer. It utilized the k-nearest neighbor (KNN) classifier to categorize the WDBC features efficiently with a reduced one feature (1C) and 30 features. It computed the performance with different matrices and attained 91% accuracy [16]. Later, this study was further improved by Rajaguru et al. (2019), who tackled the breast cancer prediction challenge by implementing the KNN and decision tree (DT) machine learning algorithms to classify the WDBC features. It used a traditional principal component analysis (PCA) feature selection method for the feature categorization and found that KNN outperformed the DT [18]. In another study conducted by Yang and Xu et al. (2019), KNN achieved 96.4% accuracy with the same feature selection method (PCA) [27]. Recently, work has involved considering KNN efficiency by the k values and many distance functions of KNN to find its effectiveness with two different breast cancer datasets. It involves the three different types of the experiment: KNN without feature selection, with linear SVM, and with Chi-square-based features. It indicated that the third technique, Chi-square-based feature selection, succeeded in accomplishing the highest accuracy on both datasets with Manhattan or Canberra distance functions [19].

As for the fourth prediction model, named ensemble classifier (EC) with the voting technique, few studies consider this approach for breast cancer prediction. For instance, M. Abdar et al. (2020) proposed an ensemble method by vote/voting classifier to detect benign tumors from malignant breast cancer. It established a two-layer voting classifier for two or three different machine learning algorithms. The results of these voting techniques disclosed the adequate performance of the simple classification algorithm [5]. From these studies, we got the motivation to conduct experiments based on voting classifiers with different machine learning techniques. However, none of the above approaches has utilized the feature correlation and elimination for the given breast cancer dataset to the best of our knowledge. These studies conducted experiments to classify the cancer features, which is still a challenging issue. Recently, in Nature Cancer, a study presented an approach to classify cancer into normal and tumor tissues [28]. Meanwhile, many studies have utilized the SVM classifier for breast cancer prediction, while a few of them used only one classifier in experiments. However, there is still a demand to explore the efficient classifier for breast cancer prediction with more effective methods [5,14,15,18]. This study performed four different prediction models with sufficient data mining exploratory techniques to diagnose breast cancer.

3. Preliminary

This section deliberates data information and evaluation matrices for this study.

3.1. Data Description

In this research, the experiments were performed on two different datasets: WDBC and BCCD. The selection reason for these datasets is it is extensively used in numerous studies [16,28–30]. Moreover, those ML models that deliver adequate accuracy with the binary dataset were trained. The detailed introduction and particular selection reason of these datasets are given below:

Wisconsin Diagnostic Breast Cancer (WDBC): The WDBC dataset consists of 10 features of breast tumor, and the result in the data were taken from 569 patients. Dr. William H. Wolberg distributed it at the General Surgery Department, University of Wisconsin-Madison, USA. It can be obtained via the file transfer protocol (FTP) from this link (https://ftp.cs.wisc.edu/math-prog/cpo-dataset/machine-learn/cancer/WDBC/ (accessed on 11 November 2021)). This dataset was created using fluid samples taken from patients' solid breast masses. Then, software called Xcyt was used to perform cytological feature analysis based on the digital scan. This software applies a curve-fitting algorithm to calculate ten features by returning each feature's mean value, worst value, and standard error (SE) value. Thus, there were 30 values in total for each sample, to which we have added an ID column to differentiate these samples. Finally, the diagnosis result of each sample, which consisted of malignant (M) and benign (B), was also added. In conclusion, the dataset contained 32 attributes (ID, diagnosis, and 30 input features) and 569 instances. Features of each sample were radius (mean of distances from the center to points on the perimeter), texture (standard deviation of gray-scale values), perimeter, area, smoothness (local variation in radius lengths), compactness (calculated by, $\frac{perimeter^2}{area-1}$ concavity (severity of concave portions of the contour), concave points (number of concave portions of the contour), symmetry, and fractal dimension (calculated by coastline approximation -1).

The first column of the dataset, ID, was not considered and was dropped from the analysis. The second column, which is the diagnosis, will become the target of the study. The third to the thirty-second column contains the mean, SE, and worst values of each feature, shown in Table 1. For instance, feature number 2 is Texture means; feature number 12 is Texture SE; and feature number 22 is Texture worst.

Breast Cancer Coimbra Dataset (BCCD): This dataset consists of nine predictors and a binary dependent variable indicating the presence or absence of breast cancer. It can be downloaded from this link (https://archive.ics.uci.edu/ml/datasets/Breast+Cancer+Coimbra (accessed on 11 November 2021)). The predictors are simple parameters that can be collected from routine blood analysis. The nine predictors are Age (years), BMI (kg/m^2), Glucose (mg/dL), Insulin (µU/mL), Homeostasis Model Assessment (HOMA), Serum value of Leptin (ng/mL), Adiponectin (µg/mL), Resistin (ng/mL), and Chemokine Monocyte Chemoattractant Protein 1 (MCP-1) (pg/dL). The dataset was gathered by the Gynecology Department of the University Hospital Center of Coimbra in Portugal between 2009 and 2013. It was collected from naïve data (the data were collected before the treatment) of 64 women diagnosed with breast cancer and 52 healthy women (a total of 116 instances).

Table 1. Features categorization of WDBC dataset.

No	Feature	No	Feature	No	Feature
1	Radius mean	11	Radius SE	21	Radius worst
2	Texture mean	12	Texture SE	22	Texture worst
3	Perimeter mean	13	Perimeter SE	23	Perimeter worst
4	Area mean	14	Area SE	24	Area worst
5	Smoothness mean	15	Smoothness SE	25	Smoothness worst
6	Compactness mean	16	Compactness SE	26	Compactness worst
7	Concavity mean	17	Concavity SE	27	Concavity worst
8	Concave pts. mean	18	Concave pts. SE	28	Concave pts. worst
9	Symmetry mean	19	Symmetry SE	29	Symmetry worst
10	Fractal dim. mean	20	Fractal dim. SE	30	Fractal dim. worst

3.2. Performance Evaluations Matrices

In this research, we compared four cross-validation matrices: precision, recall, F1 score, and accuracy. These matrices can be calculated by using the values in the confusion matrix, which are true positive (TP)—the prediction is yes, and the actual data is also yes; true negative (TN)—the prediction is no, and the actual data is also no; false positive (FP)—the prediction is yes, but the actual data is no; and false negative (FN)—the prediction is no, but the actual data is yes. Precision, recall, F1 score, and accuracy can be calculated as in the equations below [20]:

$$precision(P) = \frac{TP}{Tp + FP} \quad (1)$$

$$Recall(R) = \frac{TP}{Tp + FN} \quad (2)$$

$$F1score = \frac{2 \times P \times R}{P + R} \quad (3)$$

$$Accuracy(A) = \frac{TP + TN}{TP + TN + FN + FP} \quad (4)$$

4. Proposed Methodology

The proposed methodology, including data information, model architecture, ML models, and their assessment criteria, will be discussed in this section.

4.1. Novel Framework

In this work, we provide a solution to tackle the problems below for the breast cancer dataset, which we found from [16–19].

- How are the data exploratory techniques (DET) be used most efficiently utilized with the prediction models for breast cancer detection?
- How can the breast cancer features help the ML models detect cancer more precisely and more scalable?

To solve these problems, a solution is proposed, illustrated in Figure 1. This solution has nine significant different steps. The outlines of this methodology are as follows:

1. WDBC and BCCD datasets are downloaded from the machine learning repository.
2. Execute the fundamental preprocessing tasks for individual data.
3. Categorize the data into malignant and benign in WDBC and present and absent in BCCD.
4. Distribute the features into positive, negative, and random (unrelated) by calculating their correlation with each other.

5. Detect less significant features then eliminate such recursive features for effective results.
6. After exploratory data analysis, distribute the dataset into training and testing datasets.
7. Implementation of four predictive models (SVM, LR, KNN, and EC) on the datasets.
8. After the models' execution, the classifier's prediction is achieved with different matrices to evaluate the performance of the models, such as confusion matrices.
9. Finally, analyze the results and compare each model's accuracy and previous research studies.

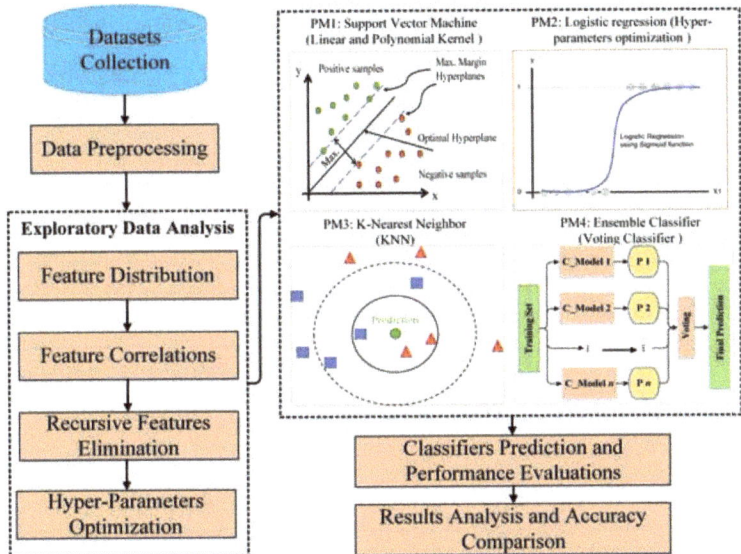

Figure 1. Schematic workflow diagram of our proposed method of breast cancer prediction with data exploratory techniques with machine learning classifiers.

4.2. Data Exploratory Techniques (DET)

DE techniques, or DET, are the processes that help understand the nature of the dataset, which will identify the outliers or correlated variables that are more accessible. Our research applied feature distribution, correlation coefficient, and recursive feature elimination as our data exploratory techniques.

- **Feature Distribution:** First, the distribution of each feature was observed to find how these features are different from each other, i.e., benign and malignant in the WDBC dataset and the presence and absence of breast cancer in the BCCD dataset. The distribution was carried out by plotting the distribution plot for each feature. The data were separated by using binary code: benign (B) = 0, malignant (M) = 1, and absence = 0, presence = 1. Then, the distribution of each feature was plotted between 0 and 1.
- **Feature Correlation:** Next, the Pearson Correlation Coefficient (r) [31] calculates the correlation coefficient between each of the two features. Then, the relationship between two features can be determined by categorizing them into three groups: positively correlated features, negatively correlated features, and uncorrelated features. The features will positively correlate ($r = +1$) if the variables move in the same direction. In contrast, if these features move in the opposite direction, they will negatively correlate ($r = -1$).
- **Recursive features elimination (RFE):** RFE is one of the essential processes of machine learning. Since the dataset has many features, selecting the number of features that give the most optimal prediction result is important for improving model performance.

Using fewer features that provide better understanding is the gist of doing RFE. It will recur the loop until it can find the optimal number of features. In this study, RFE was utilized to reduce the features from 30 to 15. It was conducted by a built-in function, *selector.fit(x, y)*, of *sklearn*. The attributes *support_*, and *ranking_* were passed to the ranking position of $i - th$ feature and mask the selected features. RFE works by searching for a subset of features by starting with all features in the training dataset and successfully removing features until the desired number remains. This is achieved by fitting the given machine learning algorithm used in the core of the model, ranking features according to their relevance, discarding the least important features, and re-fitting the model. This process is repeated until a predetermined number of features is retained.

- **Hyperparameter Optimization:** Hyperparameters optimization is a process of machine learning used for tuning a set of optimal parameters. The values of these parameters are used to control the learning process. There are many approaches for hyperparameters optimization, such as grid search, random search, Bayesian optimization, gradient-based optimization, and evolutionary and population-based optimization. In this study, we used grid search optimization due to its effective results for optimization. It applies the brute-force method to generate candidates from the grid of parameter values specified with the parameter. The grid search goal is to get the highest cross-validation metric scores. In our case, we utilized $scikit - learn$ based GridSearch K-fold CV due to the disease prediction datasets. In all prediction models, GridSearch CV was adopted to evaluate the hyperparameters. GridSearchCV uses a different combination of specified hyperparameters and their values to perform the analysis. We utilized *estimator, param_grid, scoring, verbose*, and n_jobs parameters to calculate each combination's performance.

4.3. Predictive Models

In this study, four ML classifiers were utilized as predictive models (PM) to diagnose Y-variable in the data as malignant or benign in the WDBC dataset and as the presence or absence of breast cancer in the BCCD dataset. The data were distributed into training and test sets. In experiments, we conducted this distribution by setting an integer value for the *random_state*. To tune the hyperparameter, this value can be any value, but *split_size* should be a particular value. In our scenario, we considered 20% testing sets and 80% training sets. The models were constructed on the training dataset, and then a test dataset was used to evaluate the model's performance. We chose SVM due to its highest accuracy in the previous literature, and LR had the best performance by tuning the hyperparameter. Likewise, KNN was selected due to effective results with input features. Meanwhile, we experimented with the ensemble-based classifier using voting techniques to assess its performance and compared it with other classifiers. The precise details of these models are given below:

PM1—SVM: The first model applied SVM as a predictive model. SVM is one of the robust supervised machine learning algorithms used to solve classification and regression tasks [32]. The idea of SVM is to find an optimal hyperplane that gives the maximum margin of each data class (0 and 1 in this case). The SVM approach aims to solve this quadratic problem by finding a hyperplane in the high dimensional space and the classifier in the original space, as shown in (5) [33].

$$\min_{\alpha} Q_1(\alpha) = \sum_{i=1}^{N} \alpha_i - \frac{1}{2} \sum_{i,j=1}^{N} \alpha_i \alpha_j y_i y_j K(x_i, x_j) \quad (5)$$

where $K(x_i, x_j) = (\phi(x_i), \phi(x_j))$ is called the kernel function.

In this work, SVM is applied to predict whether the data are located in class 0 or 1 based on several features and then calculates its performance. SVM has many kernel functions. For the linear dataset, it is called linear kernel SVM. For nonlinear, there are many types, such as polynomial kernel SVM, radial kernel SVM, and hyperbolic tangent

SVM. In this research, two different kinds of SVM kernels, the linear and polynomial kernel, were applied.

PM2—LR: Our second model applied LR to predict the outcomes. LR is one of the most widespread machine learning techniques. It is mainly used to predict a binary variable with a large number of independent variables. It is efficient to forecast the probability of being 0 or 1 based on predictors [34–36]. It can be expressed as (6):

$$y = \pi(X) + \varepsilon \tag{6}$$

where X is a vector that contains $x_i, i = 1, 2, \ldots, n$ independent predictor variables; $\pi(X)$ is the conditional probability of experiencing the event $Y = 1$ given the independent variable vector X; and ε is a random error term. We can express $\pi(X)$ as (7):

$$\pi(X) = P(Y = 1|X) = \frac{e^{X^T \beta}}{1 + e^{X^T \beta}} \tag{7}$$

where β is the model's parameters vector.

This study applied LR to predict whether the data are located in class 0 or 1 and then calculated the performance. LR is like an upgraded version of linear regression. However, by using linear regression to predict binary classification, some predictions will have values more than one or less than 0. A sigmoid function is employed in LR to normalize the prediction to be between 0 and 1.

PM3—KNN: The third model applied KNN as a predictive model. The KNN algorithm used in our problem considered the output a target class. The problem was solved or classified by the majority vote of its neighbors, where the value of K was taken as a small and real-valued positive integer [37,38]. There are different methods for calculating the distance: Manhattan, Euclidean, Cosine, etc [39]. However, this study applies to Euclidean distance only. Let (c_{x_j}, c_{y_j}) be the centroid and (x_i, y_i) be the data point. The Euclidean distance can be calculated by (8):

$$euclidean = \sqrt{(c_{x_j} - x_i)^2 + (c_{y_j} - y_i)^2} \tag{8}$$

From Figure 1 (the part of PM3), there are two types of data: square and triangle; each type is referred to as a datum. The circle in the middle is the prediction. K represents a numerical value for the nearest neighbors of the output. Given K = 3, the model will find the nearest three data points to the output in the small circle. It contains two triangles and one square, so the output will be a triangle because it has more than a circle. If K = 5, the model comprises three squares and two triangles. Therefore, the prediction result of K = 5 is square. Hence, this technique will be applied to predict whether an instance is malignant or benign in the WDBC dataset and the presence or absence of breast cancer in the BCCD dataset.

PM4—EC: The fourth model applies the ensemble classifier method as a predictive model. It aims to maximize the precision and recall value to detect all malignant tumors in the WDBC dataset and detect all cancer presence in the BCCD dataset. Our research applied an ensemble classifier to optimize the logistic regression model [40,41]. Ensemble classifiers have many types, i.e., bagging, boosting, and voting [42]. The kind that will be used in this research is the voting classifier. A voting classifier combines various machine learning algorithms such as SVM, LR, or KNN. Then, we ran them on the same dataset to get the prediction result of each model. Finally, it will take a majority vote to make a final prediction. For example, the voting classifier trained three algorithms; algorithm 1 resulted in "1"; algorithm 2 resulted in "0"; and algorithm 3 resulted in "0." The final result will be "0" because two of them are "0" and only one is another option.

4.4. Experimental Setup

This work was implemented in Jupiter Notebook with the Python language. We processed the following key steps that can assist the data analyst or physician in implementing this work for the breast cancer prediction in real-time:

1. Import the related Python libraries such as *pandas*, *NumPy*, and *sklearn* and execute the preprocessing steps to drop out the missing values.
2. Process and execute the four-layered data exploratory techniques on each dataset.
3. Definitions and calling of all related functions, such as the confusion matrix, the precision–recall curve, the ROC curve, the learning curve, and cross-validation metrics, and assess the models' performance.
4. Implement the proposed prediction models:
   - Starting with SVM, first, it needs to define variables and the number of test and training sets (in this case is 80% and 20%, respectively). Then, define the output results and run the model using Linear and Polynomial SVM. The results would be shown in cross-validation metrics.
   - The following model is LR; after defining the variables and splitting the data, two methods were applied to find the best hyperparameter. The first one was to use GridSearchCV, and the second one was to use Recursive Feature Elimination (RFE). Then, plot the confusion matrix, ROC curve, and learning, and find cross-validation metrics were used for both methods.
   - The 3rd prediction model was KNN; we used GridSearchCV to find the best hyperparameter to run KNN and showed the confusion matrix and cross-validation metrics.
   - The final model is EC; it applied LR with EC and the voting classifier for this work. The execution steps are similar to the previous ones. The results are shown in the confusion matrix, learning curve, and cross-validation metrics.

The experimental environment and fundamental packages for implementing proposed prediction models and DE techniques are presented in Table 2.

Table 2. Information of our experimental environment.

No	Name	Version
1	Operating System	Windows 10 Home 64-bit (10.0, Build 19042)
2	Processor	Intel® Core™ i7-9750H CPU@ 2.60 GHz
3	Python	3.6.10
4	Jupyter Notebook	6.0.3
5	Pandas	1.0.5
6	Numpy	1.17.0
7	SKlearn	0.23.1

5. Results Evaluations

This section will evaluate the findings of our proposed prediction models and DE techniques and compare them to prior research.

5.1. Exploratory Data Analysis

Data exploratory techniques were discussed in the previous section, and the DE technique presents the following significant results. Figure 2 shows the size and classes of both datasets. It is obvious that the WDBC is exponentially larger than BCCD. The WDBC has benign and malignant classes (a), while the BCCD has absence and presence classes (b). Thus, proper analysis of WDBC will provide better insight. More specifically, this study focused on means, SE, worst, and correlations for demonstrating the dataset.

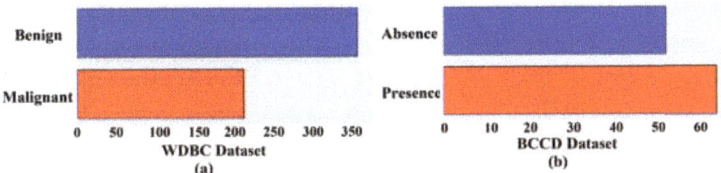

Figure 2. Class distributions of breast cancer datasets with the number of samples; (**a**) indicates WDBC classification into Benign and Malignant; (**b**) presents the BCCD classification into Absence and Presence.

For simplicity, we presented feature distribution insights from the WDBC dataset in Figure 3. We selected two random samples from each feature. For instance, the radius means (a) from both classes of WDBC (benign and malignant) are in different shapes, and benign presented the maximum intensity. While in texture mean (b), the intensity level in both classes was almost identical in shape. Likewise, it explains the SE analysis of feature sets based on concave points and smoothness. The graphs (c) of concave up and down for both benign and malignant were different, while the inflection point was crossing the up and down moments. However, in smoothness SE (d), concave down and up were approximately in the same ranges, while malignant slopes were higher than benign. It presents the worst feature (e) and (f) distribution based on Texture and area. Here Texture waves for both benign and malignant look alike in appearance. Again, in the case of the area graph, malignant cells are flatter and more prolonged.

Furthermore, we delivered the rest of the feature's curves in Note 01 in the Supplementary Materials.

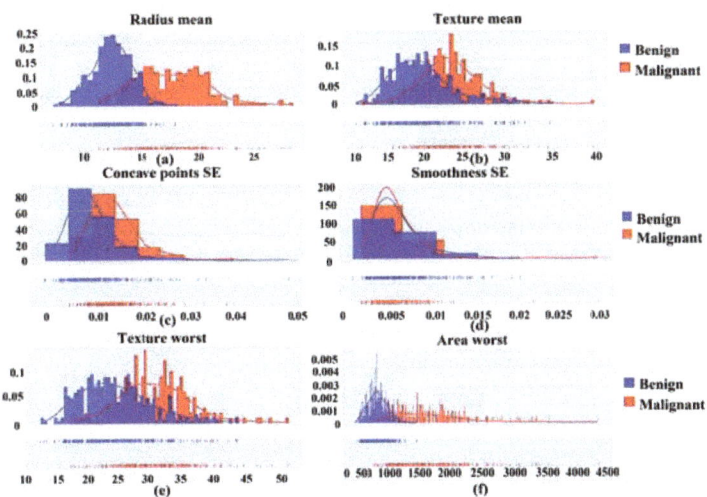

Figure 3. Feature distribution of WDBC dataset with samples of (**a**) Radius mean, (**b**) Texture mean, (**c**) Concave points SE, (**d**) Smoothness SE, (**e**) Texture worst, and (**f**) Area worst.

Furthermore, Figure 4 shows the feature correlations based on positively correlated features (proportional relationship) (a), uncorrelated features (no relationship) (b), and negatively correlated features (inversely proportional relationship) (c) among different features and samples. For instance, Texture worst and Symmetry means do not have any effective correlation (b). We presented a few features matrices due to a lack of space in this study. In conclusion, the feature distribution and correlational analysis enabled the proposed prediction models to detect the tumor more precisely. It is essential to mention that 80% of the total data set was used for training, and 20% of the data set was used for testing. The correlation matrix for all features is illustrated in Note 2 (Figures S2 and S3) in the Supplementary Materials. It shows the correlation of each pair of features by using a color and value system to distinguish between positive, uncorrelated, and negatively correlated features easily. For example, according to the WDBC dataset, area mean and radius mean are positively correlated features; Texture mean and smoothness mean are uncorrelated features; and smoothness SE and radius mean are negatively correlated features. According to the BCCD dataset, insulin and HOMA are positively correlated features; leptin and MCP.1 are uncorrelated features; and resistin and adiponectin are negatively correlated features.

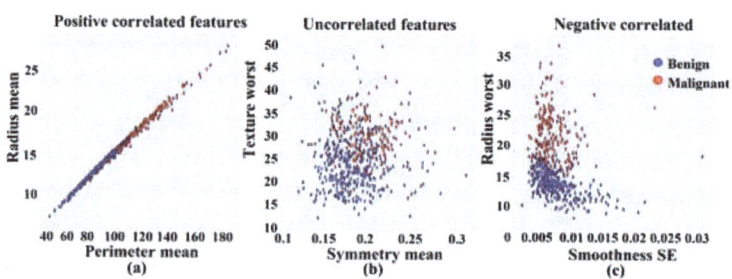

Figure 4. Feature correlation among different samples into positive, negative, and un-correlation of (**a**) Perimeter mean, (**b**) Symmetry mean, and (**c**) Smoothness SE respectively.

5.2. Predictive Model's Evaluations

The followings are the evaluations of given predictive models (PM):

PM1—SVM: This work considered two kernels for employing support vector machines, i.e., linear and polynomial kernels. Table 3 shows the performance analysis of both SVM kernels with confusion matrices in which bolder entries are the highest performances. On the WDBC data set, the polynomial kernel outperformed the linear kernel on both training and testing sets. In training sets, the polynomial kernel received an almost similar precision score to the linear kernel; however, it acquired a 99.3% F1 score and a 99.12% accuracy score. On the other hand, the linear kernel performance was also significant in training and testing datasets. Similarly, the performance of the SVM model in the BCCD data set was not up to the mark. In this dataset, linear SVM succeeded with 76.91% accuracy, while the polynomial kernel had a 76.83% F1 score, which is not significant for cancer detection. For that reason, further evaluation was excluded for the BCCD dataset; and only the WDBC dataset was considered for the rest of the experiment. As the polynomial SVM kernel performance report was superior, Figure 5 is illustrated for the comparison of both kernels' performances with four cross-validation scores with the WDBC dataset.

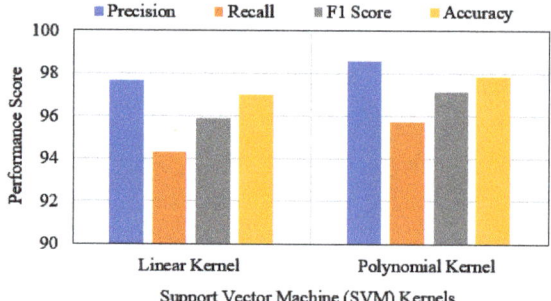

Figure 5. Performance's comparison of SVM-kernels under cross-validation.

Table 3. Performance Comparison of SVM kernels (Linear and Polynomial) on training and testing dataset of WDBC and BCCD.

Datasets Names	Data Distribution	SVM Kernels	Confusion Matrices			
			P	R	F1 Score	Accuracy
WDBC	Training Dataset	Linear SVM	98.95	98.22	98.57	98.68
		Polynomial SVM	98.62	100	**99.3**	**99.12**
	Testing Dataset	Linear SVM	97.14	95.77	96.45	95.61
		Polynomial SVM	97.26	100	98.61	98.25
BCCD	Training Dataset	Linear SVM	72.39	81.05	76.48	**76.91**
		Polynomial SVM	75.39	75.67	75.53	75.35
	Testing Dataset	Linear SVM	79.01	68.34	73.29	72.09
		Polynomial SVM	74.51	79.29	**76.83**	76.42

PM2—LR: This study utilized three types of experiments for the LR model, i.e., basic LR, LR with 100% recall, and LR with the RFE method on the WDBC dataset. However, Figure 6 shows the comparative performance of the learning curve of LR with and without the RFE method. For the small amount of data, the training scores for both models were much more significant than the cross-validation scores. However, adding more training samples will most likely increase the generalization of the training score and cross-validation score. With the more substantial number of instances, LR with the RFE model (b) improved training and cross-validation scores. Additionally, those scores were getting closer to each other than in the simple LR model (a). Table 4 shows the cross-validation performance analysis in which bolder entries are the highest performances. Among these three methods, LR with RFE received the most significant performance, with 97.36% and 98.06% of the F1 score and accuracy values, respectively. The basic LR received the second-best performance with a slightly lower matrix score. Meanwhile, LR with 100% recall received the lowest possible scores.

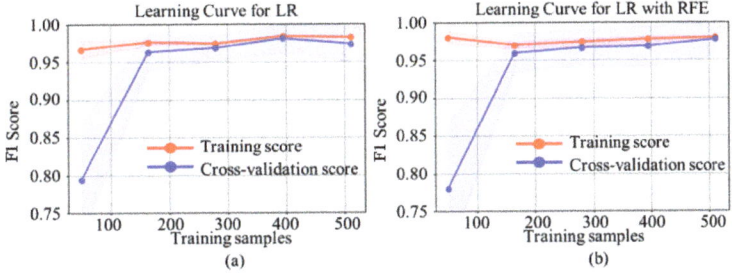

Figure 6. Comparisons of the learning curve of training and cross-validation scores for (**a**) simple LR and (**b**) LR with RFE.

Table 4. Logistic regression performance with basic LR, LR predication with 100% recall, and LR with RFE under Cross-validation.

Matrices	Basic LR	LR Predication with 100% Recall	LR with RFE
Precision	97.15	86	98.58
Recall	93.87	100	96.22
F1 score	95.45	92.5	**97.36**
Accuracy	96.66	93.9	**98.06**

PM3—KNN: The KNN predictive model has experimented on two methods, i.e., basic KNN and KNN with hyperparameter. From Figure 7, it is clear that KNN with hyperparameter showed better performance than basic KNN. Basic KNN operates automatically upon default parameters and displays results. On the other hand, hyperparameter allows parameter tuning for KNN. It represents that basic KNN acquired a 94.73% F1 score and 95.43% accuracy. Meanwhile, KNN with hyperparameter achieved a 97.35% F1 score and 97.01% accuracy.

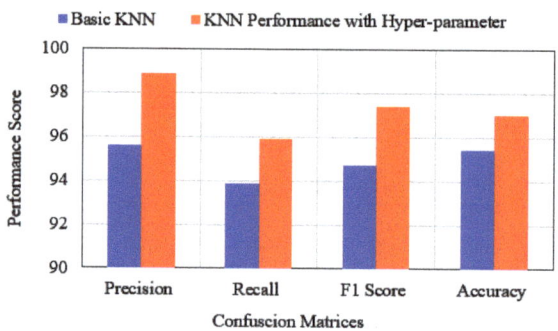

Figure 7. Comparison of KNN performance with basic KNN and KNN with hyperparameter.

PM4—EC: The performance analysis of ensemble classifiers (EC) is presented in Table 5 in which bolder entries are the highest performances. It considers three methods to evaluate the WDBC dataset: voting classifier (CV), ensemble LR, and CV prediction with 100% recall. The ensemble LR and CV achieved the highest outcomes compared to CV prediction with 100% recall. It is clear that CV successfully achieved a 96.02% F1 score while 97.61% accuracy with the given dataset. Similarly, ensemble LR performance is also significant. In contrast, CV with 100% recall values did not provide effective outcomes.

Table 5. Performance comparison of Ensemble LR, voting classifier (CV), and voting classifier prediction with 100% recall.

Matrices	CV Predication with 100% Recall	Ensemble LR	Voting Classifier
Precision	82.7	93.33	96.32
Recall	100	95.75	95.75
F1 score	90.5	95.99	**96.02**
Accuracy	92.1	97.01	**97.61**

5.3. Classifier's Comparative Analysis

After the individual classifier performance analysis, Figure 8 depicts the performance analysis of different classifiers and methods based on accuracy and F1 score with cross-validation matrices. The lowest performance was delivered by CV prediction with 100% recall, (basic) KNN, and LR prediction with 100% recall, where the F1 score and accuracy values were below 95%. In this comparison, LR with RFE outperformed other methods and achieved 98.06% accuracy and 97.36% F1 score. Meanwhile, polynomial SVM, CV, and KNN with hyperparameter performance are beneficial. Therefore, based on these analyses, it is clear that LR with RFE performance is higher than all other methods in cross-validation.

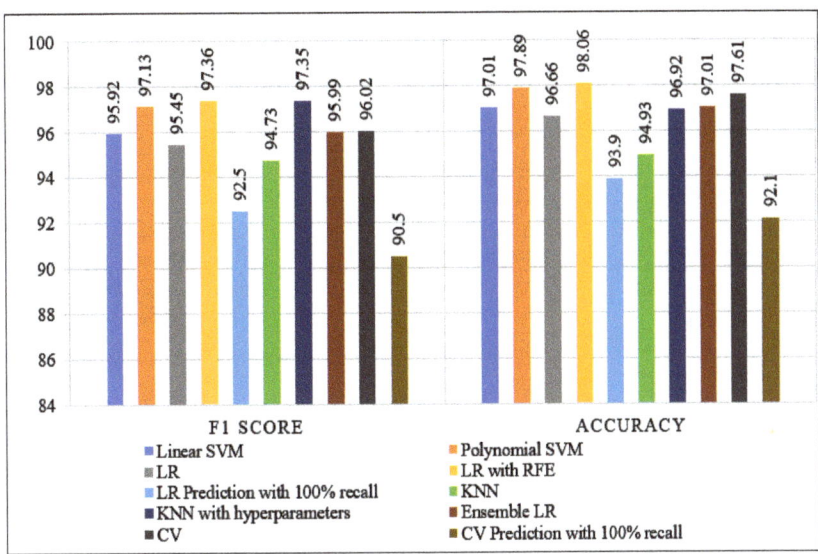

Figure 8. Comparison of all prediction models and methods under the cross-validation matrices.

Furthermore, Table 6 delivers the comparison of best-achieved accuracies along with the execution time of each classifier and bolder entries are the highest performances. It presents that polynomial SVM achieves the best accuracy (99.03%) within 0.03 s, while basic KNN performed in the shortest time but with the lowest accuracy. However, LR with the RFE method performed reasonably, which had the highest accuracy (98.06%) in cross-validation. In contrast, the execution time of KNN with hyperparameter was the longest (4.023 s), although the accuracy (97.35%) was more sophisticated.

Table 6. Execution time comparison of each model along with best-achieved accuracy.

Prediction Model (PM)	Classifiers with Proposed Approaches	Accuracy	Time (s)
PM1: SVM	Linear SVM	98.68	**0.03**
	Polynomial SVM	**99.03**	**0.03**
PM2: LR	Basic LR	96.66	0.266
	LR Predication with 100% Recall	93.9	0.87
	LR with RFE	**98.06**	0.483
PM3: KNN	Basic KNN	95.43	0.031
	KNN Performance with hyperparameter	**97.35**	4.023
PM4: Ensemble Classifier	Ensemble LR	97.01	0.634
	CV Prediction with 100% Recall	92.1	1.845
	Voting Classifier (CV)	**97.61**	0.611

5.4. Comparison with Previous Studies

The best-achieved outcomes with previous studies that used the same WDBC datasets were compared. Table 7 compares the employed models or methods and the achieved accuracies in the previous studies and our proposed prediction models and outputs. The bolder entries are the outperformed results than prior works. The proposed model, SVM polynomial kernel, gained a 99.03% of accuracy, while the LR with RFE accuracy was the nearest possible 98.06% [20]. It is evident from these comparative analyses that the proposed prediction models outperformed the previous techniques and achieved sufficient accuracy for the detection of breast cancer. The possible reason for these improvements compared to other studies is the proposed data mining techniques with the ML prediction models. The DE techniques enabled the topmost accuracy while consuming the least execution time.

Table 7. Accuracy comparison of our proposed breast cancer prediction models with previous studies that used the same WDBC dataset.

Author Name	Reference	Year	Model/Method	Best Observed Accuracy
Maglogiannis I. et al.	[43]	2007	SVM Gaussian RBF	97.54%
Mert et al.	[15]	2015	KNN	92.56%
Hazra et al.	[29]	2016	Support Vector Machine (using 19 features)	94.423%
Osman A. H. et al.	[44]	2017	SVM	95.23%
Wang et al.	[30]	2018	SVM based ensemble learning	96.67%
Abdar et al.	[16]	2018	Nested Ensemble 2-MetaClassifier (K = 5)	97.01%
Mushtaq et al.	[18]	2019	KNN with multiple distances (Correlation K = 2)	91.00%
Rajaguru & Chakravarthy	[17]	2019	KNN Euclidean distance	95.61%
Durgalakshmi & Vijayakumar	[28]	2019	SVM	73%
Khan et al.	[45]	2020	SVM	97.06%
Al-Azzam & Shatnawi	[34]	2021	LR with area under curve	96%
Proposed Prediction Models		2022	Polynomial SVM	**99.03%**
			LR with RFE	**98.06%**
			Voting Classifier (CV)	**97.61%**
			KNN Performance with hyperparameter	**97.35%**

* The bold number indicate the top performance of the classifiers.

6. Discussion

Our results evaluations mostly analyzed our findings by considering the F1 score. As in real-world classification problems, large imbalanced class distributions happened in datasets. We find some observations with significant differences between the classes in the feature distribution results. For example, the concavity mean in Supplementary Note 01 had a significant difference between the distribution of benign and malignant classes. The resampling techniques, i.e., oversampling, undersampling, and cross-validation, were adopted to balance such features. The oversampling technique duplicates the minority classes, but it creates an overfitting issue for machine learning algorithms. In contrast, the undersampling technique deletes the majority classes that discard the potential data. These disadvantages can decrease machine learning accuracy for particular problems such as fraud detection, face recognition, disease detection, etc. Therefore, we omit the oversampling and undersampling techniques in our study due to the cancer detection problem. However, the author [46] suggested the cross-validation technique as a dominant technique to overcome the imbalanced class distribution. Cross-validation utilizes different portions of the data to test and train a model. This study employed the cross-validation technique using the k-fold and GridSearchCV with prediction models to balance the benign and malignant features in the training and testing dataset. The cross-validation matrices, including F1 score, precision, and recall, were compared due to the efficient use of crucial values of TP, TN, FP, and FN to deal with actual and predicted classes. The proper definitions of these metrics are given in Section 3.2.

In the polynomial SVM implementation, we secured a 99.3% F1 score, which means our proposed prediction model successfully identified the tumor and classified the cancer features as malignant. Thus, a higher F1 score means a higher diagnostic efficiency of tumors. In Table 7, this study's F1 score and accuracy are compared with previous studies that utilized the same dataset (WDBC). These predictive models with data mining techniques would assist the data analyst in detecting the cancerous mass by analyzing the cancerous data. Similarly, Figure 8 illustrates the performance comparison of models and methods with the cross-validation techniques. As the time complexity is also a significant issue for the ML models, Table 6 presents each model's execution time with minimum but maximum accuracy. Hence, from the above analysis, our contribution with these proposed prediction models and techniques can be efficiently helpful for the cancer domain to acquire highly satisfying results for breast cancer diagnosis.

In this study, the objective was completed for detecting breast cancer with the highest accuracy of machine learning models. However, we were unable to provide the precise reason for malignant features, which needs a domain expert. It should be noted that the BCCD dataset did not yield effective results with our prediction models except for SVM; thus, we ignored those results in this study. We provided the sources/links of the datasets in the "Data Description" subsection. As these datasets belong to American patients, the results may not be similar and effective with the Asian patients' data. This is one of the limitations of this study, which could be extended in the future by a different dataset with neural network implementation.

7. Conclusions

An accurate and timely diagnosis of various diseases, i.e., breast cancer, is still a major problem for proper treatment in the healthcare field. The precise analysis of cancer features is still a time-consuming and challenging task due to the availability of massive data and the lack of DM techniques with appropriate ML classifiers. In this study, four-layered essential data exploratory techniques were proposed with four different machine learning predictive models, including SVM, LR, KNN, and ensemble classifier, to detect breast cancer tumors and classify them into benign and malignant tumors. One of the primary objectives of this study was the implementation of DE techniques before the execution of ML classifiers on the WDBC and BCCD datasets. These mining techniques enabled us to improve the prediction model's performance with a maximum F1 score and an accuracy score higher than before. The significant finding demonstrated that the first prediction model (with an SVM polynomial kernel) had acquired the highest accuracy (99.3%). Meanwhile, logistic regression with recursive features elimination also secured 98.06% accuracy, which shows that DE techniques effectively detect higher accuracy. Our outcomes depict the competence of our prediction models for breast cancer diagnosis and provide adequate results by utilizing a short time for training the model. These sophisticated models, techniques, and results would help the physician and data analyst to apply a more intelligent classifier to diagnose breast cancer features.

As the image data relating to breast cancer are available, we will use deep learning models to detect breast cancer with novel data augmentation strategies and data exploratory techniques to handle the data scarcity and diversity. In the future, we will conduct experiments on the datasets from other countries and try to answer whether or not the different area patient's data affect the model's performance.

Supplementary Materials: The following are available at https://www.mdpi.com/article/10.3390/ijerph19063211/s1, Figure S1: Feature distribution insights from the WDBC dataset into Benign and Malignant, Figure S2: The correlation matrix for all features of the WDBC dataset, Figure S3: The correlation matrix for all features of the BCCD dataset.

Author Contributions: Conceptualization, L.T.; methodology, L.T., A.R. and C.B.; software, A.R. and C.B.; validation, L.T.; formal analysis, M.R.I.; investigation, A.R., C.B. and M.R.I.; resources, L.T., Q.Q. and Q.J.; data curation, A.R. and C.B.; writing—original draft preparation, A.R. and C.B.; writing—review and editing, A.R., C.B. and M.R.I.; visualization, A.R. and C.B.; supervision, L.T.; project administration, L.T.; funding acquisition, L.T., Q.Q. and Q.J. All authors have read and agreed to the published version of the manuscript.

Funding: This work was supported in parts by the National Key Research and Development Program under Grant No. 2021YFF1200100, 2021YFF1200104 and 2020YFA0909100 and AI Innovation of Chinese Academy of Science (CAS).

Institutional Review Board Statement: Not applicable.

Informed Consent Statement: Not applicable.

Data Availability Statement: The codes are available at: https://github.com/abdul-rasool/Improved-machine-learning-based-Predictive-Models-for-Breast-Cancer-Diagnosis (accessed on 11 November 2021) and WDBC dataset at https://ftp.cs.wisc.edu/math-prog/cpo-dataset/machine-learn/cancer/WDBC/ (accessed on 11 November 2021) and BCCD dataset at https://archive.ics.uci.edu/ml/datasets/Breast+Cancer+Coimbra (accessed on 11 November 2021).

Acknowledgments: The authors would like to thank all the anonymous reviewers for their insightful comments and constructive suggestions that have obviously upgraded the quality of this manuscript. The authors would also like to acknowledge Muhammad Saqlain Aslam for sharing the idea of this work.

Conflicts of Interest: The authors declare that they have no conflict of interest.

References

1. Sung, H.; Ferlay, J.; Siegel, R.L.; Laversanne, M.; Soerjomataram, I.; Jemal, A.; Bray, F. Global cancer statistics 2020: GLOBOCAN estimates of incidence and mortality worldwide for 36 cancers in 185 countries. *CA Cancer J. Clin.* **2021**, *71*, 209–249. [CrossRef]
2. Siegel, R.L.; Miller, K.D.; Fuchs, H.E.; Jemal, A. Cancer statistics, 2022. *CA Cancer J. Clin.* **2022**, *72*, 7–33. [CrossRef]
3. Leão, D.C.M.R.; Pereira, E.R.; Pérez-Marfil, M.N.; Silva, R.M.C.R.A.; Mendonça, A.B.; Rocha, R.C.N.P.; García-Caro, M.P. The Importance of Spirituality for Women Facing Breast Cancer Diagnosis: A Qualitative Study. *Int. J. Environ. Res. Public Health* **2021**, *18*, 6415. [CrossRef]
4. Subashini, T.S.; Ramalingam, V.; Palanivel, S. Breast mass classification based on cytological patterns using RBFNN and SVM. *Expert Syst. Appl.* **2009**, *36*, 5284–5290. [CrossRef]
5. Abdar, M.; Zomorodi-Moghadam, M.; Zhou, X.; Gururajan, R.; Tao, X.; Barua, P.D.; Gururajan, R. A new nested ensemble technique for automated diagnosis of breast cancer. *Pattern Recognit. Lett.* **2020**, *132*, 123–131. [CrossRef]
6. Rasool, A.; Tao, R.; Kashif, K.; Khan, W.; Agbedanu, P.; Choudhry, N. Statistic Solution for Machine Learning to Analyze Heart Disease Data. In Proceedings of the 2020 12th International Conference on Machine Learning and Computing, Shenzhen, China, 15–17 February 2020; pp. 134–139.
7. McWilliam, A.; Faivre-Finn, C.; Kennedy, J.; Kershaw, L.; Van Herk, M.B. Data mining identifies the base of the heart as a dose-sensitive region affecting survival in lung cancer patients. *Int. J. Radiat. Oncol. Biol. Phys.* **2016**, *96*, S48–S49. [CrossRef]
8. Park, K.H.; Batbaatar, E.; Piao, Y.; Theera-Umpon, N.; Ryu, K.H. Deep Learning Feature Extraction Approach for Hematopoietic Cancer Subtype Classification. *Int. J. Environ. Res. Public Health* **2021**, *18*, 2197. [CrossRef] [PubMed]
9. Park, E.Y.; Yi, M.; Kim, H.S.; Kim, H. A Decision Tree Model for Breast Reconstruction of Women with Breast Cancer: A Mixed Method Approach. *Int. J. Environ. Res. Public Health* **2021**, *18*, 3579. [CrossRef]
10. Bicchierai, G.; Di Naro, F.; De Benedetto, D.; Cozzi, D.; Pradella, S.; Miele, V.; Nori, J. A Review of Breast Imaging for Timely Diagnosis of Disease. *Int. J. Environ. Res. Public Health* **2021**, *18*, 5509. [CrossRef]
11. Akay, M.F. Support vector machines combined with feature selection for breast cancer diagnosis. *Expert Syst. Appl.* **2009**, *36*, 3240–3247. [CrossRef]
12. Furey, T.S.; Cristianini, N.; Duffy, N.; Bednarski, D.W.; Schummer, M.; Haussler, D. Support vector machine classification and validation of cancer tissue samples using microarray expression data. *Bioinformatics* **2000**, *16*, 906–914. [CrossRef]
13. Zheng, B.; Yoon, S.W.; Lam, S.S. Breast cancer diagnosis based on feature extraction using a hybrid of K-means and support vector machine algorithms. *Expert Syst. Appl.* **2014**, *41*, 1476–1482. [CrossRef]
14. Seddik, A.F.; Shawky, D.M. Logistic regression model for breast cancer automatic diagnosis. In Proceedings of the 2015 SAI Intelligent Systems Conference (IntelliSys), London, UK, 10–11 November 2015; pp. 150–154.
15. Mert, A.; Kılıç, N; Bilgili, E.; Akan, A. Breast cancer detection with reduced feature set. *Comput. Math. Methods Med.* **2015**, *2015*, 265138. [CrossRef]
16. Abdar, M.; Yen, N.Y.; Hung, J.C.S. Improving the diagnosis of liver disease using multilayer perceptron neural network and boosted decision trees. *J. Med. Biol. Eng.* **2018**, *38*, 953–965. [CrossRef]
17. Rajaguru, H. Analysis of decision tree and k-nearest neighbor algorithm in the classification of breast cancer. *Asian Pac. J. Cancer Prev. APJCP* **2019**, *20*, 3777. [CrossRef]
18. Mushtaq, Z.; Yaqub, A.; Sani, S.; Khalid, A. Effective K-nearest neighbor classifications for Wisconsin breast cancer data sets. *J. Chin. Inst. Eng.* **2020**, *43*, 80–92. [CrossRef]
19. Kamyab, M.; Tao, R.; Mohammadi, M.H. Sentiment Analysis on Twitter. In Proceedings of the 2018 International Conference on Artificial Intelligence and Virtual Reality—AIVR 2018, Taichung, Taiwan, 10–12 December 2018. [CrossRef]

20. Brause, R.W. Medical analysis and diagnosis by neural networks. In *Proceedings of the International Symposium on Medical Data Analysis, Madrid, Spain, 8–9 October 2001*; Springer: Berlin/Heidelberg, Germany, 2001; pp. 1–13.
21. Huang, C.L.; Liao, H.C.; Chen, M.C. Prediction model building and feature selection with support vector machines in breast cancer diagnosis. *Expert Syst. Appl.* **2008**, *34*, 578–587. [CrossRef]
22. Polat, K.; Güneş, S. Breast cancer diagnosis using least square support vector machine. *Digit. Signal Process.* **2007**, *17*, 694–701. [CrossRef]
23. Prasad, Y.; Biswas, K.K.; Jain, C.K. SVM classifier based feature selection using GA, ACO and PSO for siRNA design. In *Proceedings of the International Conference in Swarm Intelligence, Beijing, China, 12–15 June 2010*; Springer: Berlin/Heidelberg, Germany, 2010; pp. 307–314.
24. Muzammal, M.; Qu, Q.; Nasrulin, B. Renovating blockchain with distributed databases: An open source system. *Future Gener. Comput. Syst.* **2019**, *90*, 105–117. [CrossRef]
25. Lim, J.; Sohn, J.; Sohn, J.; Lim, D. Breast cancer classification using optimal support vector machine. *J. Korea Soc. Health Inform. Stat.* **2013**, *38*, 108–121.
26. Yang, L.; Xu, Z. Feature extraction by PCA and diagnosis of breast tumors using SVM with DE-based parameter tuning. *Int. J. Mach. Learn. Cybern.* **2019**, *10*, 591–601. [CrossRef]
27. Fu, Y.; Jung, A.W.; Torne, R.V.; Gonzalez, S.; Vöhringer, H.; Shmatko, A.; Gerstung, M. Pan-cancer computational histopathology reveals mutations, tumor composition and prognosis. *Nat. Cancer* **2020**, *1*, 800–810. [CrossRef]
28. Durgalakshmi, B.; Vijayakumar, V. Feature selection and classification using support vector machine and decision tree. *Comput. Intell.* **2020**, *36*, 1480–1492. [CrossRef]
29. Hazra, A.; Mandal, S.K.; Gupta, A. Study and analysis of breast cancer cell detection using Naïve Bayes, SVM and ensemble algorithms. *Int. J. Comput. Appl.* **2016**, *145*, 39–45. [CrossRef]
30. Wang, H.; Zheng, B.; Yoon, S.W.; Ko, H.S. A support vector machine-based ensemble algorithm for breast cancer diagnosis. *Eur. J. Oper. Res.* **2018**, *267*, 687–699. [CrossRef]
31. Rasool, A.; Jiang, Q.; Qu, Q.; Kamyab, M.; Huang, M. HSMC: Hybrid Sentiment Method for Correlation to Analyze COVID-19 Tweets. In *Advances in Natural Computation, Fuzzy Systems and Knowledge Discovery*; Springer International Publishing: Berlin/Heidelberg, Germany, 2022; pp. 991–999. [CrossRef]
32. Huang, S.; Cai, N.; Pacheco, P.P.; Narrandes, S.; Wang, Y.; Xu, W. Applications of support vector machine (SVM) learning in cancer genomics. *Cancer Genom. Proteom.* **2018**, *15*, 41–51.
33. Tolles, J.; Meurer, W.J. Logistic regression: Relating patient characteristics to outcomes. *JAMA* **2016**, *316*, 533–534. [CrossRef]
34. Al-Azzam, N.; Shatnawi, I. Comparing supervised and semi-supervised Machine Learning Models on Diagnosing Breast Cancer. *Ann. Med. Surg.* **2021**, *62*, 53–64. [CrossRef] [PubMed]
35. Khandezamin, Z.; Naderan, M.; Rashti, M.J. Detection and classification of breast cancer using logistic regression feature selection and GMDH classifier. *J. Biomed. Inform.* **2020**, *111*, 103591. [CrossRef]
36. Hasan, A.S.M.T.; Sabah, S.; Haque, R.U.; Daria, A.; Rasool, A.; Jiang, Q. Towards Convergence of IoT and Blockchain for Secure Supply Chain Transaction. *Symmetry* **2022**, *14*, 64. [CrossRef]
37. Mejdoub, M.; Amar, C.B. Classification improvement of local feature vectors over the KNN algorithm. *Multimed. Tools Appl.* **2013**, *64*, 197–218. [CrossRef]
38. Yu, Z.; Chen, H.; Liu, J.; You, J.; Leung, H.; Han, G. Hybrid k-nearest neighbor classifier. *IEEE Trans. Cybern.* **2015**, *46*, 1263–1275. [CrossRef] [PubMed]
39. Mondéjar-Guerra, V.; Novo, J.; Rouco, J.; Penedo, M.G.; Ortega, M. Heartbeat classification fusing temporal and morphological information of ECGs via ensemble of classifiers. *Biomed. Signal Process. Control* **2019**, *47*, 41–48. [CrossRef]
40. Pławiak, P. Novel genetic ensembles of classifiers applied to myocardium dysfunction recognition based on ECG signals. *Swarm Evol. Comput.* **2018**, *39*, 192–208. [CrossRef]
41. Bunterngchit, C.; Leepaitoon, S. Simulation-Based Approach for Reducing Goods Loading Time. In *Proceedings of the 2019 8th International Conference on Modeling Simulation and Applied Optimization (ICMSAO), Manama, Bahrain, 15–17 April 2019*. [CrossRef]
42. Jafarzadeh, H.; Mahdianpari, M.; Gill, E.; Mohammadimanesh, F.; Homayouni, S. Bagging and Boosting Ensemble Classifiers for Classification of Multispectral, Hyperspectral and PolSAR Data: A Comparative Evaluation. *Remote Sens.* **2021**, *13*, 4405. [CrossRef]
43. Maglogiannis, I.; Zafiropoulos, E.; Anagnostopoulos, I. An intelligent system for automated breast cancer diagnosis and prognosis using SVM based classifiers. *Appl. Intell.* **2009**, *30*, 24–36. [CrossRef]
44. Osman, A.H. An enhanced breast cancer diagnosis scheme based on two-step-SVM technique. *Int. J. Adv. Comput. Sci. Appl.* **2017**, *8*, 158–165.
45. Khan, F.; Khan, M.A.; Abbas, S.; Athar, A.; Siddiqui, S.Y.; Khan, A.H.; Hussain, M. Cloud-based breast cancer prediction empowered with soft computing approaches. *J. Healthc. Eng.* **2020**, *2020*, 8017496. [CrossRef]
46. Kuhn, M.; Johnson, K. *Applied Predictive Modeling*; Springer: New York, NY, USA, 2013. [CrossRef]

MDPI
St. Alban-Anlage 66
4052 Basel
Switzerland
Tel. +41 61 683 77 34
Fax +41 61 302 89 18
www.mdpi.com

International Journal of Environmental Research and Public Health Editorial Office
E-mail: ijerph@mdpi.com
www.mdpi.com/journal/ijerph

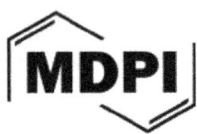

www.ingramcontent.com/pod-product-compliance
Lightning Source LLC
LaVergne TN
LVHW070740100526
838202LV00013B/1275